ESSENTIAL HYPERTENSION

AN INTERNATIONAL SYMPOSIUM

BERNE, JUNE 7th-10th, 1960
SPONSORED BY CIBA

CHAIRMAN

F. C. REUBI

BERNE

EDITED BY

K. D. BOCK

BASLE

P. T. COTTIER

BERNE

WITH 81 FIGURES

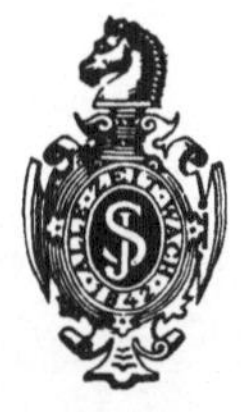

SPRINGER-VERLAG

BERLIN · GÖTTINGEN · HEIDELBERG

1960

This book has also been published in German under the title
‚ESSENTIELLE HYPERTONIE‘
Ein internationales Symposion

ISBN 978-3-642-49607-3   ISBN 978-3-642-49899-2 (eBook)
DOI 10. 1007/978-3-642-49899-2

Contents

IV   Contents

Participants in the Symposium
"ESSENTIAL HYPERTENSION"

Berne, 7th—10th June, 1960

Arnold, O. H., Medizinische Klinik der Städtischen Krankenanstalten, Essen (Germany)

Bartorelli, C., Università di Siena, Istituto di Patologia Speciale Medica e Metodologia Clinica, Siena (Italy)

Bechgaard, P., Medicinsk afdeling, Aarhus Universitet, Aarhus (Denmark)

Bock, K. D., CIBA Aktiengesellschaft, Basel (Switzerland)

Brod, J., Ústav pro Choroby Oběhu Krevního, Praha-Krč (Czechoslovakia)

Cottet, J., Médecin consultant, Paris and Evian (France)

Cottier, P. T., Medizinische Universitäts-Poliklinik, Bern (Switzerland)

Dahl, L. K., Brookhaven National Laboratory, Associated Universities, Upton, N. Y. (USA)

Ferrero, C., Centre de Cardiologie, Hôpital Cantonal, Genève (Switzerland)

Freis, E. D., Veterans Administration Hospital, Washington, D. C. (USA)

Frey, W., Oberhofen am Thunersee (Switzerland)

Genest, J., Département de recherches cliniques, Hôtel-Dieu de Montréal, Montreal (Canada)

Govaerts, P., Fondation Médicale Reine Elisabeth, Bruxelles (Belgium)

Grollman, A., University of Texas, Dallas (USA)

Gross, F., CIBA Aktiengesellschaft, Basel (Switzerland)

Hadorn, W., Medizinische Klinik der Universität, Bern (Switzerland)

Hamburger, J., Hôpital Necker, Paris (France)

Hilden, T., Diakonissestiftelsen, København (Denmark)

Hoobler, S. W., University of Michigan, Ann Arbor (USA)

Hood, B., Göteborgs Universitet, Medicinska Kliniken I, Göteborg (Sweden)

Imhof, P., Lory Spital, Bern (Switzerland)

Mach, R. S., Hôpital Cantonal, Clinique Universitaire de Thérapeutique, Genève (Switzerland)

Milliez, P., Faculté de Médecine, Paris (France)

Muller, A. F., Hôpital Cantonal, Clinique Universitaire de Thérapeutique, Genève (Switzerland)

Page, I. H., Cleveland Clinic Foundation, Cleveland, Ohio (USA)

Peart, W. S., St. Mary's Hospital, London (Great Britain)

Pickering, Sir George, University of Oxford, Oxford (Great Britain)

Platt, Sir Robert, The Royal Infirmary, Manchester (Great Britain)

Plummer, A. J., CIBA Pharmaceutical Products Inc., Summit, N. J. (USA)

Opening remarks

By

F. C. Reubi

It is a great honour for me to open this symposium, and I should like to extend to you a most cordial welcome and to thank you for accepting our invitation. I am sure you will all wish me on your behalf to express our sincere gratitude to Ciba, Basle, for financing this undertaking.

Although the question of arterial hypertension has commanded the attention of research workers ever since its existence was first discovered, we still seem to be a very long way from having solved the problem. On the other hand, while it was once true to say that medical research was confined to only a few countries, we can derive satisfaction from the knowledge that today a great deal of work has been accomplished during the past few years in both the old and the new world, in the East and in the West. For this very reason, it is becoming more and more important to ensure that results should be compared, opinions exchanged, and trends of research defined periodically on an international plane. The more widely differing the concepts presented, the more fruitful we can expect the resultant clash of ideas to prove. As men of science we have no need to concern ourselves with the battles being waged in the field of international politics. Let us therefore ignore such matters and seek to reconcile our views here in a spirit of understanding and open-mindedness. Let us banish all preconceived notions and beware of allowing ourselves to be blinded by questions of dogma, prestige, and personal pride.

Attending this symposium are some forty specialists from 12 different countries. The number of participants has deliberately been limited and the discussions will be held in private. You will all know yourselves from experience that an atmosphere conducive to a frank exchange of views — views that are sometimes diametrically opposed — can only be established if the speakers cut themselves off from the outside world. We have, however, made allowance on the programme for two sessions in public. In today's public session, we shall hear three lectures in which the problem of the pathogenesis of hypertension will be dealt with from the general aspect. The second public session — to be held at the end of the week in connection with the Annual Meeting of the Swiss Society for Internal Medicine — will take the form of a panel discussion on the treatment of hypertension. The symposium itself will be entirely devoted to the study of two specific questions, the first being the problem of the possible relationships between so-called essential hypertension and salt and water metabolism, and the second the long-term effects of anti-hypertensive therapy as regards the clinical course of hypertensive disease. We are convinced that, rather than attempt to cover the whole subject of essential hypertension, it is a sound procedure to concentrate our attention on certain particular aspects of this vast problem. Perhaps this approach will enable us to get closer to our objective and finally to reach agreement on a certain number of points — in which case we shall be in a better position to offer some practical recommendations when we come to our second public session.

You may possibly wonder why we chose these two topics for discussion in preference to others. As regards the connections between hypertension and salt and water metabolism, we have the impression that this problem has become of great current interest since the sali-diuretics were introduced in the treatment of hypertension, and that the whole question deserves to be reconsidered in the light of recent endocrinological findings. As for the long-term effects of purely hypotensive therapy on the course of the disease, the time that has elapsed since effective anti-hypertensive agents were first introduced should now be sufficient to enable us to make a preliminary assessment of the value of such treatment. Since this is a matter of major practical importance, we should certainly not wait too long before undertaking a critical analysis of the results obtained to date.

Let us hope that this symposium will prove of great help in enriching our knowledge.

The mosaic theory of hypertension

By

I. H. PAGE

It has been some years now since I proposed the mosaic theory of hypertension and it is time, I think, to review where it stands today. Has it proved useful and is it likely to continue to do so ?

The mosaic theory had its background in the fact that thirty years ago thinking in the field of infectious disease mostly prevailed, not only in its own field, but in others as well. The search was often limited to the finding of a single causative agent. If the typhoid bacillus was isolated and cultured, this was the cause of the disease and its elimination was the treatment. So those of us who worked in other fields tried to find *the* cause of hypertension and *the* cause of atherosclerosis. As a result of repeated failures, as many theories sprang up as there were investigators. The chief contender for the cause of hypertension in those days was the kidney. Many felt that after GOLDBLATT's work, the kidney was the true, and only, cause of essential hypertension. The fate of this view is an interesting story but it is diverting.

As time passed, it slowly became evident that the problems of cardiovascular disease and cancer were not likely to yield to an attack on one front. It seemed unlikely that all types of hypertension and arteriosclerosis would be explained by single mechanisms. And it seems to me that reflection on the nature of the circulation gives a clue as to why this is so. Arterial blood pressure is one of the components of the system used to perfuse tissues with blood. The problem of getting the right amount of blood to the right part of the body at the right time is an amazingly complicated and difficult one. To know where blood is available and from where it can safely be withdrawn is a major problem in itself. It is not surprising, then, that the body has developed a highly complex system for carrying out this task efficiently. We shall again put this wonderful mechanism to the test when gravitation has become but a memory in our exploration of outer space. It is my guess that man is more likely to have trouble with his cardiovascular responses to weightlessness than with his control over his actions by his brain; which is certainly a change.

I have suggested in the mosaic theory that the varied facets which compose blood pressure control are in equilibrium with one another and the final pressure level is determined by the equilibrium point. Thus, if blood volume changes, neurogenic vasomotor tone changes to keep the blood pressure at a constant level. While one facet may temporarily play a dominant role in determining the level, this does not mean that all the other facets cease functioning. Just so in the hypertensive patient one facet may be dominant, but the secondary facets are in equilibrium with it and, with the passage of time, may themselves become primary.

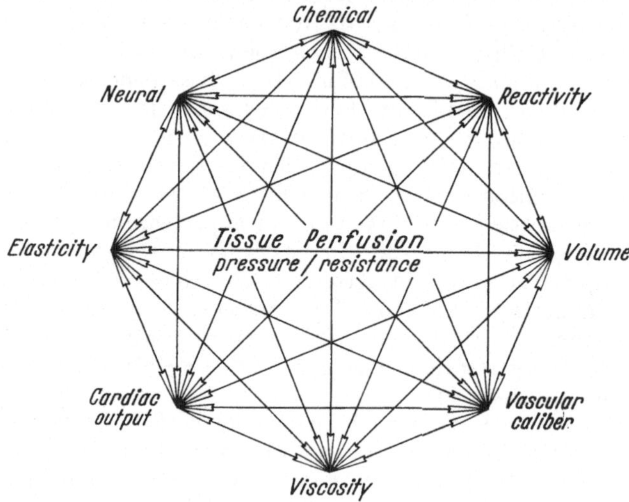

Fig. 1. The mosaic theory of hypertension showing the equilibration of the various facets of pressure control to provide for controlled tissue perfusion

This seems a simple concept indeed, with which no one should quarrel, but few physicians truly understand it. For instance, it explains why there are so many possible points at which the mechanisms of blood pressure control can be blocked, for therapeutic reasons. It explains why the clinical picture of hypertension is so variable. Not the least of its virtues is that it makes thinking about the disease orderly.

Beyond the physiological processes which I have included in the octagon, I have further divided and grouped what seem to be primary mechanisms of a variety of hypertensions. These groups are: 1. nervous, 2. endocrine, 3. cardiovascular, and 4. renal. Again, it must be recognized that while the nervous system may be predom- ·

inant on one patient, it does not mean that the endocrine, cardio-vascular and renal systems have quit their participation. It is just that they participate to a lesser degree.

Primitive and sophisticated control

I like to think of the circulation as having two levels of operation, the one primitive and largely chemically controlled, the other a more highly integrated one and nervously controlled. The prolonged slow changes in pressure and/or perfusion may be chiefly set in motion by humoral mechanisms and the fine quick changes by the autonomic and, in part, voluntary nervous system. In fact, the two systems must be closely integrated themselves to be the effective unit they actually constitute.

Even within the humoral and neurogenic mechanisms themselves there are degrees of primitiveness. For example, I have suggested that serotonin is, in some ways, a primitive norepineph-rine. In invertebrates it seems to be able to act as a neurotrans-mitter, a function largely replaced by norepinephrine in verte-brates. The endocrine secretory function of some neurones in insects is an example of the more primitive function of the nerve cell which may not be as highly developed in man. Yet there may well be important functional vestiges in higher animals which have so far been overlooked. I think until very recently we were inclined to relegate the pineal body to oblivion. Whatever its function, it is quite apparent that things of importance transpire within its orbit. I have often suspected that the pressor material cerebrotonin, which TAYLOR and I (1) showed coming from the stimulated brain, might have represented endocrine secretion of neurones. Of course, this is just a guess, which is at least better than a bad experiment.

Arterial blood pressure and tissue perfusion

Arterial blood pressure is only one of the components of the mechanism of tissue perfusion. But before I turn to consideration of some of these varied facets I would like to mention the discussion going on between those who believe that the increase in peripheral resistance which occurs in hypertension is due chiefly to humoral and neurogenic mechanisms and those who look upon it as princi-pally anatomical and biophysical due to the swelling and over-growth of the arteriolar wall or to the inherent physical properties of vascular smooth muscle. Probably all are involved. The question, rather, is how much of each.

We assume that if the sympathetic nerves are cut this removes all tonic vasomotor impulses. What vascular tone remains must then be due to blood-borne vasoconstrictors or to the anatomy of the blood vessels. It has been further assumed that complete relaxation of the blood vessels may be achieved with such drugs as acetylcholine, ATP or nitrites. The degree to which various vascular areas are under sympathetic control varies enormously as Celander and Folkow (2) have shown. The relative importance of the composition of the bathing medium for the tone of denervated blood vessels has not, so far as I know, been adequately studied. In this composition I would include both the usual constituents of the blood and any humoral agents that may be secreted into it. Such an experimental demonstration is difficult because of the subtlety of the possible compositional changes as well as the length of time required for such changes to be reflected in the tone of the blood vessels.

From the days of Cohnheim and Gull and Sutton, the notion has existed that thickening of the blood vessel wall preceded the hypertension and was the cause of it. The arguments for, and against, this concept are too well known to this audience to waste their time repeating them. Some elaboration has recently occurred in that thickening as a result of electrolyte changes in the vessel wall has been added to thickening due to hypertrophy and hyperplasia.

One more factor concerned with peripheral resistance is inherent in the vascular wall itself. Automaticity, or vasomotion, of the smooth muscle is considered one of these factors. The distending force of the blood pressure creates in smooth muscle a tendency to rebound and thereby induces some degree of vascular tone.

Applying this type of thinking to the hypertensive is no more satisfying than it is in the normotensive. Theoretically it is clearly of importance but, so far, little objective measurement of the separate components of this complex mechanism of maintenance of vascular tone is possible in patients or, indeed, in intact animals.

Whether vascular resistance when smooth muscle is completely relaxed is the same in hypertensives as in normotensives would depend at least on the stage of the disease. Early, it may well be the same, but, with time, development of vascular disease could scarcely help increasing it. The impressive thing to me is the extensive anatomical change that can occur in hypertensives and yet maintain their ability to vasodilate. Folkow (3) stresses the fact that it takes only a small decrease in the internal diameter of the maximally dilated blood vessel to cause a pronounced effect on the resistance to flow; a five percent decrease causing the resistance to be raised something of the order of 25 %. Further, it can be calculated that for any given shortening of the smooth muscle, the resistance of a hypertrophied vessel would be increased proportionately more than in normal vessels, because a larger tissue volume intrudes on the vascular lumen. At the same degree of smooth muscle tension the hypertrophied vessel, for purely mechanical reasons, exhibits a greater vasoconstrictor action than normal (4).

FOLKOW, GRIMBY and THULESIUS (5) tested this hypothesis by measuring forearm blood flow in normo- and hypertensive subjects in whom an attempt was made to elicit maximum vasodilatation by ischemia and work. Dilatation was further facilitated by heat. If, in fact, these measures yield maximal dilatation then in some well-established essential hypertensives resistance remained moderately raised. They point out that there are serious technical difficulties with this method and that the results can only be looked upon as suggestive.

Experience with the antihypertensive drugs has done much to dispel a firmly fixed notion as to the so-called "fixed hypertensive". It is relatively rare, in my experience, to see a patient in whom the supine blood pressure cannot be reduced to normal, and when it is normal, to exhibit symptoms or signs of ischemia. This is not proof that some residue of structural change in the resistance vessels is not still present, but it indicates that stronger proof of its paramount importance must be forthcoming. I would like to venture the opinion that increases in peripheral resistance as a result of structural vascular change may be important in certain specific areas such as the renal, myocardial and cerebral vessels, but that a generalized increase in resistance due to structural change is less significant, comes late in the course of the disease, and is commonly, to some degree, reversible.

Distribution of blood according to local need

Surely it is the need of organs which determines the distribution of blood. Organs undoubtedly can store blood in amounts above their need, but lack of blood is a condition essential organs do not tolerate. I say "essential", because it is well recognized that some vascular areas may be almost closed down during periods of great need in other areas. But when the heart, the brain, some endocrine glands and the kidneys need blood they usually get it.

The mechanism by which this is accomplished must be more than mere passive dilatation from local axon reflexes or locally formed metabolites allowing more blood to drain into the dilated area. I should suppose that the need is signaled by neurones and humoral messages indicating need and that, after integration, the appropriate afferent messages go to those vascular areas where blood can be spared.

In keeping with what I have said before, for quick changes in blood distribution I would expect nerve mechanisms to be chiefly involved but for prolonged changes, humoral mechanisms. Are there then such physiological mechanisms demonstrable?

The kidneys demonstrate the humoral mechanisms admirably, though I must admit that the demonstration is not rigorously proved (*58*). I shall not discuss the mechanism at this point but simply say that when the kidneys do not receive enough blood or there is a change in the pulsatile character of the blood received, a reaction is set up which raises blood pressure which may aid in overcoming blood deficit. The nerve bundles supplying the kidneys have always been a puzzle and, like those supplying the brain, seem to have only mild vasoconstrictor action and do not appear to take an important part in circulatory control except possibly under conditions of great stress. McCubbin and I (*6*) found some evidence of nervous connections with the adrenal glands which could be stimulated by the ganglion stimulating agent Dmpp, but the actual function of such connections is purely conjectural.

The brain in respect to its control of its circulation is a good deal like the kidneys. It is highly dependent on the height of the systemic blood pressure, partially on humoral agents, and with relatively little dependence on vasomotor control. On the other hand, vasoconstriction and dilatation within the brain can importantly influence vasomotor reflexes such as the reflex pressor response to occlusion of the common carotid artery. Kaneko, McCubbin and I (*7*) found that several vasoconstrictor drugs given into the cerebral lateral ventricles, as well as cooling of the cerebrospinal fluid, inhibited this reflex. The effect was opposed by central administration of vasodilator drugs or heating the cerebrospinal fluid. Vasoconstriction in the cerebral vessel was associated with a fall in systemic arterial pressure and slowing of the heart rate, while local vasodilatation opposed these central inhibitory effects. I shall discuss this phenomenon later but I want to use it now to illustrate the thesis that the blood flow to an organ can influence systemic blood pressure to an important degree. The brain, unlike the kidney, seems to exert its influence largely on the cardiovascular system by changes in neural control. But even the brain seems to have some modicum of direct chemical control if the pressor substance tentatively called "cerebrotonin" can be more closely identified and characterized. At one stage in its evolution the brain exhibited relatively highly developed endocrine function which may not have been wholly lost.

The control of blood to the myocardium seems to combine the neural and humoral mechanisms to give each clear importance. When the heart lacks blood it "cries out" for more during the familiar angina pectoris. Its afferent control is highly responsive. The efferent control affects both inotropic and chronotropic characteristics of the muscle, but it is less clear how effective the vasomotor response may be. The same may be said for the control by the blood-borne vasoactive agents, although again it is clear that both have important effects even though their quantitative relationships are not defined. We know too little of the meaning of the storage of catecholamines and other vasoactive agents in the myocardium and blood vessels to speculate profitably.

Each organ could be considered in similar fashion but enough has been discussed, I believe, to illustrate the thesis that the local need for blood is one of the critical determinants of systemic blood pressure. From this it follows that disturbances in the level of blood pressure may result from disturbances in the need for blood in single and multiple organs. The dominant mechanism employed by an organ to control its own perfusion may under some circumstances assume a primary role in controlling systemic blood pressure levels. However, the dominance of one mechanism does not insure the abrogation of all other controlling mechanisms. It is for this reason that arterial blood pressure may be affected by agents acting on such different facets of the blood pressure controlling mechanism.

1. Neurogenic participation

Clinical	*Experimental*
Poliomyelitis of brain stem	Cerebral ischemia
Porphyria, chronic	
Increased intracranial pressure	Cushing's experiment
Sclerosis of carotid sinus	Resection of sinus and aortic depressor nerves
Resection öf glossopharyngeal nerve	
Emotion	Hypertension from audiogenic stimulus

As I promised, I shall touch only superficially on a few topics of special interest to illustrate my thesis; there will be no marshalling of evidence to show the important participation of the nervous system in the mechanisms of hypertension. We have already done this in outline form recently (59). I shall first consider the problem of the resetting of the carotid sinus and similar buffer mechanisms when renal hypertension develops, merely as an example of the behavior of the nervous system under the changed conditions of hypertension.

Blood pressure regulatory mechanisms and the level of their "set"

Physicians have been puzzled for many years because of the fact that pressure on the carotid sinus area elicited the same circulatory response in hypertensive subjects as in normotensive ones. It had been taught that the sinus mechanism was one of the most powerful modulators of blood pressure levels. When blood pressure is raised by injection of pressor drugs, baroceptors are stimulated and reflexly diminish, or eliminate, neurogenic vasoconstriction from the vasomotor centers in an effort to lower blood pressure. But when the pressure rises during the course of essential or malignant hypertension the sinus mechanism seems to fail. Indeed, it seems to operate to maintain the elevated pressure.

McCubbin, Green and I (8) studied this problem using electroneurographic techniques to measure baroceptor activity in normotensive states and then after production of acute and chronic renal hypertension. The observation that in chronically hypertensive dogs baroceptors fire intermittently at supernormal pressure levels — which elicits continuous firing in normotensive animals — indicates that the regulating mechanism has been set to buffer arterial pressure at higher levels. The carotid sinus buffer mechanism has shifted its threshold and range of response upward so that it perceives, so to speak, the hypertensive levels as normal ones. The regulator has been reset upwards. After the resetting, it naturally acts to maintain arterial pressure at the higher levels rather than normal ones.

Clearly, even hypertension of primarily renal origin has an important neurogenic component and it is, in my opinion, the reason that patients with such hypertension respond to neuroplegic drugs in many cases as well as patients with essential hypertension in whom the renal component is less clearly defined. The resetting phenomenon can be used as an explanation for many of the pharmacological and clinical phenomena associated with hypertension.

For example, it may explain why nephrectomy lowers pressure in the acute stage of renal hypertension but not in the chronic. It might be a factor in the occasional patient in whom the hypertension persists after removal of a pheochromocytoma and in

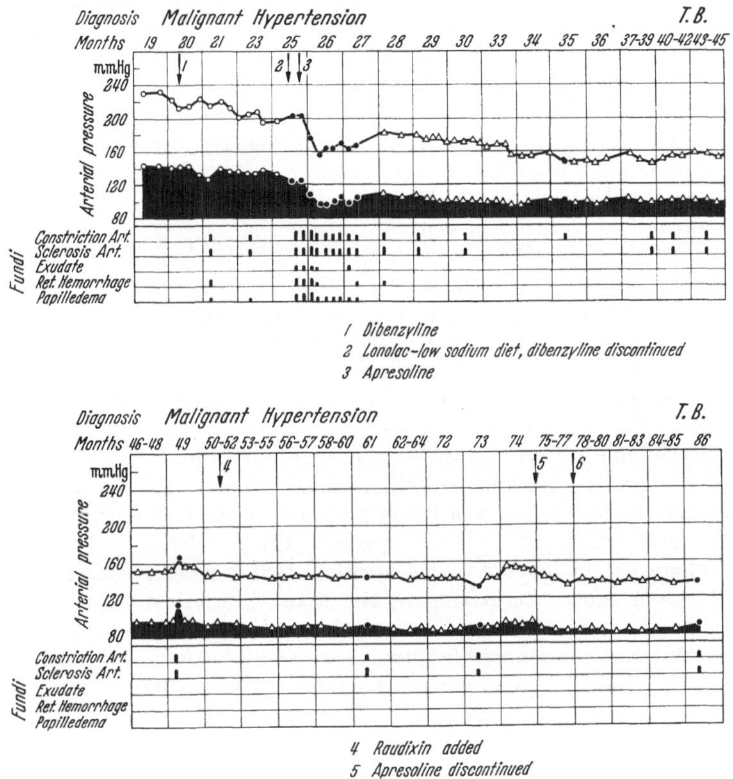

Fig. 2. Patient with malignant hypertension treated successfully with hydralazine for 5 years. When the drug was withdrawn blood pressure did not rise. Blood pressures as depicted by dots represent average of 4 measurements a day for one week. Triangles represent average taken at home or in our out-patient clinic. Eyegrounds are graded on a 1—4 scale. Failure of the sympathetic blocking agent Dibenzyline to lower arterial pressure is shown at arrow 1

the group of patients we have found to become normotensive after years of antihypertensive therapy. An example of such a patient is shown in Fig. 2.

The carotid sinus mechanism is only one of several nervous mechanisms which can control blood pressure in a discriminating fashion. Much work has shown the highly selective action of various parts in the hypothalamus. For example, MANNING and PEISS (*60*) showed that in cats electrical stimulation of various parts of the diencephalon elicited vasoconstriction, augmentation of myocardial contraction and cardioacceleration. These types of response may occur singly or, more commonly, as various combinations. The major component of a pressor response was often the result of increased force of myocardial contraction rather than vasoconstriction. FOLKOW, JOHANSSON and ÖBERG (*61*) found a restricted hypothalamic area, stimulation of which caused inhibition of sympathetic vasomotor activity. They suggest that this is a hypothalamic relay station for cortical inhibitory pathways to subordinated sympathetic structures chiefly affecting discharge of the medullary vasomotor center.

Still another possible nervous control mechanism is the chemoreceptors which seem to be in the brain. TAYLOR and I (*62*) found that the vascular responses in the body were often reversed from what might be usually expected when the vasoactive substance was injected into the perfused brain joined to the body only by the nervous system. Thus epinephrine and norepinephrine lowered, instead of raising, blood pressure and histamine and acetyl-beta-methylcholine raised it. Baroceptors were not found.

Enough examples have, I think, been given to show how complex the nervous control of blood pressure may be. It should serve as a warning against a glib approach to the problem.

There are believed to be still other buffer mechanisms in the body than those originating in the carotid sinus and aorta, but they have not been adequately enough studied to receive more than mention. But their possible importance should not be overlooked, since the resetting phenomenon may be a general one and not at all limited to the carotid sinus buffer mechanism.

Relatively much more attention has been given to baroceptors than chemoceptors. There is good reason to suspect that the latter are also concerned with regulation of blood pressure and perfusion. Control of perfusion must then almost surely be regulated by both pressure and chemical sensing elements of the nervous system. Still another mechanism may be such elements that respond not through the nervous system but by direct liberation of vasoactive agents; examples may be the juxtaglomerular apparatus, the adrenal medulla and the pituitary gland.

The central action of reserpine

Many of the drugs that have powerful effects on the hypertensive's blood pressure act primarily on the central nervous system. Reserpine is an excellent example. It is known to have a strong central cardiovascular action but the mechanism is not known. Recently Drs. McCubbin, Kaneko and I (9) studied this problem in dogs. Both serotonin and norepinephrine are released from the bound to free form in the brain by reserpine. Both inhibit central synaptic transmission. It is, therefore, possible that the central effects of reserpine on vasomotor activity depend upon release of these two amines, and it should be possible to reproduce these effects by injecting them directly into the cerebrospinal fluid, since reserpine is effective when given in this way. We tested both serotonin and norepinephrine and their respective precursors.

All of these substances had qualitatively the same effects in that they lowered arterial pressure, usually caused bradycardia despite prior vagus nerve section, and caused marked inhibition of the pressor response to occlusion of the common carotid arteries. The same result was obtained in anesthetized and unanesthetized dogs. These results are all consistent with the premise that the acute cardiovascular effects of reserpine are mediated centrally by serotonin and/or norepinephrine, either released from a bound and inactive to a free and active form, or formed by decarboxylation of their respective amino acids.

But how might they do this ? We found that not only reserpine but several vasoconstrictor drugs given into the cerebral ventricles inhibited the carotid occlusion pressor reflex. This effect was opposed by central administration of vasodilator drugs. Cooling of the cerebrospinal fluid, which presumably caused local vasoconstriction, also caused inhibition of the carotid reflex, hypotension and bradycardia — effects counteracted by central injection of vasodilator drugs. Warming the cerebrospinal fluid did just the opposite. It would appear then that these effects on vasomotor activity depend upon changes in local blood flow. It follows that the cardiovascular effects of reserpine are probably due to local decrease of tissue perfusion caused by release of serotonin, norepinephrine or other vasoconstrictor agents.

From this and the example taken from the resetting phenomenon in the carotid sinus mechanism one begins to feel the power and complexity of the nervous control of arterial blood pressure and tissue perfusion.

2. Cardiovascular participation

Clinical	_Experimental_
Coarctation of aorta	Clamping of aorta above renal
Heart failure	vessels
Arteriovenous fistula	
Arteriosclerosis	

I have already discussed the problem of increased resistance resulting from anatomical change in the resistance vessels, whether it be temporary and reversible due to edema or due to more permanent structural change. In either case it has become increasingly clear that blood pressure can usually be lowered successfully in such patients without evident deleterious effects. I was brought up on the view that when hypertension went from a functional to a structural stage, it was irreversible and the hypertension would be persistent. I still hear this explanation for therapeutic failure delivered with much assurance and authority; indeed, in direct proportion to lack of knowledge and experience.

The problem of cardiovascular reactivity is currently a complex mess. Twenty years ago I became interested because it seemed to me that the response of the substrate on which nervous impulses, or humoral agents, work should be as important as the intensity of the stimulus. We had somehow always come to think of the hypertensive patient as a jumpy, hyperirritable individual. In the light of better studies we now know this is far from true. Dr. McCubbin and I (*10*) studied the blood pressure response in a large series of normal and of experimentally hypertensive animals. The upshot of this work established several things:

1. Dogs with buffer nerves sectioned and hypertensive were exquisitely sensitive to ganglioplegics and certain other hypotensive agents. Further, serotonin was strongly depressor in them and it was extremely difficult to block the sympathetic ganglia with ganglion blocking agents. This pattern was so characteristic we believed we could readily identify this particular neurogenic hypertensive mechanism by these responses. There are several other types of experimental neurogenic hypertension not having the same mechanism for which we have found no pharmacological key.

2. Dogs with experimental renal hypertension, whether due to a clamp on the renal artery or a Cellophane fibrocollagenous hull around the parenchyma, in our hands at least, behaved as normotensive dogs. We found no characteristic change that could be brought out by the different cardiovascular responses which we elicited.

3. We have had less experience with the cardiovascular reactivity patterns of endocrine types of hypertension. But from a careful study of the literature, it is evident that there is little agreement among various investigators. Most seem to find a slight augmentation of the pressor response to norepinephrine after repeated administration of desoxycorticosterone acetate, but even this is unimpressive.

4. The problem of reactivity of patients with hypertension is in complete confusion. For many years the literature has abounded with claims and counterclaims. The cold-pressor test is one that received much attention at one time. Epinephrine and norepinephrine have been widely used and the responses to tetraethylammoniumchloride as well. As it now stands, it is impossible to form any clear notion of whether there is, or is not, increased reactivity. We have studied the problem extensively but are still uncertain in our minds about the results. Much, it seems to me, hinges on the selection of the proper stimulant to bring out differences in mechanism.

The subject is becoming increasingly more important because of the florescence of a number of theories concerned with changes in the electrolyte and enzyme content of the blood vessels themselves.

Another aspect of cardiovascular participation has recently received much attention, chiefly because of the introduction of safer forms of aortography. This is the demonstration that many patients with hypertension have obstructive lesions in the renal vessels. It is possible that the same may be true of the cerebral blood supply. I mention this at this point simply to call attention to this as another aspect of the participation of the blood vessels in the mechanism of hypertension.

3. Endocrine participation

Clinical	Experimental
Acromegaly	Anterior pituitary (growth)
	Adrenal cortical
Cushing's syndrome	Exogenous
Adreno-genital syndrome	Cortisone: hydrocortisone
Aldosteronism	Desoxycorticosterone + NaCl
Pheochromocytoma	Aldosterone + NaCl
	Endogenous
Toxemia of pregnancy	Adrenal enucleation + NaCl
	NaCl alone

The problem of endocrine participation in hypertension is far too complex for casual description here. I shall have to content myself with discussion of a few recent observations which may illustrate the broad principles concerned in the mosaic theory. In most cases the effects of the endocrine glands on the level of blood pressure are what the very up-to-date physiologist calls "permissive". For example, hypertension of a not very impressive sort can be produced in animals subjected to adrenalectomy but treated with salt. We found the same to be true after hypophysectomy. I had the notion then that most endocrine glands kept the body sufficiently normal that it could react with vigorous hypertension. A weak, flabby one usually did not.

The recent experience with adrenalectomy in the treatment of hypertension largely initiated by Wolferth et al. (*11*) in Philadelphia is another example of what appears to be a permissive role of the adrenal cortex. By no means all patients responded with a satisfactory fall in blood pressure.

A patient of ours illustrates what may happen (Cleveland Clinic Hospital No. 621—642). This man failed to improve on a rice diet; hydralazine was ineffective and, since at that time no other drugs were available, total adrenalectomy was performed. He was maintained on 50 mg of cortisone a day, 20 mg of ACTH and 6 g of sodium chloride. The blood pressure simply did not come down except during periods when maintenance of corticoid was temporarily discontinued and an Addisonian crisis was imminent. When hexamethonium became available we found that 25 mg intramuscularly effectively lowered blood pressure. At autopsy, malignant nephrosclerosis with necrotizing arteriolitis and secondary parathyroid hyperplasia was found. In view of the suggested part the adrenal glands may play in malignant vascular disease it is interesting to note it was present in the absence of the glands.

Many patients, unlike this one, could be kept in a zone of maintenance therapy where blood pressure was well controlled yet they were not suffering from overt hypoadrenalism. Clearly we have no proof that the adrenal glands are only permissive. It could just as well be that they are essential for some types of hypertension and permissive in others.

Adrenal regeneration hypertension

Skelton (*12*) discovered a type of experimental hypertension associated with regeneration of the adrenal cortex but not the medulla. Present evidence suggests that neither corticosterone nor aldosterone are secreted in sufficient quantity by regenerating adrenals to account for the production of hypertension. The hypertensive vascular disease occurs in young rats during the regeneration of the adrenal cortex when the mass of renal tissue has been reduced by uninephrectomy and intake of salt increased. In the absence of any one of these factors, the syndrome fails to develop. The similarity of this syndrome with that induced by exogenoussteroid administration under the same experimental conditions has been noted by Skelton. Once hypertension has been established, neither removal of the regenerated adrenal nor substitution of water for saline drinking fluid brings about a return of blood pressure to normal. SKELTON thinks that the association between severe renal vascular lesions and the persistence of elevated blood pressure suggests that the hypertension is maintained by some renal mechanism.

Aldosterone and hypertension

One of the most recent contributions to understanding of the mechanisms of endocrine participation in hypertension centers around aldosterone. It seems as if, as each new adrenal corticoid is discovered, it takes its place, along with the others, as still another "cause" of hypertension.

Hypertension seems commonly to be associated with primary aldosteronism usually resulting from an aldosterone-secreting adenoma of the adrenal cortex or adrenal hyperplasia (*13, 14, 21*). Administration of aldosterone in animals does not usually produce impressive hypertension.

GAUNT et al. (*15*) were unable to produce it in rats treated for 7 months with small doses. GROSS and SCHMIDT (*16*) did not observe it in rabbits given large doses for 18 days, but previously (*17*) had found hypertension in uninephrectomized rats receiving saline given 0.5 mg aldosterone acetate for 4 weeks. With 0.25 mg no change in blood pressure occurred. Daily doses of 2.5 mg of desoxycorticosterone acetate produced the same degree of hypertension. The daily uptake of fluid and of salt was about twice as great with DOCA as with aldosterone. But in the maintenance of water and electrolyte balance it is believed to be twenty times, or more, as potent as desoxycorticosterone.

An interesting aspect of the problem of the relationship of adrenal steroids to hypertension comes from the study by COOPER et al. (*18*) of steroid formation by slices of adrenal glands of hypertensive patients. The rate of steroid formation decreased per unit weight with increasing diastolic pressure. But in the less advanced hypertension the rate of formation of all steroids with the exception of delta-4-androstene-11-beta-ol-3,17-dione, was about twice that of the normotensive cancer group which acted as controls. The weight of the adrenal glands increased with increasing diastolic pressure and this compensated only in part for the reduction in the rate of steroid formation.

Hypertension and vascular disease elicited by DCA, salt and uninephrectomy does not seem to be currently under active study. Since DCA is not a normally occurring substance or at least, if it occurs, then only in minute amounts, the problem seems to have lost some interest despite the fact that cortisone has some of the properties of DCA. Gross et al. (*19*) showed that, in doses equieffective as regards sodium retention, DCA produced hypertension and severe vascular changes while aldosterone was without effect.

Recently Genest et al. (*20*) studied the excretion of aldosterone in hypertensives. They found an increased excretion in about 53% of patients. The difference between malignant hypertensives and normal controls was great. They stress the great variability of excretion, and this may be seen even in prehypertensive subjects.

Laragh et al. (*22*) utilized an isotope-dilution technique to measure levels of aldosterone secreted by the glands in relation to changes in sodium intake. They found aldosterone secretion uniformly within normal limits in essential hypertension while it was significantly increased with renal or vascular complications. Most striking was the marked increase in 11 of 12 patients with malignant hypertension. Hypersecretion of aldosterone is by no means a constant finding. Indeed, the highest values are found in cases with liver disease and nephrosis in whom hypertension is not present. Much remains to be done before aldosterone can be assigned to its role in the mechanism of essential or malignant hypertension. It is possible that the greatly differing results of various investigators may be due to the variability of excretion of aldosterone.

In 1950 we (*23*) had formulated a unifying concept which tended to reconcile some inadequacies of current theories concerned with adrenal participation in renal hypertension.

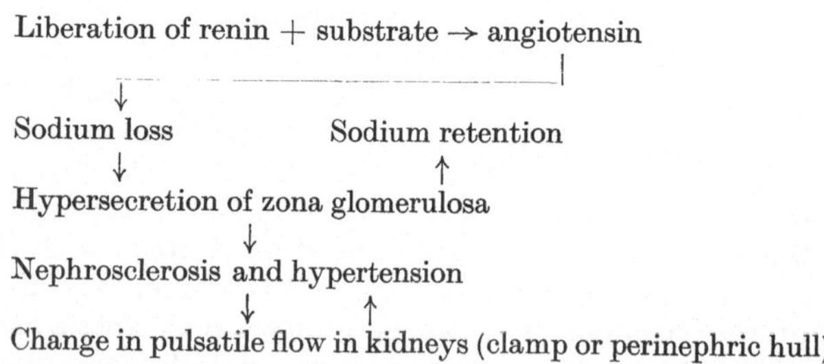

We at first observed a similarity between vascular lesions in renal and desoxycorticosterone hypertension. Then it was noted by Deane and Masson (*24*) that the zona glomerulosa was hypertrophied in rats treated with pressor renal extracts. This zone, presumed source of salt active corticosteroids, was regulated by changes in Na/K ratio of the body fluids. Thus, we had two factors having opposite effects on sodium metabolism: on the one hand, renin and angiotensin causing sodium loss and, on the other, desoxycorticoids causing sodium retention. Hypertrophy of the zona glomerulosa caused by renin and renal hypertension could then be a homeostatic response to the loss of sodium. The resulting increase in the desoxycorticosteroids originating from the glomerulosa would increase hypertension and vascular lesions and therefore renal damage; thus a vicious circle would be established. At the symposium on hypertension in 1950 at the University of Minnesota we observed that "perhaps the greatest usefulness of this rather fanciful hypothesis is that it demands the demonstration of the hypersecretion of desoxycorticosteroids from the zona glomerulosa". An equivalent of them has been demonstrated by EISENSTEIN and HARTROFT (*25*) who found hypersecretion of aldosterone in rats with induced sodium deficiency.

Clearly this is a field fraught with many conflicting experimental results and clinical observations. Whether other adrenal steroids, normal or abnormal, will be found to be more concerned with the mechanisms of hypertension remains to be seen. As it now stands, the adrenal corticoids seem to be chiefly concerned with the maintenance of the sodium and potassium content of tissues, which, in turn, seems to have some even less well-defined relationship to hypertension. Even though these relationships are not clearly defined, they seem none the less to be real and important.

4. Renal participation

Clinical	*Experimental*
Glomerulonephritis	Antikidney serum nephritis
Obstruction of renal vessels	Mechanical constriction of renal
Posttraumatic (hematoma)	artery or vein
Pyelonephritis	Cellophane perinephritis
Polycystic kidneys	Renoprival state
Acute renal failure	
Periarteritis nodosa	
Leucemic infiltration	
Wilm's tumor	
Nephrosclerosis	

It is now 21 years since angiotensin was discovered, and we still are not clear on its function in hypertension. The several steps in its formation have since then largely been elucidated. The most recent advance was the concurrent synthesis of the octapeptide in our laboratory (*26*) and in the CIBA laboratories (*27*), based on the amino acid sequence found by ELLIOTT and PEART (*28*). BRAUN-MENENDEZ and I, shortly before his tragic death, agreed on a method of ending the confusing nomenclature situation by combining angiotonin and hypertensin to make "angiotensin" (*29*). This happy solution should, and is, being widely adopted. It would be a pity to continue the now unnecessary confusion by using either of the two older names.

The fact that so many years had to elapse before the completion of the job was due to many factors, the chief of which was that it is only recently that the field of hypertension has received any large interest or financial support. Angiotensin is clearly a key substance in the mechanism of renal hypertension; yet our tiny group was the only one until recently that had any interest in isolating and synthesizing it. I do not hesitate to recognize the magnificent contributions in the past few years of others such as PEART, SCHWYZER, SKEGGS and others, but I do want you to remember the long arid years when providing the barest intellectual and financial support for the work required most of what we had.

Now that synthetic octa- and deca-peptides are available for widespread use, a number of studies on their pharmacology have appeared. So far nothing has been discovered to suggest that the studies made on the older semipurified natural product were not satisfactory.

HELMER'S (*30*) observation that during renal hypertension a substance can be demonstrated in the renal vein blood that contracts an aortic strip is of much interest. The vasoconstrictor substance has many of the properties of angiotensin, possibly bound to a larger protein. This work is obviously of much importance and for that reason I will have little to say about it in detail at this time. We, probably like others, are studying the matter to be sure that no artefacts have inadvertently been introduced to confuse the issue.

The problem of the renin content of the kidneys is also a vexed one and has been under investigation almost from the beginning of the study of renin itself. The trouble has been that no quantitative method has been developed for measurement of this proteolytic enzyme. Indeed, the enzyme itself has received little enough study. PLENTL and I (*31*) showed in 1944 that even the most purified renin preparations of that time exhibited carboxypeptidase, pepsinase, trypsinase and aminopeptidase activities. The carboxypeptidase and pepsinase activities did not appear to be a necessary part of the specific renin action. HAAS, LAMFROM and GOLDBLATT (*32*) attempted to obtain pure renin with no success.

Theirs is doubtless the purest to date. So when saline extracts are made of kidney tissue and these crude extracts studied for pressor content it should be clear that almost any result might be expected. And this is exactly what has been happening. Different investigators' results have been so erratic that it is impossible to be sure of any of them. So far, I have only been impressed with some of the experiments of GROSS and his associates (*33, 34*) and MASSON and OMAE (*35*) in our laboratory, where renin seems to have been demonstrated to disappear in rats under treatment with salt, DCA, and after renal infarction. The results of BLAQUIER, GOMEZ and HOOBLER (*36*) are of great interest. They showed that transplanting a normal kidney to the hind limb of a hypertensive rat resulted in a reduction of blood pressure. Clamping the artery to the transplanted kidney restored the hypertension. Hypertension caused by infusion of renin or angiotensin into an arenal rat was not lowered by a transplant. Renin inactivation was not therefore the mechanism of lowering blood pressure.

OMAE, MASSON and PAGE (*35*) have shown that grafting a normal kidney causes a sharp rise in pressure in a 24 hr nephrectomized rat, followed by a further slow increase. Infarcted and encapsulated kidneys, as well as those from rats with hormonal hypertension, or as a result of high salt diets, did not release any pressor material. But in hypertension due to a clip on the renal artery, pressor material was released, but not from the contralateral "normal" kidney. These observations seem to me to be of interest but I submit that, until much more is known, it would be premature to base any important conclusions on them. The next step will be to determine the rate of turnover of the renin in the kidneys. The failure of release could mean that the secretory mechanism has been blocked or that the release had been so active that little or none was actually stored so that it could be washed out when the kidney was perfused.

KOLFF and I transplanted normal kidneys into dogs with Cellophane perinephritic hypertension and found reduction of blood pressure in 6 of 15 dogs. This work is still incomplete. The transplantation of normal kidneys into hypertensive patients with subsequent removal of the diseased kidney by MERRILL, MURRAY and HARRISON (*36*) in a few cases of identical twins has resulted in normal blood pressure. This seems to me to be an important validation of the experimental work. Dr. MERRILL tells me that 6 years after the first operation the patient's blood pressure is still normal. It seems that the removal of the diseased kidneys is a necessary part of the procedure. In one patient in whom this was not done the normal transplanted kidneys developed the same vascular lesions of malignant hypertension as did the diseased kidneys. Fall in blood pressure as long as the kidney functions has also been observed by them in transplants between persons who were not twins.

Except for this sort of study, little has been learned about the quantitative aspects of renin. And until respectable assay methods for this enzyme are elaborated and thoroughly validated, I believe it a great mistake to base theory of mechanism on the current wholly inadequate methods.

After much work we still don't know the exact distribution of renin in the kidneys. Some found it in the tubules, others in the glomeruli and still others in the juxtaglomerular cells. Most recent work suggests it is in the glomerular zone [BING and WIBERG (*37*)] but not in the glomerular capillary loops. If I am not mistaken, COOK and PICKERING (*38*) have localized it in the glomerular pole. NAIRN et al. (*39*) suggest, from fluorescent antibody studies, that it is in the glomerular epithelial cells. One half of the renin activity is said to be in the mitochondrial fraction [DENGLER and REICHEL (*40*)].

It almost appears as though renin were strategically placed where pressure effects from the blood could affect its release. The angiotensin formed may well act locally on the kidney just as some of the tissue kinins are believed to act. The local and general systemic effects of angiotensin need untangling.

The assay of angiotensin has been just as troublesome. KAHN et al. (*41*) thought they had demonstrated a large excess of angiotensin in patients with malignant hypertension. GOLLAN, RICHARDSON and GOLDBLATT (*42*) found much the same in dogs with experimental renal hypertension. Neither of these investigations has seemed convincing to most workers.

The participation of the kidney in the mechanism of hypertension by inactivating an extrarenal pressor mechanism

Probably the beginning of the idea that normal kidney tissue was somehow important in the mechanism of hypertension was the observation made by many of us who worked early in the field that the removal of the normal kidney in an animal with a clamp on the other renal artery made the hypertension much worse. I have seen this in patients, dogs and rats on many occasions. Then followed a series of attempts by HARRISON and GROLLMAN and our group, at that time in Indianapolis, to prepare kidney extracts which could use this property to lower blood pressure therapeutically.

We were not sufficiently successful to carry conviction, although I think Dr. GROLLMAN and I personally still think there is an antihypertensive substance present in kidneys. Perhaps this is just the stubbornness of the ageing mind.

GROLLMAN (*43*) then showed that hypertension followed some days after total nephrectomy. The suggestion was not long in coming that renoprival hypertension proved that the kidneys were not the source of a pressor substance responsible for hypertension. If the excretory function of the kidneys is thwarted by implanting the ureters into the vena cava, hypertension does not develop. By exclusion, hypertension would seem to be due to the action of a pressor substance produced elsewhere but normally destroyed by the kidneys. Hypertension of renal origin could then be due to a defect in the function, rather than the circulation, of the kidneys. KOLFF and I (*44*) found that renoprival hypertension disappeared if a pair of normal kidneys was transplanted into the dog's neck. Using the same technique, a pair of hind legs or spleen was ineffective. This suggested that normal kidneys exert a protective effect against renoprival hypertension.

FLOYER (*45*) suggested, from studies in hypertensive rats, that the kidney maintains normal blood pressure by inhibiting an extrarenal pressor system. Nephrectomy or partial renal arterial constriction was thought to prevent the kidneys from exercising this function and resulted in hypertension. FLOYER thinks the hypothetical extrarenal pressor system operates in the early as well as later stage of experimental renal hypertension, although he grants that a renal pressor factor may be responsible for the pressure rise during the first few days. He too finds, along with others [GROLLMAN (*43*), KOLFF (*46*)], that the kidney maintains normal blood pressure by renal inactivation of the extrarenal pressor mechanism by some process independent of excretion.

There has been much discussion, and disagreement, as to whether total nephrectomy does, or does not, abolish experimental renal hypertension. Most agree that early in its course hypertension is abolished, but after several months the results are highly irregular. KOLFF and I (*47*) studied the problem by using the artificial kidney to keep the dogs alive and in reasonably good health. In former studies the animals had died in from 3—6 days, often in miserable condition. We found that hypertension persisted after nephrectomy. As another working hypothesis, we suggested that angiotensin acts in the early stage as a pressor agent but that in the chronic phase it acts to blunt or destroy the kidney's ability to maintain arterial pressure at normal levels. Both renoprival and chronic renal hypertension under this hypothesis are due to loss of this specific renal function. These are all interesting suggestions, but so far no definitive evidence has appeared to support them. Further, it should be recognized that most of the experiments on which they are based are not as secure as they sound. There are many variables in this kind of experimentation and at this juncture we can afford to be wary. For example, no one has yet found an "extrarenal pressor system" to be inactivated by the kidneys, though it must be admitted that no one seems to have looked very hard.

Plasma from hypertensive renoprival rats was found by RON-DELL, McVAUGH and BOHR (*48*) to have increased constrictor action on rat's aorta strips, but it had no pressor action in acutely nephrec-tomized rats cross-circulated with the hypertensive animals. They are not yet certain that increased constrictor action is not an artefact. If it is not, they suggest that its action is on arterioles sensitized by the chronic arenal state.

Renotrophin as a cause of renal hypertension

BRAUN-MENENDEZ (*49*) proposed the hypothesis that the size of the kidney and its functional capacity is determined by the con-centration of trophic substances in the blood which the kidney eliminates. When the production of these renotrophins is increased, the kidneys enlarge and function increases until a new equilibrium is reached between production and elimination of renotrophin. Thus, if nutritional and humoral conditions are kept constant and the amount of renal substance reduced by nephrectomy, the concentration of renotrophin should increase, stimulating growth of the remaining kidney until equilibrium is re-established. Hyper-tension occurs when the remaining renal tissue is unable to respond to the stimulus of normal, or increased amounts, of renotrophin present in the blood. According to this hypothesis, blood pressure of animals with experimental renal hypertension should be reduced if (1) the rate of renotrophin production is reduced (hypophys-ectomy, thyroidectomy, low protein diet), (2) the functional renal mass is increased (kidney transplant, parabiosis). Conversely, hypertension should appear if (1) the rate is increased (thyroid hormone, somatotrophin, testosterone, protein rich diets) or (2) the functional renal mass is reduced (sensitizing actions of uni-lateral nephrectomy).

Most of the methods for producing experimental renal hyper-tension involve reduction in the amount of functional renal tissue, according to BRAUN-MENENDEZ (*50*). While this may be questioned still the ideas involved in the theory are cogent ones. It is greatly to be hoped that the hypothesis will provide an orderly framework to aid in clarifying this diverse and confused aspect of hypertension. Knowing EDUARDO BRAUN-MENENDEZ as well as I did, I am sure this is precisely what he hoped it would do.

Hypertension of renal vascular origin

I have reviewed elsewhere (*51, 52*) the history of the endeavor to involve the kidneys in the mechanism of hypertension. Suffice it to say here that angiograms are now in ever more widespread use for the detection of renal vascular lesions and that enough surgical vascular repair has been performed to convince us that this is an aspect of hypertension of the greatest importance.

The usual cause of narrowing of the renal artery is atherosclerosis followed in frequency by thrombosis and congenital stenosis. The lesions may be unilateral or bilateral. Unlike the results in animals, surgical correction seems commonly to be followed by return of blood pressure to normal or near normal levels. It does not happen in everyone. We have no assurance in all cases that the proper correction of the difficulty has been accomplished.

It has been our experience that, if patients are carefully selected for further more penetrating study of the mechanism of their hypertension, something of the order of 25% will be found with clearly demonstrable renal vascular and parenchymal lesions. This by no means indicates anything like this number in the total hypertensive population. Unfortunately we have no control series of normotensive patients who have had aortograms. Further, it is unlikely that we will have such for many years, as there are few normal people who care to have aortography performed in order to become a statistic among controls.

The problem of nephrectomy in the treatment of hypertension can now be much more intelligently approached. In general every effort should be made to conserve healthy, or potentially healthy, renal tissue. If the lesion is segmental within the renal parenchyma, resection should be considered. In most cases vascular surgery can correct lesions of the larger blood vessels. If these fail, and there is clear evidence that the opposite kidney is "reasonably" normal, then nephrectomy may be performed. The unknown in this procedure is what constitutes a "reasonably" normal kidney. I am afraid we will not know until we know how the kidney is concerned in the production of hypertension and how to measure this participation.

I wish I could give you a list of signs and symptoms which would with reasonable assurance tell you whether an aortogram should be done. I have made up such a list and here it is, but I would warn you that it is far from a reliable guide.

Diagnosis of renal vascular disease

1. Young patients without family history of hypertension.
2. Elderly hypertensives whose hypertension suddenly becomes malignant.
3. Malignant hypertension arising de novo.
4. Those of any age with long-standing hypertension which suddenly becomes more severe.
5. Disparity of size or function shown by I. V. urogram.
6. Aortograph and split renal function test.

For instance, much stress has been put on the importance of heredity, and it is stated with much confidence that hypertension under the age of 30 is certainly not essential. Unfortunately this isn't true in particular but is true in general. It just isn't true enough to rely on it.

I know from my travels that many people are fearful of aortograms. Some years ago I shared that fear, but no longer. Dr. E. Poutasse and Dr. A. Humphries at the Cleveland Clinic have done more than 1,500 without morbidity or mortality. If they can do these, others can too. I have little patience with the assertion that this sort of record can only be gotten in Cleveland. I suspect this is a faint suggestion that we are exaggerating.

The aortogram is currently essential to us in making the diagnosis and providing the surgeon with the necessary information to decide whether corrective surgery should be done. Much has been made of the so-called Howard test (*55*) which measures fluid and salt excretion from each kidney. What is not emphasized is that this is a test which requires infinite care to be carried out successfully and even if it is, is far from infallible. If surgery is contemplated an aortogram must be done as well. Perhaps, then, it might as well have been done in the first place.

This aspect of hypertension seems unusually shrouded by clinical lore. You all remember the rules some years ago about nephrectomy curing a patient if the hypertension had not been present for longer than 2 years. It was believed after 7 years it was hopeless. Then there is a more recent one that the majority of young patients have bilateral disease and for them the only treatment is hypotensive drugs. This is patently a half-truth. I wonder why such statements recur with such regularity. I suppose it is because we all like aphorisms; they are to physicians what slogans are to politicians.

The initiation of renal hypertension

It is clear that there are some patients with renal vascular or parenchymal lesions in whom it is altogether reasonable to believe that the lesions are initiating the hypertension. But what about the rest ? We do not know whether subtle changes in the character of pulsatile flow to the kidneys can initiate hypertension. CORCORAN and I (*53, 54*) convinced ourselves, if not others, that hypertension could be produced in dogs by enclosing the kidneys in Cellophane without reduction in blood flow. Even a Goldblatt clamp could be put on in such a way as to change the pulse characteristics in the renal artery without reducing blood flow significantly. This is why we suggested that "an intrarenal hemodynamic change" was the immediate cause of the hypertension and that this was followed by reduction in blood flow. It is evident that eliciting hypertension is not wholly accounted for by reduction in blood flow, else renal ischemia would always be followed by hypertension. A variety of clinical experience shows this to be untrue.

There are those who believe that widespread vascular disease precedes the hypertension in human beings. GOLDBLATT is one of the chief proponents of this view. Most others in the field take the contrary view that the hypertension causes the vascular disease, and to this I subscribe. This does not preclude the possibility that functional changes in the renal vasculature may not occur such as to influence the pulsatile characteristics of the renal blood flow and to initiate hypertension. But so far there is no evidence for, or against, such a view.

Antirenin and experimental renal hypertension

The problem of antirenin is an important one. When GEORGE WAKERLIN first demonstrated the occurrence of these antibodies there was a good deal of justifiable skepticism. But later GOLDBLATT confirmed most of this work. One of the important arguments in favor of the renin-angiotensin hypothesis was the demonstration that antirenin lowered the blood pressure to normal in dogs with experimental renal hypertension. That there may be a difference in mechanism between experimental renal hypertension and renoprival hypertension follows from KOLFF's and my demonstration (*56*) that the latter is unaffected by antirenin. Further, R. E. SHIPLEY showed, in one dog with chronic renal hypertension, that removal of both kidneys failed to lower blood pressure. Injection of a high antirenin titer serum failed to lower blood pressure. Since only one experiment was done, too much weight cannot be given it.

Whether it will be possible to treat hypertension, or to determine its mechanism, by immune methods, remains one of the fascinating and relatively undeveloped fields. I hope the next decade will show great activity in this approach, since more and more pure compounds which may be involved in the mechanism of hypertension are becoming available in quantity.

The structure of angiotensin II and its biological activity

A fairly large number of angiotensin analogues have now been prepared. In our own laboratory, Drs. BUMPUS, SMEBY and KHAIRALLAH (57) have shown that at least 3 groups are essential

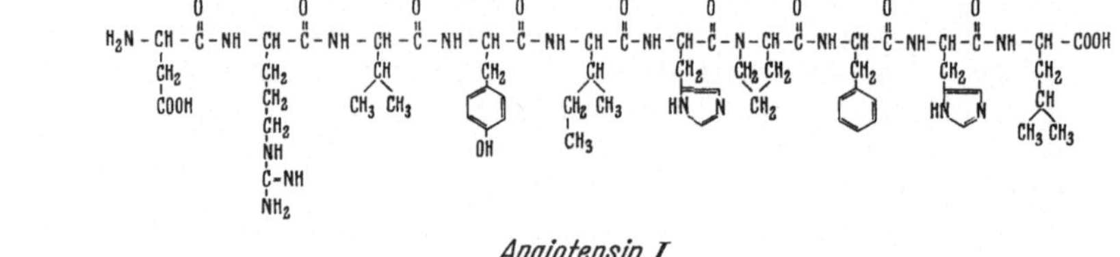
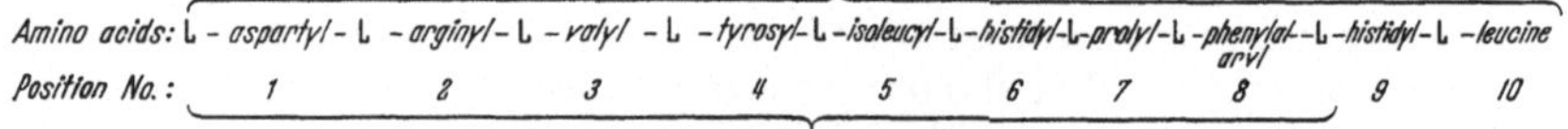

Fig. 3. Structure of angiotensin

for pressor and oxytocic activity: 1. the C-terminal amino acid must be L-phenylalanine, 2. the terminal carboxyl group must be free, 3. tyrosine must be present, and 4. the peptide must contain at least amino acids numbered 3 to 8. This peptide can be inactivated by urea and arginine, compounds well known to break peptide hydrogen bonds, and thereby destroy a particular configuration. The suggestion has been made by us that the smallest peptide capable of assuming this configuration is the hexapeptide (amino acids 3—8) and that this is the basic unit required for activity. The additional amino acids would function only to stabilize the proper spatial form.

It is possible to construct a helical model of angiotensin II which has the 3 necessary groups, the carboxyl and phenyl groups of L-phenylalanine and the phenolic group of tyrosine, arranged close together. The isoleucine side-chain, which has some effect on activity, is positional directly adjacent to these groups. In this peptide there seems to be a portion of the molecule in which the shape, or ionic character, is highly specific for biological activity, while the rest of the molecule is relatively non-specific. This implies that the receptor site in muscle also exhibits similar specificity. It must be of such ionic and spatial character that it will specifically interact with the C-terminal L-phenylalanine and a phenolic group.

Clearly, we are still far from our goal of understanding the mechanism of renal hypertension, although we now are much closer to it in that we fully recognize the importance of the participation of the kidneys and the nervous system, not merely as a hunch, or on an emotional basis, but on relatively rigorous scientific evidence. The participation of the endocrine system is still tantalizing, especially since the work of SELYE and the more recent contributions on aldosterone. DAHL has fostered the notion of the importance of salt. Our Russian colleagues, MYASNIKOV and SPERANSKY, are strongly impressed by the contribution of the "thinking brain". This seems to me to be one of those situations where almost everbody is right — it is largely a matter of degree.

Conclusion

I have tried to persuade you that arterial blood pressure functions as a part of a complicated mechanism to control tissue perfusion. It is compounded of a large variety of facets which are in constant equilibrium with one another: a mosaic if you will. When one facet is changed, all change to restore equilibrium. At one time one facet or another may become dominant, but those mechanisms which are thereby made secondary do not abrogate their function.

But the directive of blood pressure comes from the local needs of the tissues. It is their signaled demand for blood which determines blood pressure levels and the mechanisms by which it will be controlled. The set and resetting of the mechanisms which control this organ perfusion may importantly affect the long-term average blood pressure level.

Arterial hypertension itself, therefore, results from a constellation of facets, one or even none being more or less dominant. For this reason, I have included in the application of the "mosaic theory" to clinical and experimental hypertension an artificial, but useful, division into four groups divided according to supposed primacy: 1. nervous, 2. endocrine, 3. cardiovascular, and 4. renal. Under each of these categories I have discussed some recent advances in knowledge which serve to illustrate their individual significance.

References

1. TAYLOR, R. D., I. H. PAGE, and A. C. CORCORAN: A. M. A. Arch. Int. Med. 88, 1 (1951).
2. CELANDER, O., and B. FOLKOW: Acta physiol. Scand. 29, 241 (1953).
3. FOLKOW, B.: Structural, myogenic, humoral and nervous factors controlling peripheral resistance. In: Hypotensive drugs. Ed.: M. HARINGTON. London 1956.
4. FOLKOW, B., and B. ÖBERG: Acta physiol. Scand. 47, 131 (1959).

5. Folkow, B., G. Grimby, and O. Thulesius: Acta physiol. Scand. **44**, 255 (1958).
6. Page, I. H., and J. W. McCubbin: Amer. J. Med. **15**, 675 (1953).
7. Kaneko, Y., J. W. McCubbin, and I. H. Page: Circulation Res. (U.S.A.) (In press).
8. McCubbin, J. W., J. W. Green, and I. H. Page: Circulation Res. (U.S.A.) **4**, 205 (1956).
9. McCubbin, J. W., Y. Kaneko, and I. H. Page: Circulation Res. (U.S.A.) (In press).
10. Page, I. H., and J. W. McCubbin: Circulation (U.S.A.) **4**, 70 (1951).
11. Wolferth, C. C., W. T. Fitts, W. A. Jeffers, and A. M. Sellars: Bull. N. Y. Acad. Med. **33**, 151 (1957).
12. Skelton, F. R.: Physiol. Rev. (U.S.A.) **39**, 162 (1959).
13. Chalmers, T. M., M. G. Fitzgerald, A. H. James, and H. Scarborough: Lancet (G. B.) **1956/I**, 127.
14. Holten, C., and V. Posborg Petersen: Lancet (G. B.) **1956/II**, 918.
15. Gaunt, R., G. J. Ulsamer, and J. J. Chart: Arch. int. pharmacodyn. thérap. (Belg.) **110**, 114 (1957).
16. Gross, F., and H. Schmidt: Acta endocrin. (Den.) **28**, 467 (1958).
17. Gross, F., P. Loustalot, and R. Meier: Acta endocrin. (Den.) **26**, 417 (1957).
18. Cooper, D. Y., J. C. Touchstone, J. M. Roberts, W. S. Blakemore, and O. Rosenthal: J. Clin. Invest. (U.S.A.) **37**, 1524 (1958).
19. Gross, F., P. Loustalot, and R. Meier: Experientia (Switz.) **11**, 67 (1955).
20. Genest, J., E. Koiw, W. Nowaczynski, and G. Leboeuf: Proc. Soc. Exper. Biol. Med. (U.S.A.) **97**, 676 (1958).
21. Buchem, F. S. van, H. Doorenbos, and H. S. Elings: Lancet (G. B.) **1956/II**, 335.
22. Laragh, J., S. Ulick, W. Januszewicz, Q. B. Deming, W. G. Kelly, and S. Lieberman: Aldosterone secretion and arterial hypertension. Proc. 32nd Scien. Sessions, Amer. Heart Ass., p. 725. Philadelphia 1959.
23. Page, I. H.: The renin-angiotonin system. In: Hypertension — A Symposium, p. 48. Ed.: E. T. Bell. Minneapolis 1950.
24. Deane, H. W., and G. M. C. Masson: J. Clin. Endocr. (U.S.A.) **11**, 193 (1951).
25. Eisenstein, A. B., and P. M. Hartroft: Endocrinology (U.S.A.) **60**, 634 (1957).
26. Schwarz, H., F. M. Bumpus, and I. H. Page: J. Amer. Chem. Soc. **79**, 5,697 (1957).
27. Rittel, W., B. Iselin, H. Kappeler, B. Riniker, and R. Schwyzer: Helvet. chim. acta **40**, 614 (1957).
28. Elliott, D. F., and W. S. Peart: Biochem. J. (U.S.A.) **65**, 246 (1957).
29. Braun-Menendez, E., and I. H. Page: Science (U.S.A.) **127**, 242 (1958).
30. Helmer, O. M., and W. E. Judson: The presence of vasoconstrictor activity in renal vein plasma of patients with arterial hypertension. In Hypertension, Vol. VIII, Proc. Council for High Blood Pressure Res. (In press).
31. Plentl, A. A., and I. H. Page: J. Biol. Chem. (U.S.A.) **155**, 363 (1944).
32. Haas, E., H. Lamfrom, and H. Goldblatt: Arch. Biochem. (U.S.A.) **42**, 368 (1953).
33. Gross, F., and P. Lichtlen: Amer. J. Physiol. **195**, 543 (1958).
34. Gross, F., and F. Sulser: Arch. exper. Path. u. Pharmakol. (G.) **229**, 374 (1956).

35. OMAE, T., G. M. C. MASSON, and I. H. PAGE: Amer. J. Physiol. (In press).
36. MURRAY, J. E., J. P. MERRILL, and J. H. HARRISON: Ann. Surg. (U.S.A.) **148**, 343 (1958).
37. BING, J., and B. WIBERG: Acta pathol. microbiol. Scand. **44**, 138 (1958).
38. COOK, W. F., and G. W. PICKERING: J. Physiol. (G. B.) **143**,78 P (1958).
39. NAIRN, R. C., K. B. FRASER, and C. S. CHADWICK: Brit. J. Exper. Path. **30**, 155 (1959).
40. DENGLER, H., and G. REICHEL: Experientia (Switz.) **16**, 37 (1960).
41. KAHN, J. R., L. T. SKEGGS jr., N. P. SHUMWAY, and P. E. WISEN-BAUGH: J. Exper. Med. (U.S.A.) **95**, 523 (1952).
42. GOLLAN, F., E. RICHARDSON, and H. GOLDBLATT: J. Exper. Med. (U.S.A.) **88**, 389 (1948).
43. GROLLMAN, A., E. E. MUIRHEAD, and J. VANATTA: Amer. J. Physiol. **151**, 21 (1949).
44. KOLFF, W. J., and I. H. PAGE: Amer. J. Physiol. **178**, 75 (1954).
45. FLOYER, M. A.: Clin. Sc. (G. B.) **14**, 163 (1955).
46. KOLFF, W. J., I. H. PAGE, and A. C. CORCORAN: Amer. J. Physiol. **178**, 237 (1954).
47. KOLFF, W. J., and I. H. PAGE: Amer. J. Physiol. **182**, 531 (1955).
48. RONDELL, P. A., R. B. McVAUGH, and D. F. BOHR: Circulation (U.S.A.) **17**, 708 (1958).
49. BRAUN-MENENDEZ, E.: Acta physiol. latinoam. (Arg.) **2**, 2 (1952).
50. BRAUN-MENENDEZ, E.: Circulation (U.S.A.) **17**, 696 (1958).
51. PAGE, I. H., H. P. DUSTAN, and E. POUTASSE: Ann. Int. Med. (U.S.A.) **51**, 196 (1959).
52. DUSTAN, H. P., I. H. PAGE, and E. P. POUTASSE: N. England J. Med. **261**, 647 (1959).
53. CORCORAN, A. C., and I. H. PAGE: Amer. J. Physiol. **129**, 698 (1940).
54. CORCORAN, A. C., and I. H. PAGE: Amer. J. Physiol. **130**, 335 (1940).
55. HOWARD, J. E., M. BERTHRONG, D. M. GOULD, and E. R. YENDT: Bull. Johns Hopkins Hosp. (U.S.A.) **94**, 51 (1954).
56. KOLFF, W. J., and I. H. PAGE: Amer. J. Physiol. **181**, 575 (1955).
57. BUMPUS, F. M., P. A. KHAIRALLAH, I. H. PAGE, and R. R. SMEBY: The relationship of structure to pressor and oxytocic actions of isoleucine 5 angiotensin octapeptide and various analogues.
58. PAGE, I. H., and J. W. McCUBBIN: Amer. J. Physiol. **173**, 411 (1953).
59. PAGE, I. H., J. W. McCUBBIN, and A. C. CORCORAN: Perspect. Biol. Med. **1**, 307 (1958).
60. MANNING, J. W., and C. N. PEISS: Amer. J. Physiol. **198**, 366 (1960).
61. FOLKOW, B., B. JOHANSSON, and B. ÖBERG: Acta physiol. Scand. **47**, 262 (1959).
62. TAYLOR, R. D., and I. H. PAGE: Circulation (U.S.A.) **4**, 563 (1951).

Inheritance of high blood pressure

By

G. W. PICKERING

Let me begin by reminding you of two elementary facts, usually overlooked when this question is discussed. The first concerns the definition of essential hypertension. Essential hypertension represents no more than elevated blood pressure without a known cause, and the consequences of the raised pressure. Despite what anyone may say at this gathering, any division between normal and elevated pressure is purely arbitrary. There is no unequivocal evidence known to me for any natural division. The artificiality of a division into normal and raised pressure is further emphasized by the diurnal fluctuation of blood pressure which all subjects experience, though some more than others. The second elementary fact is that blood pressure is a quantity and should be studied as a quantity by the accepted methods of biometrics.

The modern study of inheritance of human characteristics began with FRANCIS GALTON (1889). As a result of his enquiries, GALTON concluded that there were two kinds of human inheritance, namely alternative and blended. The first, of which eye colour is an example, we now know to be largely a manifestation of single genes. The latter has been agreed to be a manifestation of the interaction of several genes; in fact, to represent polygenic inheritance. GALTON's example of blended inheritance was stature, and it is most instructive to look at his data and his conclusions, since they both bear some resemblance to the state of affairs in regard to arterial pressure.

GALTON collected data concerning stature on adults from as many families as possible. In interpreting them, he met a difficulty. Women are shorter than men. He saw that if he was to deal with the data mathematically, he had to allow for this. He did so by multiplying female heights by 1.08, the ratio between the mean values for stature in the two sexes in a given population. Having thus transmuted female heights to figures comparable with those of males, he was able to calculate the mid-parental stature. When he arranged the parents in order of ascending mid-parental stature, the children were found to show a series of frequency distributions which moved upwards with the statures of their parents. This slide shows three such frequency distribution curves. When the mean heights of the children were plotted against the mid-parental height, the points fell on a straight line but exhibited regression towards the mean for the population; thus, the children of the tallest parents tended, on the whole, to be less tall, and the children of the shortest parents tended to be less short, than their parents. However, the important thing is that throughout the range investigated, there is a linear relationship between the mean heights of children and parents. The resemblance between children and parents is quantitative. This is now accepted as meaning graded inheritance through the interaction of many genes. As GALTON himself remarked, this might have been anticipated, since stature is the result of many different bones and tissues in the human frame.

Now let us turn to arterial pressure. I wish to describe to you the investigations made with my colleagues HAMILTON, ROBERTS and SOWRY, and published in full in Clinical Science in 1954. I was led to begin this work because of my previous interest in the mechanism of hypertension. At that time the best evidence suggested that essential hypertension was the manifestation of a single gene inherited as a Mendelian dominant. Accepting the one-gene-one substance hypothesis, this meant that a specific chemical abnormality should form the basis of essential hypertension and its discovery would be a matter of patience and persistence. I will not go into the evidence for this hypothesis, but it was clear to me that it was based on a number of assumptions which were not necessarily true.

In our work we started from the beginning and the only assumption we made was in choosing our propositi. Here, I should explain that propositus (plural propositi) is, in the language of genetics, the subject from whom the family investigation begins. The data consist of single measurements of casual arterial pressure made with the subjects seated for 5 to 10 min. in three groups of subjects:

1. A sample of the general population. This consisted of about 2,000 men and women attending poli-clinics at St. Mary's Hospital for diseases not known to be associated with hypertension, namely clinics for skin diseases, for varicose veins, orthopaedics, fractures and dental treatment.

2. First-degree relatives of propositi with essential hypertension. These propositi had diastoloic pressures of 100 mm Hg or more. Secondary hypertension was excluded. First-degree relatives include parents, siblings and offspring.

3. First-degree relatives of propositi without essential hypertension. These patients all had diastolic pressures of 85 mm Hg or less.

I shall first deal with the population sample. The slide shows you the means for systolic and diastolic pressures for each 5-year age group for females and males. The lines are the fitted curves. These curves are cubics, but straight lines adequately fit the data relating diastolic pressure to age. The fitted curves had been used to obtain the norm for any age and either sex, which is the first step in calculating the age-adjusted score, which I will describe later. You will note that the curves are different for the two sexes. In particular, arterial pressure rises with age faster in women than in men after the age of 40. You will also note that pulse pressure rises conspicuously with age.

The next slide shows you the frequency distribution curves for systolic and diastolic pressures for each 10-year age group from the second to the eighth decade for women. The height of each rectangle represents the percentage of subjects having that particular arterial pressure. You will note that at the young ages the distribution curves are compact. As age increases, the curves move to the right and spread out. High values appear for the first time and become more frequent. At the other end of the scale, low values tend to diminish in frequency, but only the lowest disappear.

Several lessons may be learned from these curves. In the first place, variation appears to be continuous. The dotted lines have been drawn at pressures of 150 systolic and 100 diastolic, one of the most popular divisions between normal pressure and hypertension. You will note that there is no natural division into two populations at this or at any other point. Secondly, you will observe that the blood pressure tends to rise with age, but that it rises more in some subjects than in others. Evidence which I hope to present in a few minutes suggests that these different rates of rise depend on environmental rather than genetic factors.

By far the most important suggestion that emerges from the distribution curves is, however, that essential hypertension, as a well-defined entity, disappears. It is a name given by us to that section of the population whose pressures are above a level selected on arbitrary grounds and who have no specific lesion to which these high pressures can be attributed. I find it difficult to emphasize how important this conclusion is. It has changed my way of thinking about the problem of essential hypertension.

This conclusion is well-illustrated by this slide, in which I have followed current practice and separated the two halves of the distribution curves and labelled them normal and hypertension. You will see that these are obviously artefacts; each distribution curve ends and begins in a precipice. You will also notice how many of the features of the natural history of "essential hypertension" are displayed here. First, it is rare in the young and increases as age advances. As we know clinically, hypertension in young subjects is nearly always secondary. Secondly, the higher the subject's pressure, the more likely is it that he crosses the division from the normal to hypertension in the next decade. Thirdly, if the pressure occasionally rises above 150 (transient hypertension), then it is likely that in 5 or 10 years' time it may be usually above 150 (permanent hypertension). Nor is there any justification for the division into normal and pathological from a study of expectation of life. Mortality steadily rises with diastolic pressure from 63 to 103. There is no sudden break.

Now let us turn to the relatives of the propositi with and without so-called essential hypertension. I am now going to show you the frequency distribution curves for diastolic pressures in females of the two sets of relatives compared with the population sample. The next slide shows this for age group 10 to 19. The black rectangles refer to the relatives of hypertensive propositi, the hatched columns to the relatives of control propositi, and the open columns to the population sample. You will note that, even in the second decade, the relatives of the hypertensives tend to have higher pressures. The same features are noted in all the succeeding decades. The significance of these curves is best displayed by the regression lines, that is to say, the best straight lines that can be drawn for each sample to show the relationship between blood pressure and age. You will note that the lines for the relatives of propositi without hypertension are indistinguishable from those of the population sample. The lines for the hypertensive relatives are parallel to the other two but at a higher level. In other words, the arterial pressures of parents, siblings and children of patients with essential hypertension tend to be higher at all ages, but the rate of rise of blood pressure with age is not abnormal. I would suggest, therefore, that the differences in the rates at which blood pressure rises in different individuals may be due chiefly to environmental factors.

A detailed genetic analysis of these data was rendered difficult by the effects of age and sex. To overcome this, my colleague, Dr. FRASER ROBERTS, devised a score which adjusted for the effects of age and sex on arterial pressure. In allotting a score, the first step is to calculate the deviation of the observed blood pressure in mm Hg from the norm for that age and sex. How we obtained the norms has been described already. Since, however, at young ages the distribution curves are narrow and at older ages broad, a given deviation at, say, age 60 has not the same significance as the same deviation at age 20. The next step is to allow for variance. This is done by multiplying the deviation by a factor derived from dividing the standard deviation at age 60 by the standard deviation at observed age. Thus, the final score represents the expected deviation from the norm at age 60, had the subject survived that long and had the rate of rise of arterial pressure approximated to that observed in the general population. While the individual significance of these scores is low, owing to the assumptions made, they can be applied to groups of subjects with greater confidence. This was tested on the largest constituent of our population sample, the skin clinic, in which the scores were corrected entirely for sex, and nearly entirely for age. I shall now show you the calculation of score for three blood pressures, 120/80, 150/100, and 250/150 at ages 25 and 60. Table 1 summarises the scores, from which you can see the profound effects of age. Now I said earlier that these scores represented the expected deviations from the norm at age 60. Thus, systolic pressure of 250 at age 25 would imply at age 60 a systolic pressure of 155, the norm, plus 275, the age-adjusted score, a total of 430, a value which is far outside the range of that observed.

Table 1. *Age-adjusted score*

Blood pressure	Age 25		Age 60	
	S	D	S	D
120/80	+ 5	—35	—35	—10
150/100	+ 40	— 5	— 5	+10
250/150	+120	+95	+95	+60

So far as I know, however, unless effective treatment has been employed, an arterial pressure of 250 systolic at age 25 is incompatible with survival to age 60.

Using these scores, we found:

1. That the scores of first-degree relatives of control propositi had a small + value but were not significantly different from zero.

2. That the scores of hypertensive relatives were raised. The rise was similar in siblings, parents and children and there was no sex association.

3. That the scores of the relatives of hypertensive propositi obtained by SOBYE in Copenhagen were identical with ours.

4. That if our hypertensive propositi were arranged in order of increasing score, the score of the relatives likewise increased. Thus, there are degrees of hypertension and these degrees are faithfully repeated by the relatives.

5. That the degree of resemblance between propositi and their relatives or between sibs in the hypertensive series is indicated by a regression coefficient of 0.2. That is to say, if the arterial pressure of one member of a family is raised above the norm by 10 mm Hg, the pressures of the first-degree relatives will be raised on an average by 2 mm Hg.

When we selected our propositi we selected them on the basis of their arterial pressures and irrespective of their ages. We now know that a given pressure at young age represents a greater departure from the norm than at an advanced age. Table 2 shows the propositi and their relatives arranged in four groups by age. Note that the arterial pressures of the propositi are nearly the same in each age group. The scores fall with age. The scores of the relatives also fall with age. And the regression coefficient stays nearly constant at 0.2.

Table 2. *Analysis by age of hypertensive propositi*

Age of propositus	No. of propositi	Actual mean B.P. propositi	Mean AAS propositi	No. of relatives	Mean AAS relatives	Regressions[1]	
						Systolic	Diastolic
20—34	20	190/119	136/70	61	28.7/14.3	0.21	0.20
35—49	49	214/129	111/58	171	25.0/13.7	0.23	0.24
50—64	34	225/129	87/45	126	20.0/10.6	0.23	0.24
65—79	7	200/118	26/24	29	10.3/6.2	0.40	0.26

These were the conclusions we reached in 1954. However, we realised that our data were not entirely satisfactory from the biometric point of view. Our propositi had been chosen on the basis of their arterial pressures and were in this way selected by the very factor which we sought to investigate. This defect was rectified by MIALL and OLDHAM, who had COCHRANE's population in the Rhondda Fach, a mining valley, at their disposal. This was later amplified by that of the Vale of Glamorgan, an agricultural area. They took as propositi a 1 in 90 sample of the population and they measured a single arterial pressure in them and in over 95% of their first-degree relatives living within a restricted radius. In this population they found very much the same behaviour of blood pressure with age using the same age and sex adjusted score. They showed that there was a linear relationship between the blood pressures of the first-degree relatives and those of their propositi, that this relationship was independent of the blood pressure of

---

[1] Between sample regressions obtained by dividing mean age-adjusted score of relatives by mean age-adjusted score (AAS) of propositi (unweighted).

the propositus, and that the slope of the line was the same whether the blood pressure of the propositus was greater or less than the norm. Their regression coefficients were 0.224 (standard error $\pm$ 0.022) for systolic pressure and 1.078 (standard error $\pm$ 0.024) for diastolic pressure. These regression coefficients are almost exactly those which we found for our hypertensive families. The conclusion thus plainly emerges that blood pressure is inherited like height as a graded character, that the inheritance is probably multifactorial, and that the inheritance is of the same kind and the same degree over the whole blood pressure range.

From this it follows that any attempt to separate essential hypertension and normal pressure by a sharp dividing line is an artefact. This artefact is to my mind the basis of the erroneous concept of the nature of essential hypertension. The old concept, which nearly all still accept, is that essential hypertension represents a qualitative deviation from the norm; the new concept emerging from this work is that the deviation is quantitative. If we are to understand essential hypertension, we must reorientate our minds and we must accept the idea, which indeed might seem self-evident, that in some diseases the deviation from the norm is quantitative and not qualitative.

The conclusions drawn by us from these studies seem in general acceptable to biometricians and geneticists. They seem in general to be unacceptable to physicians. This is understandable, since the new concept of essential hypertension as a quantitative deviation from the norm is in conflict with the concept of disease as a qualitative disorder. The alternative interpretations of the genetic data are as follows.

The first is that resemblance between close relatives may be due not to inheritance but to the tendency of close relatives to share the same environment. The greater resemblance between the blood pressures of identical as compared with non-identical twins, demonstrated by Stocks, can for example also be interpreted as representing merely a nearer identity of environments. This, while possible, is not generally thought to be a probable explanation, and partly because the few environmental factors thus far recognised are of small size.

A much more popular explanation is that inheritance is that of a single gene behaving as a Mendelian dominant. Since arterial pressure is the resultant of many factors, this explanation does not seem very likely on general biological principles. Its chief attraction lies in its conformity with the general belief that disease represents a qualitative deviation from the norm. My colleagues and I have recently examined the evidence put forward for Mendelian dominant inheritance and found it wanting. The hypothesis implies that the population consists of two contrasting types of people, well described by PLATT as follows: "This concept of essential hypertension as an inherited tendency to develop high blood pressure in middle life presumes that there are two populations, one in which blood pressure rises significantly in middle age, often reaching heights at which it seriously contributes to mortality, and another population in which blood pressure rises only very little if at all with advancing years."

Now population samples do not in general show evidence of bimodality. Their distribution curves are positively skewed, but as GADDUM showed clearly for ALVAREZ' data, the curves tend to be normal when the arterial pressure is plotted on a logarithmic scale. However, PLATT pointed out that the distribution curves of the sibs aged 45 to 59 of subjects of similar age do seem to be bimodal, showing dips at 150 systolic and 90 diastolic. Re-examining the evidence showed features of these distribution curves which suggested that digit discrimination was a more likely cause of the dips in SOBYE's and our series. No dips were found in MIALL and OLDHAM's sibs selected on a similar basis. Moreover, a comparison between MIALL and OLDHAM's and our series in respect to relatives and propositi severally, showed features that could only be explained by there being a quantitative resemblance between first-degree relatives. We therefore concluded that the evidence for two populations, even in the middle-aged sibs of middle-aged propositi with hypertension, is unconvincing. Nor is there any evidence for separation into two populations as regards expectation of life, heart size or vascular disease. In all these the relationship with arterial pressure is quantitative and continuous.

The remaining evidence depends on the assumption, which we believe is groundless, that a sharp division into normal and abnormal is possible. Accepting the role of advocatus diaboli and making this assumption, then three pieces of evidence for dominant gene inheritance have been brought forward. The first is the presence of the disease, as indicated by studies of family histories in three generations. Accepting a systolic pressure of 160 or over in middle life as evidence of hypertension, and making no assumptions concerning inheritance, essential hypertension would be expected to occur in a parent and corresponding grandparent in about one-third of families, a frequency more than four times as great as that adduced as evidence for Mendelian dominant inheritance. The second evidence is the equality in numbers of affected and unaffected elder sibs found by Weitz by taking 160 mm Hg as the dividing line. A similar equality in numbers above and below this division is found in women in the seventh decade in the population at large.

Finally, calculations of gene frequency unfortunately fail to distinguish between multifactorial and dominant inheritance and are rendered almost valueless by the rapid rise in the proportion of those with pressures of 160 mm Hg and over in the population at large in the sixth decade and later.

I then present you with these conclusions:

1. Blood pressure is inherited as a graded character over the whole range, from less than the norm to so-called essential hypertension. The degree of resemblance between first-degree relatives is a little over 0.2. Inheritance is probably multifactorial or polygenic.

2. Blood pressure tends to rise with age and differently in the two sexes. The rate of rise with age is not an inherited quality but probably depends on environmental factors.

3. The practice of sharply dividing arterial pressure into normal and abnormal is an artefact.

4. Essential hypertension represents a form of disease not previously recognized, in which the deviation is quantitative, not qualitative.

The figures mentioned here are mainly to be found in the following:
1. Pickering, G. W. (1955), High Blood Pressure, London: Churchill.
2. Significant Trends in Medical Research. CIBA Foundation Symposium, 1959, p. 273. London: Churchill.

The nature of essential hypertension

By

R. PLATT

When HAMILTON, PICKERING, FRASER ROBERTS and SOWRY published their four papers in 1954 I accepted the authority of PICKERING and was blinded by the treatment of mathematical data to 8 places of decimals. It never occurred to me to question either the reliability of their data or the validity of their treatment of them, and I accepted for several years their theory of the continuous distribution of hypertension with the corollary that what we call essential hypertension is no more than the tail end of a distribution curve.

Gradually I became less and less convinced for two reasons. First, that in common with other clinicians I had difficulty in believing that the numerous patients I see with alarmingly high blood pressures differ in no way but quantitatively from the general population; how could they have reached these pressures if the regressions of blood pressure on age of the PICKERING group had any real meaning? And, secondly, because my clinical experience seemed to reveal a hereditary factor in essential hypertension much stronger than that which the PICKERING data appear to show.

I remembered that about 7 years before the publications of the PICKERING group I had published 2 papers which had a bearing on this subject. One (1947) seemed to show a difference between the heredity of essential hypertension on the one hand and of secondary hypertension on the other. The second (1948) showed that when younger people aged below 40 and especially below 35 had severe hypertension it was secondary in the great majority of cases. I examined the reliability of the PICKERING data with these points in mind and found that they admitted that they had not in all their cases taken steps to exclude secondary hypertension and that one-third of their cases of so-called essential hypertension were under 40 or over 60, ages at which the diagnosis is at least suspect. Furthermore they had treated the relatives of their hypertensives as if they were a homogeneous population, which of course, if it were due to a single gene, they would not be. The treatment of their data in fact involved the assumption of a continuous distribution. It occurred to me that the heredity of Huntington's chorea might never have been established if a considerable proportion of the propositi were not Huntington's chorea at all and if the age of onset had been disregarded.

So I thought we might take a look at the siblings aged 45—60 of Pickering's hypertensives aged 45 to 60, for at that age hypertension is more likely to be "essential" and the siblings more likely to have developed it. I got clearly bimodal curves for the distribution of blood pressure in these siblings. Numbers were small and

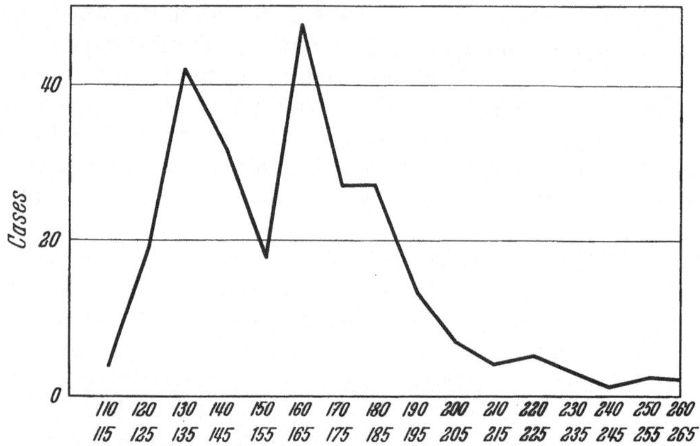

Fig. 1. Frequency distribution of relatives of hypertensives (see text)

I added the data of Sobye which Pickering had also used and which showed the same bimodality. I show here only one curve (Fig. 1); the others were published by me in 1959.

Pickering (see Oldham et al., 1960) has tried to explain away these curves by observer error, but even if one accepts this explanation, they are bimodal curves and had been concealed for 5 years in data which had been supposed to support the continuous distribution theory. The mathematical treatment by the Pickering group was therefore shown to be inappropriate to revealing bimodality. So I became rather bolder and examined the first fundamental major premise of the Pickering theory, namely that their frequency distributions for blood pressure in the general population are continuous or unimodal. I set up a model (Fig. 2) of how most people look at essential hypertension, namely that in middle age there are two groups of people, each varying around a mode, and probably overlapping to some degree. Inheritance of "normal" blood pressure would no doubt be multifactorial and both would be affected by environment. The high-blood-pressure group in my diagrams are 25% of the whole. Fig. 3 shows what happens when these two groups are treated as if they were one, and Fig. 4 is one of the distribution curves from the data of HAMILTON, PICKERING, FRASER ROBERTS and SOWRY. You will see that, far from showing a continuous distribution, it is strongly in

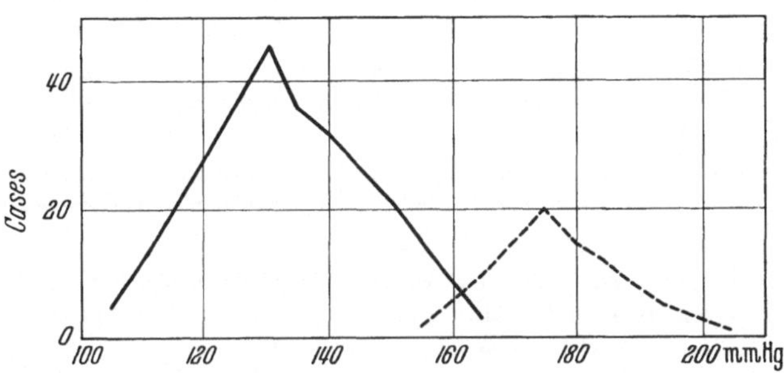

Fig. 2. Model of two hypothetical populations

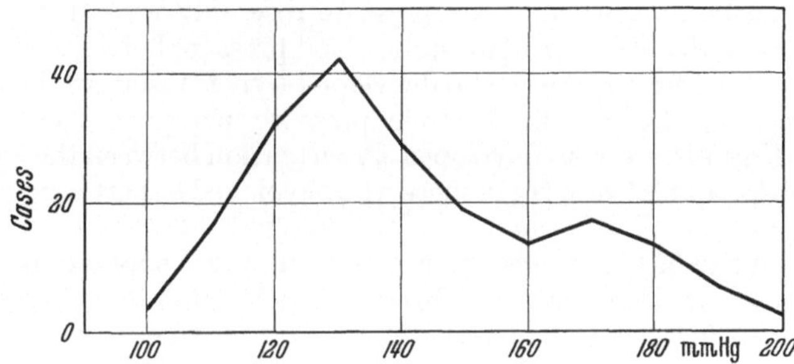

Fig. 3. The same expressed as a single curve

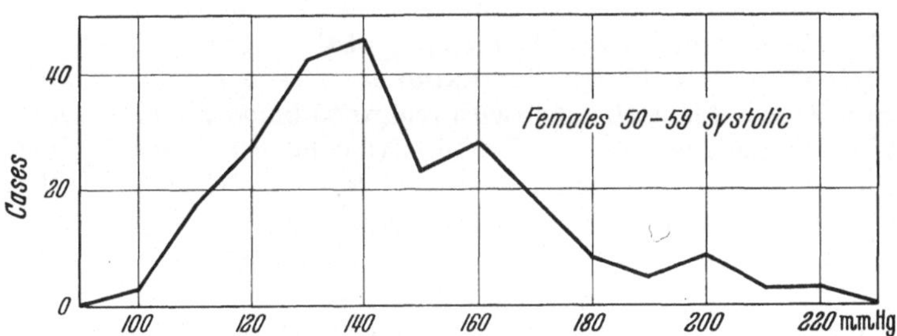

Fig. 4. Frequency distribution from data of HAMILTON, PICKERING, ROBERTS and SOWRY

favour of there being two (or perhaps three) populations, which behave differently with regard to their blood pressure.

If essential hypertension is an entity — something which you either have got or have not got — if in fact there are two populations and not one as regards blood pressure, then we would expect to find that in the one population the blood pressure rose fairly steeply in middle age, and in the other population very little if at all. Strangely enough, the evidence on this is still inadequate. Nobody has followed for 10, 15 or 20 years individual blood pressures in a large enough population, but such evidence as there is suggests that the concept of two populations is correct. JEFFERSON THOMSON (1950), who studied employees of the Metropolitan Life Insurance Company of New York, and followed their blood pressures for many years, noted the age of onset of diastolic hypertension (defined as a blood pressure of 90 or over). This change towards diastolic hypertension most commonly occurs between 45 and 54, and is less common after that age. In other words, it is something which occurs at middle age in a certain proportion of the population, and is not a general effect of ageing. CRUZ-COKE (1959), from the study of a large number of persons, showed that in those who remained normotensive, blood pressure rose only very slowly, less than 1 mm Hg per year of diastolic blood pressure between the ages of 30 and 69, but in those who developed hypertension while under observation, the rise in diastolic pressure per year was nearly 6 mm Hg in those who developed hypertension between the ages of 30 and 49, and 3.5 mm Hg in those who developed hypertension after the age of 50. This seems to be striking evidence that regressions based on rise of blood pressure with age in mixed populations have little meaning. MORRISON and MORRIS, in an unpublished investigation to which they have kindly given me access, show from PICKERING's data that the rise of pressure in middle age in the relatives of hypertensives is very different from the rise of pressure with age in the relatives of normotensives (Fig. 5).

Now a few words as to the meaning of the regression coefficient of 0.2 which is said by PICKERING to be the extent to which relatives resemble each other with regard to blood pressure. In the first place the relatives of propositi (who have not usually complained of symptoms) are likely to have lower blood pressures than the propositi (who have). Secondly, half the sibs will not (on the single-gene theory) inherit hypertension at all, and thirdly if they are not examined at appropriate ages and if, say, 25% of the propositi have not got essential hypertension at all, the resemblance will be further reduced.

Finally I must refer to the interesting studies of MIALL and OLDHAM. The most interesting thing about them is how little hypertension they found in the inbred Welsh neighbourhood where their studies were made. Of 316 males only 3 had diastolic

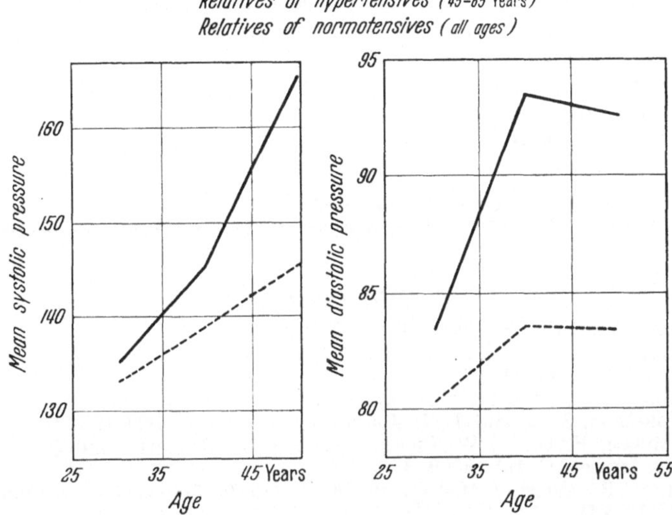

Fig. 5. Behaviour of blood pressure with age (males — see text)

blood pressures of 110 or over and none of these had siblings of appropriate age. In order to use them for a study of essential hypertension, the PICKERING group (1960) has had to use border-line cases which may well be at the tail end of a normal curve, and have used all 1st degree relatives from age 35 upwards, including the fathers and mothers, who may well be in advanced stages of arteriosclerosis. The fallacies are only too obvious.

I therefore conclude that the attractive theory of the PICKERING group is unsupported by evidence.

What is there on the positive side? There is my own demonstration of the segregation of sibs of hypertensives of appropriate age, strongly supported by the bimodal curves which MORRISON and MORRIS derived from their busmen. In these the blood pressure was taken before the family history, so they were presumably not looking out for hypertension in one group and forgetting it in another. The blood pressure was recorded to the nearest 2 mm Hg and the usual concentration at the 10's does not show in their data.

The general population of bus drivers showed distribution curves similar to those of Pickering, but when they were divided, from their family histories, into those with one or both parents dying in middle age and those with parents surviving into old age, bimodal distribution curves came out quite strikingly in the former but not in the latter. There is also the strong evidence of a difference of behaviour in middle age between two groups of the population.

I conclude therefore:

That the evidence against the continuous distribution theory is overwhelming.

That the evidence of two (or more) distinct populations is very strong indeed.

That the single-gene theory of essential hypertension is by no means proved but the evidence in its favour is highly suggestive.

References

Cruz-Coke, R.: Lancet (G. B.) **1959/II**, 853.

Hamilton, M., G. W. Pickering, J. A. F. Roberts, and G. S. C. Sowry: Clin. Sc. (G. B.) **13**, 11, 37, and 273 (1954).

Miall, W. E., and P. D. Oldham: Clin. Sc. (G. B.) **14**, 459 (1955).

Morrison, S. L., and J. N. Morris: Lancet (G. B.) **1959/II**, 864.

Oldham, P. D., G. W. Pickering, J. A. F. Roberts, and G. S. C. Sowry: Lancet (G. B.) **1960/I**, 1085.

Platt, R.: Quart. J. Med. (G. B.) **16**, 111 (1947); **17**, 83 (1948). — Lancet (G. B.) **1959/II**, 55.

Sobye, P.: Copenhagen 1948.

Thomson, K. J.: Proceedings of the 38th Annual Meeting of the Medical Section of the American Life Convention (1950).

Discussion

REUBI: I should like to open the discussion on the problem introduced this morning by Dr. PICKERING and Dr. PLATT.

Perhaps Dr. PICKERING could now answer some objections raised by Dr. PLATT.

PICKERING (drawing on the blackboard and demonstrating slides): Well, may I say how very grateful I am to ROBERT PLATT for raising these queries, because I think unless there are two sides to a question it never deserves full attention. May I try and develop some of the doubts which PLATT has in his own mind, and which you have in your minds, and which I also have in mine. And the first relates to the contrast of what you might call the mean value of a large population with which I was dealing this morning and individual behaviours. One of the points which bothered PLATT as a clinician was the patient with very high pressures. Of course, I am a clinician, too, and I see the same kind of problem. I do not know exactly what has happened to each individual; we need observations on the way in which blood pressure changes with time in individuals, and we want to put these all together to see what they may add up to. But supposing this axis is blood pressure and this axis is age, we know that around about 20, most people are somewhere between 150 and 100 systolic. And if you take an individual like the speaker, he began at 100 and ends at 100, and if you take an individual like the speaker's wife, she began at 150 and 25 years later is 160. Now, if you like, you can call this hypertension, and you can call this normotension, and she, of course, might be a labile hypertensive in the initial stage, and you might say she is still a labile hypertensive; anyhow, the point is that these are two individual patterns that I know about. Others end down here — or up there; HOLMGEN's results suggest that the way blood pressure changes with age is very different in different individuals. These individual patterns of the change of blood pressure with age obviously have to be studied and are not in any way expressed by the kind of regression lines that have been demonstrated this morning. So I hope that there is no real disagreement between us on that point.

The second thing is whether there are two populations or one or more than two. And I think that we are not really so greatly in disagreement. I do not think that there is a single homogenous population; I also do not think there are just two populations; I think there is a very large number of populations as regards blood pressure, and I will show you what I mean by some slides.

These are three of GALTON's distribution curves. A point I want to make is that these dips in distribution curves can occur by chance when the numbers are not very large. And curiously enough, these three dips are in the same place. Now, I work with two mathematicians, and my mathematical friends tell me it is extremely difficult to say when a curve is truly unimodal or truly bimodal and it is particularly difficult when the peaks are near together. When you have large numbers of subjects — about 90,000 in this instance, I think you get a truly normal distribution curve for height. You might say that there is one population, but in fact it is not one. It is a collection of a large number of different populations. Please look back to GALTON's distribution curves. If you break down your population according to the heights of their mid-parents, you can see that you have a whole series of distribution curves. So that the normal GAUSSIAN curve which was obtained from a large population is really the summation of a number of separate populations (slide). If you isolate the constituents you can show that these populations are different. This you have seen already, but may I remind you that this curve is the population sample and that curve the relatives of the patients with hypertension. You may say, well, here obviously there are two distribution curves; these are two different frequency distribution curves. If you added them together you would get the humped curve that ROBERT PLATT showed you this morning. And that may be so, but I think it is much more complicated. This slide suggests that in fact you can break down the population into a large number of distribution curves which, if added together, would make the familiar GAUSSIAN curve, each differing slightly from the other. It is not two populations, it is a very large number. This is really where I differ from PLATT. I do not think there are two populations, I think there is a large number of populations.

REUBI: Five years ago, I asked Dr. PICKERING, who had just been developing his new conception on high blood pressure at a meeting of the Belgian Cardiological Society, what he could say about a disease like diabetes mellitus. This point was raised again a fortnight ago in Prague by Dr. PERERA. I agree that it is difficult to find a sharp dividing line between normal and high blood pressure. But if you want to define diabetes mellitus in terms of blood sugar, what is the normal limit for blood sugar? If you want to define jaundice in terms of bilirubinaemia, where is the normal limit? How do you separate patients with a normal cardiac activity and patients with beginning heart failure? Is it in terms of venous pressure or in terms of cardiac output? I do not know, but I think you can go even further and take almost every disease. Nevertheless we all agree that diabetes, jaundice, and heart failure are diseases in themselves, so that I do not see why hypertension should not be an entity like those I mentioned.

SCHROEDER: I wonder if it is valid to pay so much attention to systolic pressure as was done by Drs. PICKERING and PLATT. Their curves show an increasing pulse pressure with age. When a clinician or a physiologist sees a patient with a large pulse pressure, he suspects that the elasticity of the aorta and some of the larger arteries is lessened. The usual basis of this disturbance is aortic atherosclerosis. Again as clinicians we define hypertension as elevated diastolic pressure. The rise with age is much less obvious. I suggest that such studies as those presented here should therefore be confined to diastolic pressure, thus partially excluding the effects of another disease. A second point: I wonder whether or not we are confusing what is normal with what is average. Many of us here have healed tuberculous lesions in our lungs from childhood infections; this is average but not normal. An examination of the arteries of almost all of the men in this room would reveal more or less atherosclerosis, certainly a disease and not a normal variation. A statistical analysis of atherosclerosis without recognizing it as a disease might suggest that it is a normal variation increasing with age. As physicians we must recognize diseases as such even if they are extremely frequent in our civilized or uncivilized populations.

GROLLMAN: It seems to me that our difficulty in deciding whether hypertension is an entity is a consequence of our egocentricity in focusing our attention on the human while disregarding the results obtained in the experimental animal. Unfortunately, the blood pressure in the human is complicated and subject to many extraneous and environmental factors. Arteriosclerosis, for example, as Dr. SCHROEDER has indicated, alters the systolic blood pressure and has not been evaluated in most statistical studies. I agree with Prof. PLATT that essential hypertension represents a distinct clinical entity with a definite familial tendency. Experimental studies on animals offer objective evidence that there is such a disease, since one can induce a disorder by a variety of procedures which is identical in all respects to that occurring spontaneously in the human. Much of the confusion in the field of hypertension might be avoided if we were to define what we mean by essential hypertension rather than use it as a synonym for "elevation of blood pressure of unknown origin". Recent studies certainly justify a more exact definition. We ought not to designate all elevations of so labile a hemodynamic function as the blood pressure as "hypertension", for many are obviously of varied and known origin. Essential hypertension can be defined in terms of its known clinical course, definite hemodynamic features (increased diastolic pressure, increased peripheral resistance and normal cardiac output), and demonstrable pathologic changes (arteriolosclerosis, cardiac hypertrophy, etc.). We would exclude by this definition such conditions as "systolic hypertension" secondary to arteriosclerosis, hyperthyroidism, arteriovenous fistula, the elevation in blood pressure observed in coarctation of the aorta, phaeochromocytoma, adrenal cortical tumors, poliomyelitis, etc.

There is adequate evidence to justify the conclusion that essential hypertension, as defined above, is of renal origin and a consequence of some functional defect in the kidney not morphologically obvious by our present methods of examination. If so-called essential hypertension is a congenital disorder of renal origin one would anticipate that a similar disease might also be acquired by a variety of disturbances which interfere with that function of the kidney concerned in the maintenance of the normotensive state. These forms of hypertension secondary to nephritis, vascular lesions of the kidney, etc. are generally accepted as being of renal origin. The presently available evidence would indicate that essential hypertension as well as so-called "renoprival" hypertension are also of renal origin and that all have the same pathogenesis. This would not deny the existence of disturbances characterized by elevations in blood pressure resulting from other mechanisms. Such is certainly the case in so-called "unilateral" hypertension secondary to infarction of the kidney, ureteral ligation, or a plaque on the renal artery, in which presumably some circulating pressor agent mediates the observed rise in blood pressure. However, these are rarely encountered and from a practical clinical point of view it would be a pity if we were to allow ourselves to become preoccupied with these rather than with the great group of patients suffering from essential hypertension and its consequences.

PEART: I think I'd like to disagree with Dr. GROLLMAN, because if we followed his ideas we would end up in great confusion, for the following reason: I would like to know by what criteria you recognise hypertension except by the level of the blood pressure. Well, one knows that the blood pressure varies under the influence of various factors, but if one talks of hypertension as a specific disease, that carries further implications. You define it by the word and from there you go on and a lot of confusion ensues, as it seems to me, about the consequences of the rise of blood pressure. One talks vaguely of atherosclerosis as a definite disease; I wonder if it is. Surely, you have got to discriminate once and for all between high blood pressure and its effects. We are talking of a subject which is altogether defined by exclusion. It is essential or idiopathic in the case of hypertension, and basically we cannot define it, as far as I know, at the present time, except by measuring the blood pressure. If one confuses the issue, it seems to me, by talking about a disease and its consequences and its causes when nobody has got the evidence for it, I think we will create further confusion. I would suggest that we stick to disagreements about the actual measurements and the meanings of the measurements of blood pressure, and not confuse the question by discussing the effects which it causes.

REUBI: You do not feel that arteriosclerosis is a direct consequence of an elevated blood pressure?

PEART: No, I do not think anybody knows. I feel, if we introduce this concept, what is the point of it? I mean first let us have the evidence about consequences or not consequences. I think now in discussing the two papers of this morning we are erecting a concept as a disease which I do not think will stand up at the present time.

GROLLMAN: I would take exception to Dr. PEART's contention that we cannot define hypertensive disease except in terms of blood pressure levels. The level of the blood pressure is a practical and readily available indication of the presence of the disease but represents only one manifestation of the disorder and may often be misleading and quantitatively indefinite. Certainly one can say with assurance from an examination of the heart and blood vessels as seen at autopsy that a patient had suffered from hypertension without ever having taken his blood pressure during life. On the other hand, many conditions — emotional stress, hypermetabolism, etc. — may cause elevations in blood pressure; to designate these as "hypertension" can only lead to confusion. Hypertension, as a disease, is a systemic disorder which is reflected in functional as well as chemical and other changes in many tissues and organs. The level of the blood pressure is only one hemodynamic manifestation of the disease and may in fact be absent, as for example in the patient who has suffered a myocardial infarction or cerebrovascular accident. Surely Dr. PEART would not deny that such patients were suffering from hypertensive disease despite the normal or even subnormal levels of their blood pressure at the time of their examination. This same line of reasoning should make us realize also that hypertensive disease in its early stages may be manifested by only insignificant or no elevation in blood pressure, just as diabetes mellitus may be said to exist in a patient prior to the development of significant hyperglycemia.

REUBI (to PICKERING): You do not agree?

PICKERING: Oh, I do not agree at all, no.

REUBI: Can you quickly say why?

PICKERING: Well, I feel if we are talking about, or if we are going to define, essential hypertension we ought to mean the high pressure and its consequences and not something different. Is a large left ventricle a consequence of high pressure or of something different?

REUBI: I think most of us believe that hypertension is really a disease.

TAQUINI: I would not.

REUBI: I know. But if we try to define this disease, it is a very difficult task, because we do not know its cause and there is no general agreement on the normal limits of blood pressure. Therefore I understand why Dr. GROLLMAN says we cannot take just the blood pressure into consideration and why he thinks it's valuable to consider other manifestations of what we call the hypertensive disease: for example, arteriolosclerosis. We know that in most patients with a permanently elevated blood pressure there are vascular lesions, whereas in normal individuals where the blood pressure is only accidentally elevated there are no lesions. On the other hand, it may also happen as Dr. GROLLMAN pointed out, that in essential hypertension with vascular lesions the blood pressure transiently drops. I am not sure whether we disagree. Perhaps it is just a question of terminology.

WILSON: I think that certainly we concentrate too much on the blood pressure level and not on the disease as a whole in the sense of something that has a natural history. On the other hand, I think it is unreasonable to refuse to accept essential hypertension as a disease entity simply because its only manifestation may be a change in blood pressure. After all, we have no hesitation in diagnosing diabetes mellitus on the sole evidence of a diabetic blood sugar curve. This is only a disturbance of function just as hypertension is a disturbance of function. We have not sufficiently considered the relationship of symptomatology to the development of high blood pressure. I think the patient with this condition may complain of real symptoms which are not related to the level of the blood pressure and before there is any question of arterial degeneration. Arterial degeneration is the consequence of sustained diastolic hypertension, and I think we can rule it out when considering the pathogenesis of the disease. Perhaps we are not considering sufficiently that at different stages of the disease there may be different types of physiological disturbance, not only in the peripheral blood vessels but in the heart itself and in the kidney. Nevertheless, I feel that in the stage of established hypertension, essential or otherwise, the pattern is so uniform that there must be a definable underlying functional lesion. I think it is probably a complex one and may differ qualitatively from the mechanism in the early stages of the disease. We must therefore go on looking for the cause of the disturbance of vascular tone. I think a great deal of confusion arises from the difficulty in separating primary and secondary factors, especially where disturbances of water and electrolytes are concerned.

GOVAERTS: Obviously, the expression "essential hypertension" has merely a clinical meaning, as it implies that the pathogenesis of the syndrome is unknown. Therefore, one has to proceed by exclusion and to make such a diagnosis only after considering the well-defined varieties of hypertension.

So far we know from experimental medicine the pathogenesis of at least five varieties:

1. suprarenal hypertension,
2. hypertension of central nervous origin (including cisternal occlusion),
3. carotid sinus regulation disturbances,
4. renoprival hypertension,
5. hypertension of renal origin.

Concerning the last variety, I wish to call attention to one point which for me has remained rather difficult to understand, namely the reason why the presence of even a non-functioning kidney may impede the development of hyperreactivity to renin which would develop in a dog deprived of both kidneys. The same degree of uraemia is observed in the renoprival animal as in the dog with the one remaining kidney with an artery tightly constricted and without excretory function. Nevertheless, the renoprival dog has a great increase in sensitivity to renin, while the latter has a normal response[1]. I believe that it would be worthwhile to study again the

---

[1] GOVAERTS, P., A. VERNIORY, and J. LEBRUN: Bull. Acad. Roy. Med. Belg. **15**, 375, 1950.

mechanism of changes in sensitivity to renin and that such a study could help us to understand the pathogenesis of some varieties of hypertension.

REUBI: I am sure that both Dr. PICKERING and Dr. PLATT agree that some types of hypertension, which may be called secondary, are due to known causes, and that in other cases, which might be called primary, we do not know the cause. I suggest that we limit this discussion to primary hypertension.

SARRE: Regarding the hereditary aspect of hypertension, I should like to refer briefly to some of my own investigations involving over 400 hypertensives. The mean height of the blood pressure in these cases varied significantly according to whether the case history showed no hereditary trait (I) or whether there was a history of hypertension in one parent (II), in both parents (III) or in the parents and the siblings (IV). In group I the mean blood pressure was 193/122 mm Hg, in group II 204/130 mm Hg, and in group III 210/135 mm Hg. Thus, patients with a history of hypertension in both parents showed higher blood pressure levels than the cases in which only one parent had suffered from hypertension, while the latter showed higher levels than the cases where no hereditary factors of this kind were operative. Moreover, the severity of the clinical course and the mortality also depended on the extent of the hereditary influence (see Fig.). The survival curves for the four groups from the first to seventh year differ considerably. One obvious assumption is that the severity and course of the hypertension vary according to whether the individual in question is homozygous or heterozygous. But it is also conceivable that, as stated by Dr. PICKERING, what the patient inherits is not the disease of "hypertension" as such, but a tendency to high blood pressure which is all the more marked the greater the hereditary influence and which accordingly also affects the severity of the clinical course and the mortality. It would be interesting to find out if similar observations could be made in, for example, diabetes mellitus.

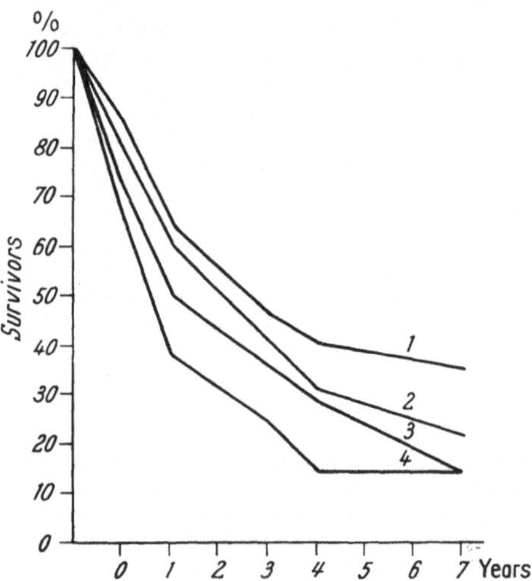

Mortality of 400 hypertensives in relation to hereditary factors (SARRE 1959)

Group 1: no hereditary predisposition
Group 2: one parent hypertensive
Group 3: both parents hypertensive
Group 4: parents and siblings hypertensive

PLATT: I would just like to say one word to Dr. SCHROEDER that whereas I agree that the diastolic pressure is a much better index, it is more difficult to take the diastolic pressure accurately and the range within which to take it is narrow, and the systolic has certain advantages for those reasons. Now, as to the argument between Dr. GROLLMAN and Dr. PEART: I believe of course that there is a group which is essential hypertension that we are beginning to define, but we are not yet ready to define it. I think we are in the position that you might have been in if there had been a method of testing the pulmonary blood pressure before there had been a method for diagnosing mitral stenosis. We should be saying, what are all these people with different degrees of pulmonary hypertension? Do some fit into a definable group which represents .a definite departure from the average? And I must say that if this were the case it would not be very greatly helped by mathematical treatment which conceals those groups completely. Dr. PICKERING has shown us with remarkable curves how in some people blood pressure may start here and rise abruptly or it may start here and remain stationary; it may even go up and come down again, and yet he showed us this morning a regression of blood pressure over age which is either a straight line or an absolutely smooth curve. It is quite meaningless. Such mathematical treatment is not appropriate to the question which we are trying to answer and I do not think that bringing in the interesting GALTON distribution of height helps us very much. We all know, or we all assume at any rate, that height is a multifactoral inheritance. But it can still be disturbed by a single factor, which might be rickets for instance, which was common in GALTON's time. It is much more interesting to me to say: these curves are peculiar — why do they not conform to a normal distribution? — than to treat them in a way which removes all their interest.

BROD: May I show a slide? About the question: is essential hypertension a qualitative change or is it just a change in quantity? We have done several studies of basic haemodynamics in essential hypertension comprising not only cardiac output and calculated peripheral vascular resistance, but estimating at the same time in one and the same individual regional resistances in the kidneys, in the splanchnic region, in the skin, and in the muscles. Now, if essential hypertension were just a quantitative change in one direction, we would expect all these regional resistances to move upwards. However, this is not so. While renal resistance, splanchnic resistance, and the skin resistance are all elevated compared with normal individuals, indicated by the dotted line, the vascular resistance in muscles is decreased. For comparison, haemodynamic responses to emotional stimulus in normotensive subjects are summarized in the second row, the dotted line indicating again the resting level in normotensive subjects. It is obvious that the haemodynamic pattern of what we call essential hypertension is very similar to the haemodynamic pattern of emotional reaction and also very similar to the haemodynamic pattern of the response to severe muscular exercise. This is much more compatible with the view that essential hypertension is a qualitative change and not only simply a quantitative change of all regional resistances in the upward direction. If I may raise a second point: repeatedly it was stated here that essential hypertension is not only a change in blood pressure, but that it is a disease with symptoms. I think Dr. WILSON stated it beautifully. But, as Dr. REUBI said: what is actually the symptomatology of the disease? It is a pity that Dr. MYASNIKOW is not here, because he probably would have been able to report a few things about the studies of various institutes in the Soviet Union of changes of conditioning in patients with essential hypertension: it was easier to establish a conditioned reflex, whereas inhibition and extinction of the reflex was more difficult. They also found changes in the function of the various sensory organs. While I have no personal experience in this field, it is known that the majority of patients in the initial stages of essential hypertension have a lot of subjective symptoms. The only difficulty we are facing is that also some normotensive people suffer from insomnia, irritability, from inability to concentrate and so on. We do not know actually what is the significance of these symptoms, as very few studies of their meaning were carried out. I think that is one gap in our knowledge which we will have to fill.

TAQUINI: In considering peripheral resistance in hypertension, a distinction has to be made between functional vasoconstriction and secondary organic narrowing of the vessels. The irregular distribution of these secondary changes may produce differences in the blood flow and resistance in different regions and especially in the kidneys at different stages in the evolution of the disease that are independent of the general vasoconstriction which characterizes essential hypertension.

PICKERING: Well, there are just a few points I should like to make on this extremely difficult subject. I think one of the difficulties is the words that we use. Dr. SCHROEDER drew your attention to the paradox between normal and average, saying that most of us have atherosclerosis; that was average, but was it normal? Could I just take that argument a little further and say that probably we are all going to die; that is average, but is it normal? Now may I look at this problem of disease from the point of view of the meaning of the word; we employ this to describe people, who, so far as we know, have a shorter expectation of life than average or who, for some reason or other, are not able to do their work. And, in general, people who have this kind of disability are said to be diseased. We classify diseases and we learn to classify them. I remember when I was a student I went through my text-book of medicine and I made a list of diseases and I looked at them to see which of them we knew the causes of and which we did not. We are rather apt to think that all these diseases are just as distinct as the buttercup and the daisy, and I sometimes wonder whether they are. And I think what Dr. PAGE said this morning is right. The first diseases that we got to know anything about were the infective diseases, and I detect in the speakers this afternoon an urge to make essential hypertension just as definite a thing as an infective disease such as typhoid, for example. I am not convinced that this symptomatology is quite characteristic of essential hypertension. I have worked on this subject for some 30 years; I have always had a very keen interest in the mechanism of symptoms, and the only symptom I know which is characteristic of hypertension is the intense headache which occurs on waking in the morning, and even that also occurs in cerebral tumour. So I rather think we are in danger of manufacturing something that seems a good deal more definite than in fact it is. Now to the question of Dr. BROD's muscular resistance as evidence of qualitative change. Well it may be, but I'd like to know a bit more about why it has happened; for this reason, I like just as much the definition of hypertension that Dr. PEART produced in Prague, which suggested that we should agree that hypertension was present when there was an increase of sodium and water excretion in response to an infusion of angiotensin. I think we have had a jolly good discussion and I'd like to say thank you.

Possible role of salt intake in the development of essential hypertension[1]

By

L. K. Dahl

Introduction

Although the practice of adding salt to food is an ancient one, there seems to be little doubt that until relatively modern times its widespread use as a condiment was uncommon. At present, the practice is a ubiquitous one and, in the United States at least, salt may be added at any stage before, during or after food-processing as well as before, during or after cooking. And sometimes salting takes place during each of these steps!

The ancient valuation of salt as a precious possession (*1*) may have contributed to the modern notion that the addition of salt to food is necessary or even beneficial (*2*). Nonetheless, during the 20th century, there has been evidence accumulating which suggests a possible relationship between salt ingestion and hypertension in man (*3*). In this paper we will review the sum total of the evidence, which we have been gathering since 1954 (*1, 4—14*). The original papers should be consulted both for the primary data as well as for correlation with the experiences of others in this field. These studies are in line with the modern effort against subtle lethal agents as, for example, fall-out, carcinogens and atherogenic factors.

Salt need, salt intake, salt appetite

We have dealt with these considerations at some length elsewhere (*9—14*).

Need. There is no doubt that some salt is required by man, and estimates of normal daily requirements for adults have ranged up to 15 g per day. For the most part, such estimates were arrived at by a circular argument in which, over any given period, the amount of salt excreted in the urine was equated with the need for ingestion of an equal amount in order to maintain metabolic

---

[1] This work was supported by the United States Atomic Energy Commission.

balance. As opposed to such opinion there are numerous careful metabolic studies which indicate unequivocally that in people with normal renal function, salt balance can be maintained easily on daily intakes well below 1 g. Our own group has studied many individuals who were limited to 100—375 mg for periods of 3 to 12 months (*15—18*). We have reported 3 subjects whose intake was proven to have been restricted to 250—375 mg NaCl continuously for periods ranging from about 2 to 5 years (*13*). We recently studied a 17-year-old girl for several months who easily maintained salt balance while her daily intake was only 10—12 mg of salt. We do not imply that such low intakes are either necessary or advisable, but we do suggest that under ordinary circumstances the adaptive mechanisms of the body are so exquisitely effective in conserving salt that intakes of only 1 or 2 g a day are more than sufficient for metabolic needs, including periods of growth (*1*).

Intake. There are — *were* is perhaps more accurate today — many vigorous peoples which for countless generations added no salt to their food and ate only that which was present naturally. Among such groups are the Eskimos, some of the northwest American Indians, and the Masai of Africa. Analysis of the diets among such groups or maximal estimates based on the rather constant salt content of foods in their natural state indicate maximal daily intakes of not more than 5 g, with some eating 1 g or less (*1*). Calculations based on the analyzed sodium content of known foods indicate that salt intake rarely could exceed 4 or 5 g per day without the addition of salt to food, save in areas where drinking water had a high salinity.

Determinations of actual as contrasted with estimated salt consumption are remarkably few in all societies, and no less so in western than in other societies. Measurement of 24 hr urinary excretion is a reliable index of *minimal* salt intake. Except when sweat losses are significant it is even an accurate index of total intake (*1*) in normal people. In view of the ubiquitous sources of salt in modern diets the errors of this technique are in my opinion less than those of any other method. There are two criticisms of this means of evaluating salt consumption: 1. losses from the skin as well as inevitable losses from lack of total co-operation will cause underestimation of salt intake in some subjects; and 2. salt consumption may vary so widely from day to day that a single or even several consecutive 24 hr collections will hardly give an accurate index of a person's average intake. These criticisms are more applicable when determining *maximal* consumptions but less so when *minimal* consumptions are being investigated.

Similar problems have existed in estimating the exact consumption by a single individual of such common items as fat, cigarettes, or alcohol, but excesses are well recognized here, whether committed by an individual or a nation. I suggest that this be also applied to salt: single 24 hr urine collections may be inaccurate, but my own considerable experience during the last ten years with five different peoples in five different parts of the world indicates that this method is an excellent index of average salt consumption by a group as well as by individuals. It has been checked against known national and community salt purchases in Japan, where salt is controlled by a monopoly; against actual 24 to 48 hr diet collections in Japan, in the United States, and among natives of the Marshall Islands in the Pacific; and finally against known salt content of natural foods eaten by Alaskan Eskimos.

By the use of such methods my associates and I have found that Eskimos were consuming an average of less than 4 g of salt per day, Marshall Islanders about 7, white male Americans about 10, and Southern Japanese farmers and laborers about 14 g. Northern Japanese farmers were found to average 26.3 g by my Japanese friend and investigator, Dr. FUKUDA of Chiba University. Studies on Eskimos, Marshallese, and Americans (including the southern negro) are still in progress and shall be periodically reported.

These group averages indicate that salt intakes may and do vary widely among different peoples. However, these figures will be misleading if they are interpreted to mean that all individuals in such communities are consuming equivalent amounts of salt, since we have observed a wide diversity in individual salt consumption if salt is readily available. Just as data based on average alcohol consumption fail to indicate either the total abstainer or the chronic alcoholic, so average levels of salt consumption fail to show that, among individual members of the communities we have studied, some people habitually eat very little salt while others consume it gluttonously.

Table 1. *Average daily salt intake (based on 24 hr urine excretion) in several societies*

Group	Year	Sex	Salt Intake Average (g/d)	Range (g/d)
Alaskan Eskimo	1958, 1960	both	4	1—10
Marshall Islander (Pacific Ocean)	1958	both	7	1.5—13
United States (Brookhaven) .	1954—1956	male	10	4—24
Japan				
Hiroshima (South. Japan)	1958	male	14	4—29
Akita (North. Japan)	1954	both	26	5—55

The accompanying table (Table 1) summarizes these data up to the present time: the variable *range* of values in the several communities may be as informative as the variation in *averages*. Comparison of these data on salt intake with the earlier estimates of metabolic need indicates a very considerable excess of intake over need in some societies. The importance of this disparity is basic to the thesis of this paper.

I have often been asked whether an average difference of only a few grams of salt per day could be important. In this regard, it is critical to remember that "grams per day" defines a *rate* as opposed to a *quantity*. Relatively small rate differentials operating over long periods of time can yield striking disparities in end result, as the fable of the tortoise and the hare aptly illustrates. From some data now in preparation for publication, our group has found by means of Na^{22} turnover studies that the biological half-life of sodium in humans is a clear-cut function of salt intake. There is more than a two-fold difference in turnover rate between intakes of 2 and 5 g, or between 5 and 10 g; there is a five-fold difference between the effect of 2 and 10 g, and a ten-fold difference between 2 and 30 g. The thesis that such marked differences are without physiological implication appears untenable.

Appetite. Detailed consideration of the role of salt *appetite* as it relates to salt *intake* is beyond the scope of this paper. There is no doubt that salt appetites exist, as every reader can personally testify. The issue is whether salt appetites are innate or acquired. Among animals, the long treks to salt-licks are well known; less well known is the fact that the herbivores rather than the carnivores do this. Whether the high dietary K/Na ratio of about 20 : 1 in the herbivores as contrasted with the 5 : 1 ratio in the diet of the carnivores is important is not known.

We have never seen evidence of salt-craving in our subjects whose salt-intakes were drastically reduced for months or years. Reports by Stefansson (*19*) and Holmberg (*20*) show that the primitive Eskimos and Bolivian Indians, with whom they were associated respectively, did not like salt initially, although they could grow to like it rapidly. Within my own family, where the children were reared without added salt, there was no evidence of a salt appetite until it was induced by well-meaning friends. Furthermore, it seems clear that if an innate appetite exists it is surprisingly easy to change, in contrast to some of the better-established ones. In our patients who were on diets containing only 100 to 250 mg of NaCl per day, the addition of as little as 0.5 to 1 g to their total daily intakes evoked initial comments of "too salty", although later adaptation occurred. In sharp contrast, among subjects on 10 to 20 g per day, the addition of 5 or 10 g went unnoticed. Thus it seems evident that salt appetite is induced rather than innate. This is fundamental, since having shown that salt *intake* bears no necessary relationship to salt requirement, it now seems highly likely that salt *appetite* is also unrelated to requirement.

Evidence that salt ingestion may be related to hypertension

A) Experimental hypertension

In several forms of experimental hypertension, the simultaneous ingestion of excess salt appears to be necessary. GROLLMAN and his associates were the first to demonstrate that various sterols were hypertensogenic only if additional salt was provided (*21*). The effectiveness of desoxycorticosterone acetate in producing hypertension with the addition of extra salt is well known (*22, 23*). Salt feeding with fluid restriction by means of hypertonic saline as the sole source of liquid has been used to produce hypertension in the chick (*24*), rat (*25*) and rabbit (*26*). Finally, MENEELY and his collaborators have shown that chronic ingestion of excess sodium chloride *alone* will produce a hypertension in rats which mimics human hypertension morphologically (*27—30*). We have been using this same technique in our laboratory for some years and have confirmed the potential of chronic salt-feeding to produce hypertension. I suspect that inability to confirm MENEELY's work may be caused by failure to engage in long-term, chronic experiments. To investigators whose previous experience has been with the rapidly evolving varieties of experimental hypertension, that which follows chronic salt-feeding will seem negligible or non-existent because of its slow onset. Nonetheless, from extensive personal experience I would like to state unqualifiedly that hypertension ultimately will result in most rats that are chronically fed extra salt. Its onset may occur at different intervals following the onset of salt-feeding; its character may vary from mild to severe; however, once present, it rarely if ever disappears if salt-feeding is continued. It is usually slowly progressive, but may reach only a modest level and remain on this plateau for the remainder of the animal's life; in contrast we see animals whose disease is marked by early onset, rapid severe elevation of blood pressure and death within a few months. In all of these respects it must be conceded that it resembles the picture of the human disease more closely than the commoner varieties of experimental hypertension.

Hence, chronic salt-feeding in rats can produce a picture resembling human essential hypertension. Furthermore, the evidence is unequivocal that, as the *amount* of salt ingested daily is increased, both *incidence* and *severity* of the hypertension will be increased.

B) Human hypertension

Let us now turn to man. Here, salt restriction has long been used as part of the therapeutic regimen against established hypertension. Much of the early work either failed to separate sodium from chloride or frankly ascribed the results to chloride. In 1945 GROLLMAN and his associates clearly demonstrated that it was the sodium restriction which was important (*31*). This idea is today so widely accepted and used that dilation would belabor the obvious.

Although there were a number of carefully controlled metabolic studies which had established the usefulness of sodium restriction in hypertension, widespread acceptance of this fact came only after the recent development of effective, relatively non-toxic natriuretic agents such a chlorothiazide. Here, too, salt ingestion seems to modify the response, since a high salt diet appears to limit or even block the hypotensive response to chlorothiazide (*32*).

In our experience, which is now much more extensive than the early report (*15*), addition of salt to the diets of individuals who have responded to its restriction generally results in a return of the elevated blood pressure. Furthermore we have found a few reports indicating that the addition of salt to the diet of *normotensive* individuals for short periods of time has resulted in significant elevations of pressure. McQUARRIE (*33, 34*) reported that some diabetic children rapidly became hypertensive when salt was presented, and McDONOUGH and WILHELMJ (*35*) made similar observations on a normal young adult male.

Failure to observe a rise in blood pressure on short-term salt-feeding is not surprising to me for two reasons: 1. If it be granted that excess salt ingestion plays a primary role in the etiology of human hypertension, then the paucity of essential hypertension before the 4th decade would suggest that the salt effect must operate over a considerable span of time, possibly starting well before maturity is reached. Both our own experience as well as that of MENEELY's group (*27—30*) indicates younger animals are more susceptible and that the development of significant disease ordinarily requires a third or more of the animals' expected life-time. 2. Even if salt-feeding is continued throughout the life of a colony, some 20% of the rats remain normotensive: this variability in response to salt-feeding, exhibited by a relatively inbred species like the Sprague-Dawley rat, must operate to a much higher degree in an animal with the mixed ancestry of man. It is intriguing to speculate on the possibility that a susceptibility to salt could be bred in or out of isolated communities depending upon the original make-up of the members.

It will be recalled that earlier in this paper we stated unless drinking water had a high salinity it was unlikely that on the average more than 4 or 5 g of NaCl per day would be ingested from foods not salted by man; ordinarily it would be less, particularly among people who were largely vegetarians. Since hypertension appeared to be *uncommon* among groups which did not add salt to their food, we though that it might be *common* among groups which did add it and that the higher the salt consumption, the higher the incidence of hypertension. This would have been in agreement with our experimental animal data as well as those of MENEELY and collaborators (*27—30*). The remainder of this paper will be devoted to exploring the studies which we have made to test this hypothesis.

Preliminary to epidemiological investigations, we considered a pilot method of estimating average salt intakes in an effort to judge whether this hypothesis warranted the time and expense of a formal study. In our milieu, salt shakers are ubiquitously available. Therefore some inferences might be made from an individual's use of salt at the table. We arrived at the following 3 classifications: 1. Low intake — did not add and never had added salt to food at all; 2. Average intake — added salt to food only if, after prior tasting, it was insufficiently salty for the palate; 3. High intake — added salt to foods routinely without prior tasting for degree of saltiness.

We were aware then, as we are now, of the defects in such a classification: 1. It is qualitative and not quantitative; 2. No allowance is made for addition of salt to food prior to its arrival at the table; 3. No provision is made for differences in sensitivity to saltiness among different individuals or even the same individual at different times. In spite of all these reservations the pilot technique proved to be a useful one in our hands. Nevertheless there was no suggestion then, nor is there now, that it is a generally applicable technique, for it clearly is dependent upon salt-eating practices in a community. We have evidence that salt-adding customs may be very different in the northern area, where the original study was made, from those in the deep south of the United States, where a small rural community is now under study. This technique would have been misleading in Japan, where salt consumption is high, but where I found that the salt ordinarily was added to foods and sauces prior to reaching the table.

It would be unfortunate if this pilot study were interpreted to mean that we were or are interested in salt-shakers. On the contrary, let me state categorically that what we *are* interested in is *actual salt consumption*, whatever its source and however it gets into the gastro-intestinal tract.

With the use of the pilot technique we obtained information which was suggestive of a relationship between salt consumption and hypertension. Upon completion it indicated that further expense and effort were warranted in exploring this area. During the years 1953—1956, Dr. Robert A. Love, at Brookhaven Laboratory, kindly queried for me all employees upon whom he made a physical examination as to their customary salt-adding habits, according to the classification above. The incidence of hypertension among these 3 groups was significantly different from random distribution (p< .001). Those classified as having been on low intakes throughout their lives showed significantly less hypertension (p < .01) and those classified as having been on high intakes showed significantly more hypertension (p < .02) than would have been predicted by chance alone (*8*). We have assessed the validity of this method of estimating salt intake in a series of 28 males who were willing to collect 24 hr urines for from 6 to 38 days and found that the average of those classified as "Low" was significantly lower (p < .01) than those who had been classified as "High" (*7*). More importantly, the non-hypertensives appeared to be eating significantly less (p < .01) salt than the hypertensives. We have pointed out (*36*) that in this relatively young group of males (40.3 ± 10.6 years) even the non-hypertensive individuals classified as being in the "Low" category were consuming on the average about nine and a half grams per day. On the basis of such intakes I expect some of these men to develop hypertension later in life.

These data indicate the probability of a *group* developing hypertension. It would be most fallacious to surmise that a *person* who consumed a given amount of salt would carry the same probability as the *group*. An individual obviously would have, as a rule, either a higher or a lower probability than the group, depending upon the type of distribution defining his particular group.

We were encouraged by these results to explore actual salt intake among groups in which the prevalence of hypertension is variable. These data are summarized briefly in Table 2, which is an extension of Table 1, as well as in the accompanying graph (Fig. 1). These data suggest in conformity with the animal data that with higher average salt consumption there is higher prevalence of hypertension. It will be of interest to compare these data with those from other areas as they become available. The small number of Eskimos that have been studied obviously requires the amplification in which we are

Table 2. *Salt intake (measured by urinary salt excretion) compared with prevalence of hypertension in five geographic areas*

Group	Year	Sex	No.	Age (average)	Salt intake average (g/d)	Salt intake range (g/d)	% HT (140/90 or over)
Alaskan Eskimo	1958, 1960	both	20	38	4	1—10	0
Marshall Islanders (Pacific)	1958	both	231	41	7	1.5—13	6.9
United States (Brookhaven)	1954—1956	male	1124	36	10	4—24	8.6
Japan							
Hiroshima (South. Japan)	1958	male	456	43	14	4—29	21
Akita (North. Japan)	1954	both	5301	45	26	5—55	39[1]

now engaged. However, most experience with Eskimos suggests that hypertension was uncommon or rare among those who were on a truly native diet and therefore did not add salt to the food (*37—40*).

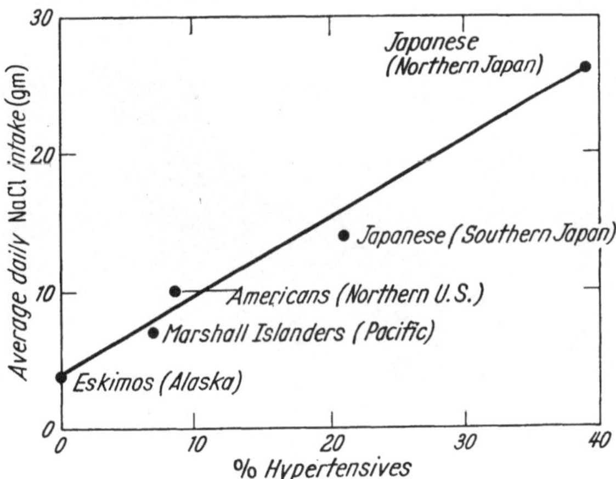

Fig. 1.   Correlation of average daily salt (NaCl) intakes with prevalence of hypertension in different geographic areas and among different races

The recent report by SCOTT et al. (*41*) is in contrast to the earlier reports on Eskimos in that hypertension was found to be as prevalent among them as among men in the United States. This report may be of great pertinence to the present work: these Eskimos were not primitives any longer, since they were all

---

[1] Systolic and diastolic pressures reported separately. This number (39%) based on diastolic pressure of 90 mm Hg or more.

sufficiently civilized to join the Alaska National Guard. No details on their salt intakes are available, however.

In Japan, hypertension is a common disease. Average levels of salt intake are high, and interestingly, appear to decrease from north to south (*42*). In association with this, both the incidence of hypertension and the incidence of cerebrovascular accidents decrease from north to south. In Fig. 2, we have summarized the

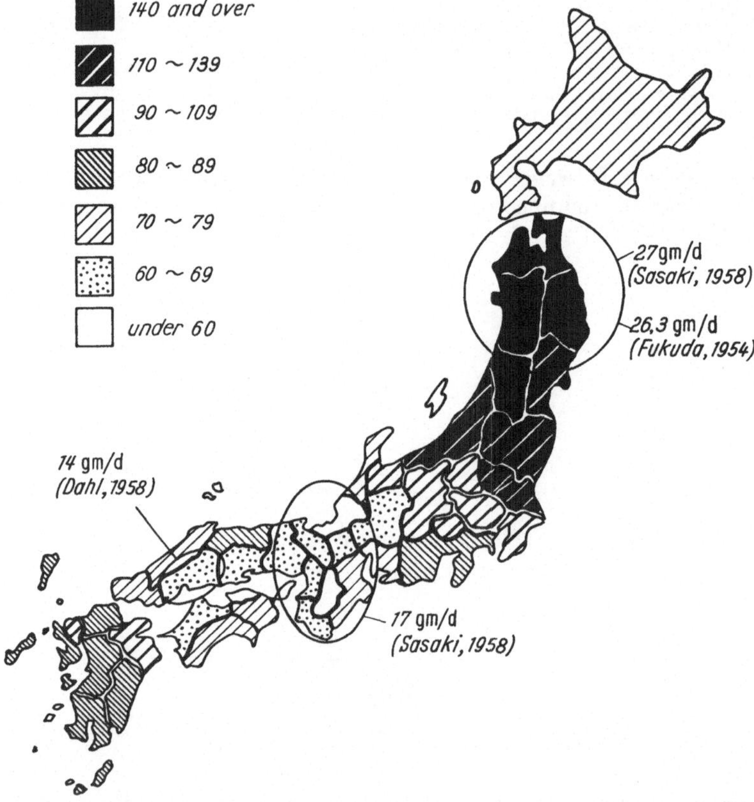

Fig. 2. Distribution of death rate (per 100,000 males aged 30—59 years) from cerebral hemorrhage, in various regions of Japan. Average daily salt intakes of farmers in 4 regions added to original. (Taken, with additions, from TAKAHASHI et al., Human Biol. (U.S.A.) 29, 139 (1957)

known data on average salt intakes and death rate from cerebral hemorrhage in Japan. Since 1951, cerebrovascular complications of hypertension have been the leading cause of death in Japan, as well as one of the leading causes of death in that country during the 20th century (*42*).

What of factors other than salt? The highly sophisticated members of this symposium will be aware that other possible factors have been omitted from this discussion. Among several, one which is most intriguing to us is the likelihood of an interaction between salt and susceptible tissues, that is, the interaction of environment with heredity: the environmental factor in this instance is represented by dietary salt levels.

There is considerable evidence which suggests that hereditary factors operate in human hypertension. This has been well reviewed by BECHGAARD (*43*), PLATT (*44*), SOBYE (*45*), SCHROEDER (*46*), and PICKERING (*47*), among modern authors. In an earlier publication we discussed this possibility citing rheumatic fever as a disease in which hereditary susceptibility is important, but a concomitant streptococcic infection (*8*) is necessary for development of the disease. There are many similar examples of which only a few will be cited. The ease with which certain families develop hay-fever after exposure to rag-weed suggests an inherited susceptibility to this allergen, but in the absence of rag-weed pollen hay-fever will not develop. Parkinson-like syndromes have been seen in miners inhaling manganese dusts but, in spite of the specific chemical agent, illness of a given individual indicated to RODIER (*48*) that it would develop subsequently more readily in relatives than in a general population that was similarly exposed. Furthermore, the susceptibility to Parkinsonism which develops as a toxic complication in about 7—10% of individuals chronically treated with chlorpromazine (*49*) was recently linked to prevalence of "spontaneous" Parkinsonism in the individuals' families (*50*).

These considerations lead us to evaluate the concept of a *lethal dose* as it might relate to salt intake and the development of hypertension. An LD_{50} dose of a toxic or infective agent is premised on the established fact that biological responsiveness is inconstant even within highly inbred organisms. One might cite the variable response of members of the same strain of bacteria to antibiotics or of mosquitoes to DDT. Obviously much greater variability in response must be possible in any single individual human under the usual conditions of enforced out-breeding in man. In the most virulent epidemics some people survive unharmed. Many individuals who smoke 2 or more packs of cigarettes per day will survive to old age without evidence of bronchogenic carcinoma. We venture to say that the same applies to chronic excessive salt intake. The failure of some or indeed most individuals to develop hypertension following chronic excessive salt intakes is, in my opinion, comparable to the failure of most individuals to develop other common diseases in which chronic exposure to the etiological agent is established as a requisite. It does not mean that salt is not involved but rather that not *only* salt is involved.

Summary

We wish to reiterate what we have said before (*11*): Among societies or groups habitually consuming low salt diets (perhaps 5 g of NaCl per person per day or less) essential hypertension will be uncommon. Among societies or groups consuming high amounts of salt (in excess of 10—15 g per person per day) essential hypertension will be common. Individual susceptibility will determine which one individual in a group will develop the disease.

Résumé

L'hypertension essentielle se rencontre plus rarement dans les sociétés ou communautés consommant d'ordinaire des rations alimentaires pauvres en sel (par exemple 5 g ou moins de NaCl par personne et par jour) que chez celles qui en consomment de grandes quantités (plus de 10—15 g par personne et par jour). La susceptibilité individuelle reste le facteur essentiel pour déterminer l'apparition de la maladie.

Bibliography

1. Dahl, L. K.: N. England J. Med. **258**, 1152 and 1205, 1958.
2. Kaunitz, H.: Nature (G. B.) **178**, 1141, 1956.
3. Meneely, G. R.: Amer. J. Med. **16**, 1, 1954.
4. Dahl, L. K., and R. A. Love: Fed. Proc. (U.S.A.) **13**, 426, 1954.
5. Dahl, L. K., and R. A. Love: A.M.A. Arch. Int. Med. **94**, 525, 1954.
6. Dahl, L. K., and R. A. Love: Fed. Proc. (U.S.A.) **15**, 513, 1956.
7. Dahl, L. K.: Proc. Soc. Exper. Biol. Med. (U.S.A.) **94**, 23, 1957.
8. Dahl, L. K., and R. A. Love: J. Amer. Med. Ass. **164**, 397, 1957.
9. Dahl, L. K., L. Silver, and R. W. Christie: N. England J. Med. **258**, 1186, 1958.
10. Dahl, L. K.: Amer. J. Clin. Nutr. **6**, 1, 1958.
11. Dahl, L. K.: Nature (G. B.) **181**, 989, 1958.
12. Dahl, L. K.: Sodium as an Etiologic Factor in Hypertension. In Hypertension. The First Hahnemann Symposium on Hypertensive Disease. Ed.: John H. Moyer. Philadelphia 1959, p. 262.
13. Dahl, L. K., L. Silver, R. W. Christie, and J. Genest: Nature (G. B.) **185**, 110, 1960.
14. Dahl, L. K.: Nutr. Rev. **18**, 97, 1960.
15. Dole, V. P., L. K. Dahl, G. C. Cotzias, H. A. Eder, and M. E. Krebs: J. Clin. Invest. (U.S.A.) **29**, 1189, 1950.
16. Dole, V. P., L. K. Dahl, G. C. Cotzias, D. D. Dziewiatkowski, and C. Harris: J. Clin. Invest. (U.S.A.) **30**, 584, 1951.
17. Dahl, L. K., B. G. Stall, and G. C. Cotzias: J. Clin. Invest. (U.S.A.) **33**, 1397, 1954.
18. Dahl, L. K., B. G. Stall, and G. C. Cotzias: J. Clin. Invest. (U.S.A.) **34**, 462, 1955.

19. STEFANSSON, V. (ed.): Not by Bread Alone. New York, 1946, p. 50.
20. HOLMBERG, A. R.: Nomads of the Long Bow: The Siriono of Eastern Bolivia. (Smithsonian Institute of Social Anthropology, Publication No. 10.), Washington, D. C., 1950, p. 35.
21. GROLLMAN, A., T. R. HARRISON, and J. R. WILLIAMS Jr.: J. Pharmacol. Exper. Therap. (U.S.A.) **69**, 149, 1940.
22. SELYE, H., C. E. HALL, and E. M. ROWLEY: Canad. Med. Ass. J. **49**, 88, 1943.
23. KNOWLTON, A. I., E. N. LOEB, H. C. STOERK, and B. C. SEEGAL: J. Exper. Med. (U.S.A.) **85**, 187, 1947.
24. LENEL, R., L. N. KATZ, and S. RODBARD: Amer. J. Physiol. **152**, 557, 1948.
25. SAPIRSTEIN, L. A., W. L. BRANDT, and D. R. DRURY: Proc. Soc. Exper. Biol. Med. (U.S.A.) **73**, 82, 1950.
26. FUKUDA, T.: Union méd. Canada **80**, 1278, 1951.
27. MENEELY, G. R., R. G. TUCKER, W. J. DARBY, and S. H. AUERBACH: J. Exper. Med. (U.S.A.) **98**, 71, 1953.
28. MENEELY, G. R., et al.: Amer. J. Med. **16**, 599, 1954.
29. BALL, C. O. T., and G. R. MENEELY: J. Amer. Diet. Ass. **33**, 366, 1957.
30. TUCKER, R. G., et al.: J. Geront. (U.S.A.) **12**, 182, 1957.
31. GROLLMAN, A., T. R. HARRISON, J. BAXTER, J. CRAMPTON, and F. REICHSMAN: J. Amer. Med. Ass. **19**, 533, 1945.
32. MOSER, M.: The Effect of a High Salt Intake on the Treatment of Hypertension. In Hypertension. The First Hahnemann Symposium on Hypertensive Disease. Ed.: J. H. MOYER. Philadelphia, 1959, p. 512.
33. McQUARRIE, I.: Proc. Staff Meet. Mayo Clin. (U.S.A.) **10**, 239, 1935.
34. McQUARRIE, I., N. H. THOMPSON, and J. A. ANDERSON: J. Nutr. (U.S.A.) **11**, 77, 1936.
35. McDONOUGH, J., and C. M. WILHELMJ: Amer. J. Digest. Dis. **21**, 180, 1954.
36. DAHL, L. K.: J. Amer. Diet. Ass. **34**, 585, 1958.
37. THOMAS, W. A.: J. Amer. Med. Ass. **88**, 1559, 1927.
38. HOYGAARD, A.: Studies on the Nutrition and Physio-pathology of Eskimos. Undertaken at Angmagssalik East Greenland, 1936—1937. Oslo: I Kommisjon Hos Jacob Dybwad 1941, p. 176.
39. EHRSTROM, R.: Acta med. Scand. **140**, 239, 1951.
40. RODAHL, K.: Observations on Blood Pressure in Eskimos. Norsk Polarinstitutet, Skrifter No. 102, 1954, pp. 53—65.
41. SCOTT, E. M., I. V. GRIFFITH, D. D. HOSKINS, and R. D. WHALEY: Lancet (G. B.) 1958/**II**, 667.
42. BECHGAARD, P.: Arterial Hypertension. A Follow-up Study of one Thousand Hypertonics. Copenhagen: NYT Nordisk Forlag, Arnold Busck 1946, pp. 102—105.
43. PLATT, R.: Quart. J. Med. (U.S.A.) **16**, 111, 1947.
44. SOBYE, P.: Heredity in Essential Hypertension and Nephrosclerosis. A Genetic-Clinical Study of 200 Propositi Suffering from Nephrosclerosis. Copenhagen: NYT Nordisk Forlag, Arnold Busck 1948, p. 225.
45. SCHROEDER, H. A.: Hypertensive diseases, causes and control. Philadelphia, 1953, p. 39.
46. PICKERING, G. W.: High blood pressure. New York, 1955, pp. 184—203.
47. RODIER, J.: Brit. J. Industr. Med. **12**, 21, 1955.
48. Current concepts in therapy. II. Phenothiazine, 2. N. England J. Med. **260**, 231, 1959.
49. MYRIANTHOPOULOS, N. C.: Symposium on Current Status of Parkinson's Disease. Parkinsons Disease Foundation (Ed.), New York. In press.

Renal hemodynamics, water and electrolyte excretion in essential hypertension

By

P. T. Cottier

The fact that patients with essential hypertension show an altered renal excretory response to sodium chloride loading or under water and mannitol diuresis has been well established by several authors (*1, 2, 4, 6, 7, 8, 11, 16, 17, 18*) since the original study of Farnsworth and Barker (*15, 16*) was published in 1943. Hypertensive patients acutely eliminate a greater proportion of a salt and water load than do normotensive subjects. This renal abnormality appears to be due to an augmented tubular rejection of sodium, chloride, and water. It is still a matter of controversy whether this kind of excretory pattern is specific for essential hypertension. Of paramount importance is the question whether the phenomenon of exaggerated natriuresis in hypertensives reflects a disorder in water and mineral metabolism, which would be of interest with regard to the pathogenesis of essential hypertension, or whether hypernatriuresis is solely a consequence of the elevated arterial blood pressure. It is my purpose to review the data we have collected during the last few years, and to discuss the arguments in favour of our opinion that hypernatriuresis is a non-specific feature of essential hypertension and that it is due to the effect of high blood pressure on renal function found in arterial hypertension of any kind.

In respect to this main problem we have attempted to solve the following questions:

1. Is the abnormal excretory pattern of water and electrolytes already detectable during basal excretion and how does basal excretion correlate with excretion under intravenous sodium chloride load ?

2. What is the plasma concentration of sodium, chloride, and potassium in patients with various degrees of arterial hypertension and how does it correlate with the urinary excretion of these electrolytes ?

3. How does the excretion of urine, sodium, and potassium following the more physiologic oral administration of salt and water compare with that following an intravenous load ?

4. Are there any correlations between renal hemodynamics and sodium excretion ?

5. Studying the possible pathogenetic factors responsible for hypernatriuresis in hypertension, we had to consider extrarenal and renal factors:

Extrarenal factors: a) extracellular fluid volume
b) exchangeable sodium
c) aldosterone
d) extrarenal hemodynamic factors
e) volume receptors.

Renal factors: f) glomerular filtration rate
g) renal plasma flow
h) filtration fraction
i) renal vascular resistance
k) renal arterial pressure.

6. Is hypernatriuresis specific for essential hypertension? We approached this problem by comparing natriuresis in patients with essential hypertension and those suffering from arteriosclerotic or renal hypertension.

7. We were also interested in finding out to what extent hypotensive therapy of any kind (drug therapy, sympathectomy and nephrectomy) may decrease natriuresis.

The patients studied were usually placed on a low-sodium diet with 2.0 g of sodium chloride added daily for 3 weeks prior to the clearance study. The hypertensive patients were grouped as mild, moderately severe, and severe hypertensives. Height of blood pressure and vascular changes of the target organs (eye fundus, heart, kidney function, and state of cerebral function) were graded and taken as the basis for this classification.

1. Basal excretion of urine, sodium, and potassium, and its correlation with the excretion under intravenous saline load

Diuresis and the electrolyte clearances were studied during a 12 hr night period. In several cases the period lasted 24 hrs. In 30 normotensives and 87 hypertensives 176 analyses were performed. The correlated blood pressure measurement was taken in the morning following the urine collecting period, after 5 min of rest. Diuresis did not differ in the normotensive and hypertensive groups (Fig. 1). The mean sodium clearance of hypertensives with a mean arterial blood pressure $\left(\dfrac{\text{systolic} + \text{diastolic}}{2} \right)$ of 120 to 140 mm Hg was slightly higher (0.86 ml/min/1.73 sq m) than in normotensives

(0.45 ml/min) and patients with severe hypertension (0.49 ml/min).
Although there is no statistically significant difference because of
the considerable individual scattering, there appears to be a blood-
pressure dependent excretory pattern for sodium, whereas potassium
excretion was the same for all groups. Under these circumstances
the patients with mild or moderately severe hypertension exhibit

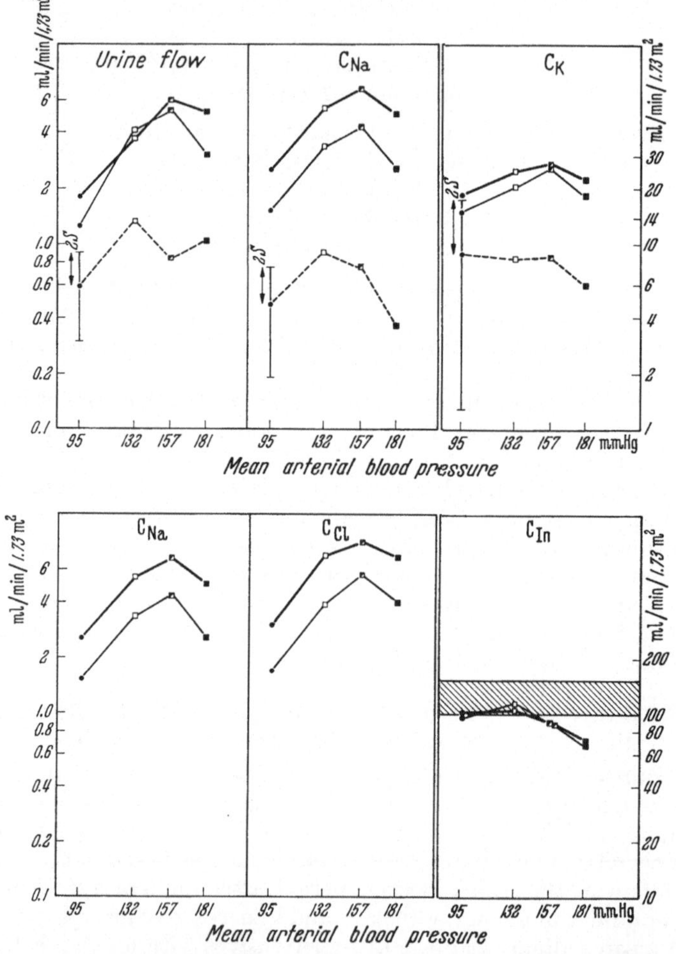

Fig. 1. Urine flow and clearances of Na, Cl, K, and inulin during the basal period and under
isotonic and hypertonic (2.5 %) saline infusion in normotensives (·), mild (□), moderately
severe (▨), and severe (■) hypertensives (10 individuals in each group). ··· Basal period
(12—24 hrs), — infusion with 0.9% NaCl (3 periods, 15 minutes each), —infusion with 2.5 %
NaCl (4 periods, 15 minutes each), 2 S: double standard deviation, ▨: normal range of C_{In}

higher excretory rates for sodium than those with severe hypertension. Further studies are necessary to permit a definite conclusion to be drawn.

We then compared diuresis, as well as sodium and potassium clearances under basal conditions and during isotonic and hypertonic (2.5%) saline infusion in 30 hypertensive patients, grouped as mild (10 patients with a mean blood pressure of 132 mm Hg), moderately severe (10 patients with a mean blood pressure of 157 mm Hg) and severe hypertensives (10 patients with a mean blood pressure of 181 mm Hg), and 9 normotensive individuals (mean blood pressure 95 mm Hg). The urine volume during the basal period was lowest in the group of normotensive subjects (average 0.59 ml/min/1.73 sq m) and higher in the 3 hypertensive groups .The highest mean value was found in the group of mild hypertension (1.30 ml/min). The mean diuretic response under isotonic and hypertonic saline infusion was similar in all groups except for the patients with severe hypertension, whose diuresis augmented from 3.0 to 5.0 ml/min under hypertonic saline infusion (Fig. 2).

It is worthwhile noting that the percentage difference of the mean urine volume between the group of normotensives and the mildly hypertensives is similar during the basal state and the load periods. Under load the group of moderately severe hypertensives attains the highest urine volume (5.9 ml/min).

A similar pattern is observed with regard to sodium clearance. The basal sodium clearance is highest in the group with mild hypertension. Under load with isotonic and hypertonic saline the group with moderately severe hypertension attains the maximal values of sodium clearance. The normotensive group exhibits significantly lower values with regard to sodium clearance under load. The patients with severe hypertension were found to have a sodium clearance under load slightly below the values of those with mild hypertension.

Potassium clearance during basal excretion is similar for the normotensive, mildly hypertensive and moderately severe hypertensive group (8.1—9.0 ml/min). The lowest basal potassium excretion was encountered in cases with severe hypertension (C_K 6 ml/min). Loading with isotonic and hypertonic saline did increase potassium excretion in all 4 groups, but no statistically significant difference between groups could be detected, although the qualitative excretory pattern is comparable with that of water, sodium, and chloride.

The glomerular filtration rate (C_{In}) for the normotensive and mildly hypertensive group was within the normal range (99 ml/min

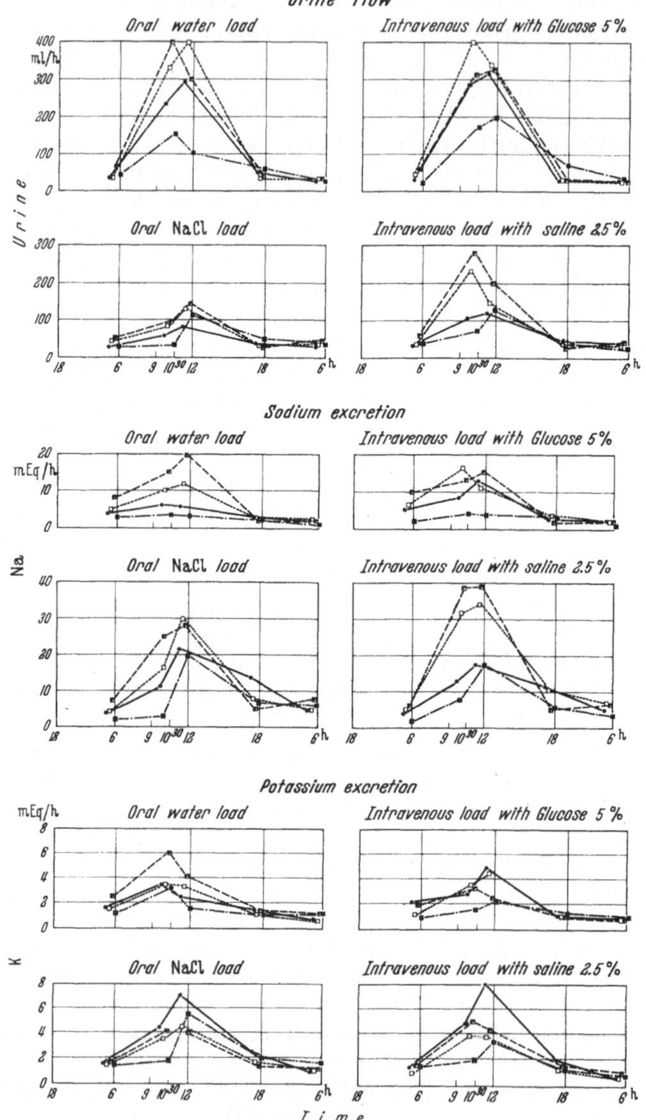

Fig. 2. Urine flow, Na, and K excretion prior to and following various loads [1000 ml/1.73 sq. m. of tea or 1000 ml/1.73 sq. m. of a salted bouillon (12.5 g NaCl) orally or 500 ml/1.73 sq. m. of 5% glucose or 2.5% NaCl intravenously following the oral intake of 500 ml/1.73 sq.m. of tea] in normotensives (●), mild (▢), moderately severe (◪) and severe hypertensives (■)

and 111 ml/min, respectively) and slightly reduced in the moderately severe hypertensives (90 ml/min) (Fig. 2). The severely hypertensive group had a mean filtration rate of 66 ml/min, which corresponds to a reduction of 50%. Glomerular filtration rate showed no increase in any of the groups during loading with hypertonic saline (2.5% sodium chloride with a speed of 8 ml/min/1.73 sq m). It is, therefore, conceivable that the increased water, sodium, and chloride excretion in hypertensives under load conditions is due to increased tubular rejection rather than to augmented filtration.

2. Plasma electrolytes in essential hypertension

Since TAQUINI et al. (25) described elevated concentrations of sodium in the plasma of hypertensive patients, we determined the sodium, chloride, and potassium concentration in the plasma of patients with various degrees of hypertension. There is no doubt that we had to face the possibility that hypernatriuresis in hypertension is due to an increased filtered load of sodium as a consequence of an elevated plasma level.

Although in the groups of hypertensives studied the values were within the normal range, the mean concentrations of sodium or chloride and potassium showed slight changes in the opposite direction. Mildly hypertensives had slightly higher sodium concentrations than the normotensives, the moderately severe, and the severe hypertensives (11, 12).

3. Diuresis, sodium and potassium excretion, as well as specific gravity of urine, following oral and intravenous water and salt load

These studies were performed with the assistance of M. PEYER (19). 16 hypertensives (graded as mild, moderately severe, and severe) were compared with 13 normotensives with regard to diuresis, sodium and potassium excretion and specific gravity of the urine prior to and following the oral and intravenous administration of water and salt. The excretory pattern was followed during 21 hrs after the administration of the load, the periods of urine collection lasting from $1^1/_2$ to 6 hrs. The mild and moderately severe hypertensives showed the highest urine volumes during the 3 hrs following the various loads, the differences being most marked after an intravenous infusion of a hypertonic (2.5%) saline solution. At 6 p. m. (9 hrs after the load was started) the various groups of patients exhibited similar amounts of urine volume (Fig. 2). Sodium excretion in response to the 4 types of load was highest in the mild and moderately severe hypertensives, the differences being again most marked following hypertonic saline infusion. During the course of the first 21 hrs following the loads the normotensives and severe hypertensives did not show any delayed natriuresis.

Potassium was excreted in a rather reciprocal way to sodium. Under sodium chloride load a linear, but inverse correlation between

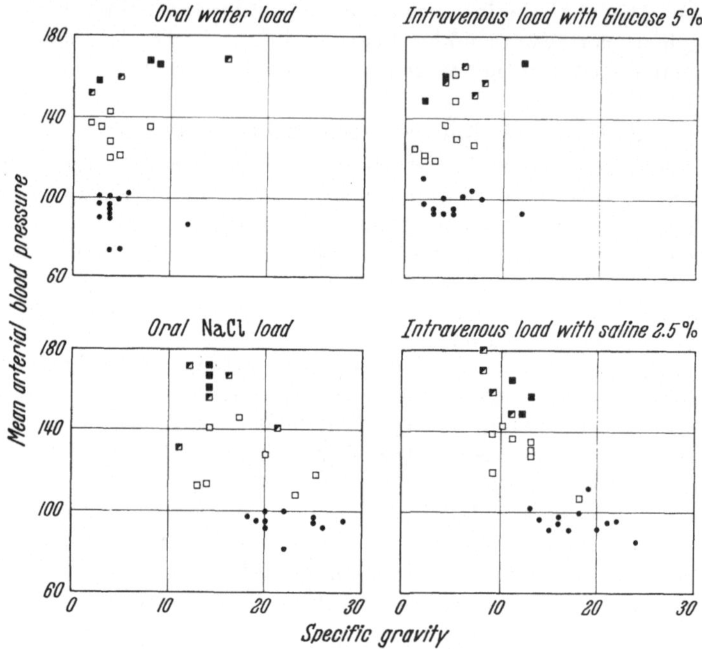

Fig. 3. Specific gravity of urine and mean arterial blood pressure following the various loads in normotensives and hypertensives of various degree

mean arterial blood pressure and specific gravity of the urine could be demonstrated, whereas under dilution (water load) a similar reduction of the specific gravity occurred in all 4 groups (Fig. 3). This permits the assumption that under sodium chloride load and increasing arterial pressure a urine of lower specific gravity, i.e. concentration, is produced.

4. Correlations between renal hemodynamics and sodium excretion

In our study with Weller and Hoobler (6, 7) we emphasized the correlation between sodium clearance and renal resistance. Since the renal extraction of Na-PAH is only slightly reduced in the hypertensive kidney, provided the blood flow is not grossly impaired (*19*), it is possible to calculate renal resistance even without performing catheterisation of the renal vein in every instance. Plotting sodium clearance or the "tubular rejection of sodium" $\left(\dfrac{C_{Na} \cdot 100}{C_{In}}\right)$ versus renal vascular resistance, we find that there is a linear correlation between these parameters up to a resistance of 18,000 dynes/sec/cm^{-5} (Fig. 4) or with a glomerular filtration rate greater than 70 ml/min. It is not yet possible to draw any conclusions regarding pathogenesis from this finding. In view of the arteriolar spasms or arteriolosclerosis representing the basic functional and morphologic process in the hypertensive kidney, one is tempted to speculate

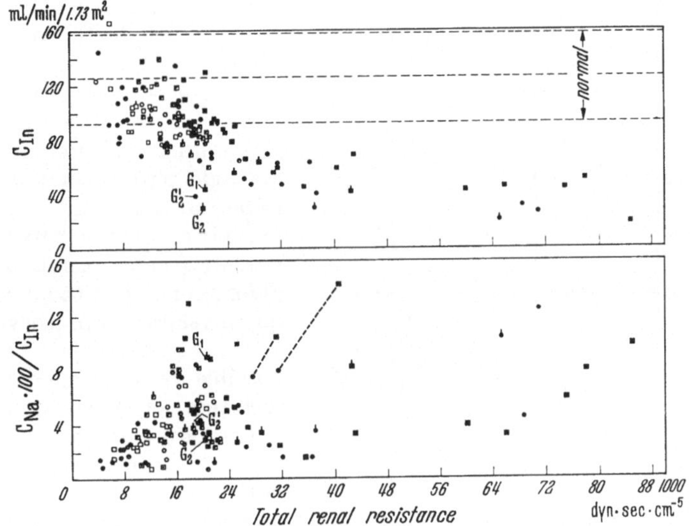

Fig. 4. Inulin clearance and tubular rejection of Na versus total renal resistance in normotensives (·) and hypertensives of various degree. ☐ mild hypertension ◻ determination of E_{PAH}, ◧ moderately severe hypertension, ■ severe hypertension, ⊡ labile hypertension, ○ hypertensives under hypotensive therapy, G: 2 patients with glomerular nephritis

that the renal resistance or an altered intrarenal distribution of vascular resistance could be of importance for the natriuresis in hypertension. At least we can assume that hypernatriuresis in hypertensives is optimal, the higher the arterial blood pressure and renal blood flow.

5. Possible pathogenetic factors responsible for hypernatriuresis in hypertension

Extrarenal factors

a) Extracellular fluid volume. We were not able to demonstrate any correlation between inulin spaces as a measure of the extracellular fluid volume (*11, 12*) and natriuresis or tubular rejection of sodium in hypertensives.

b) Exchangeable sodium. Plotting sodium clearance on a semilogarithmic scale versus body sodium (exchangeable sodium) we found an inverse correlation. "High salt excretors" had a subnormal sodium space and the "low salt excretors" were above normal range (Fig. 5). This represents an argument in favour of our view that hypernatriuresis is primary and not secondary to an elevated body sodium (*11*).

c) Aldosterone. Together with A. F. Müller (*9, 10*) we studied aldosteronuria and aldosterone secretion in hypertensives and hoped to find a correlation between natriuresis and excretion of aldosterone. But there was no correlation whatsoever. It has not so far been possible to determine the secretion of a postulated natriuretic hormone.

d) Extrarenal hemodynamic factors. With the help of A. Schmid (*10, 12*) we tried to correlate hemodynamic changes (cardiac output, end diastolic pressure in the right ventricle, pressure in the vena cava and the renal vein) with the excretory pattern of electrolytes in hypertensives. It was thought that the low salt excretors in the group of severe hypertension suffered from latent cardiac insufficiency and therefore were retaining salt. The hemodynamic parameters studied did not correlate with natriuresis.

e) Volume receptors and "natriuretic center". It could be postulated that an abnormal response of the so far postulated volume receptors or natriuretic centers is responsible for the exaggerated diuresis and natriuresis observed in hypertensives. When loading

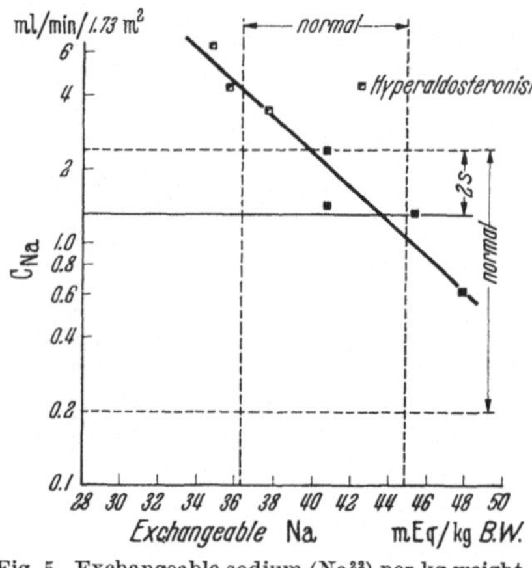

Fig. 5. Exchangeable sodium (Na²²) per kg weight and sodium clearance in 7 patients with essential hypertension of various degree, (◪ moderately severe, ■ severe)

normotensive and hypertensive individuals with equal amounts (500 ml/1.73 sq m body surface, administered with a speed of 8 ml/min/1.73 sq m body surface) of a gelatin-like plasma expander (Physiogel[1]), hypertensives even showed a smaller percentage increment of sodium clearance and tubular rejection of sodium than the normotensives (*13*) (Table 1). The mean change of plasma volume (Evan's blue) was + 16.8%. On the basis of these preliminary data we have no reason to presume that hypertensives have an increased susceptibility of the postulated natriuretic centers which are possibly sensitive to intravascular volume changes.

Renal factors

f) Glomerular filtration rate. We were not able to demonstrate any correlation between the absolute filtration rate and the natriuresis. The glomerular filtration rate, however, represents

Table 1. *Change in % following the intravenous infusion of 500 ml/1.73 sq. m. Physiogel (plasma expander)*
Rate of infusion: 8 ml/min/1.73 sq. m.

	Hypertensives (5 individuals) %	Normotensives (5 individuals) %
Mean art. pressure	+ 5.8	+ 2.9
C_{In}	+ 4.9	+ 3.9
C_{PAH}	+ 9.0	+ 10.1
Urine volume .	+50.6	+175.3
C_{Na}	+55.4	+ 75.2
$\dfrac{C_{Na}\,100}{C_{In}}$ . . .	+47.4	+ 68.3
C_{Cl}	+50.8	+ 98
$\dfrac{C_{Cl}\,100}{C_{In}}$ . . .	+43.2	+ 85.1
C_{K}	+ 8.2	— 6.2
$\dfrac{C_{K}\,100}{C_{In}}$ . . .	+ 2.0	— 5.1

in a way a permissive factor. Hypernatriuresis can only occur if the filtration rate is greater than 50—70 ml/min. The fact that patients suffering from chronic glomerulonephritis with a decreased filtration fraction, i.e. a relatively low filtration rate, may show a tubular rejection of sodium similar to that of essential hypertensives with a comparable elevation of blood pressure supports the view that the glomerular filtration rate is not a determinant factor responsible for hypernatriuresis in hypertension (*6, 8, 10, 11*).

g) Renal plasma flow. No correlation between total renal plasma flow (C_{PAH}) and natriuresis in hypertensives could be detected (*12*).

h) Filtration fraction. As long as the renal resistance does not exceed 18,000 dynes/sec/cm^{-5} the filtration fraction (glomerular

---

[1] *Physiogel* was manufactured and supplied by the Central Laboratory of the blood bank of the Swiss Red Cross.

filtration rate/renal plasma flow) may parallel natriuresis. Since patients with cardiac insufficiency — exquisite salt and water retainers — also exhibit an increased filtration fraction, it is difficult to accept the view that this factor may play a role in regulating natriuresis.

i) Renal vascular resistance. The questionable implication of renal resistance in the pathogenesis of hypernatriuresis in essential hypertension has been mentioned above.

k) Renal arterial pressure. Experimental (*23, 24*) and clinical studies (*21*) revealed that the intrarenal pressure is dependent upon the intra-arterial blood pressure. The fact that sodium clearance has a tendency to decrease beyond a critical value of renal resistance can easily be understood. We have to assume that, with the deterioration in renal blood flow due to the progressing arteriolosclerosis, the mass of functioning nephrons becomes reduced. On the other hand, it is not at all clear why the tubular rejection of Na also decreases beyond this critical value of renal resistance (18,000 dynes/ sec/cm^{-5}) or a glomerular filtration rate below 70—50 ml/min.

First of all, one could use the argument of a "glomerular tubular imbalance", as was done to explain antinatriuresis in heart failure (Merrill). It could be stated that both in heart failure and hypertensive kidney disease tubular function is affected later than in other nephropathies (for example, pyelonephritis). A marked reduction of the glomerular filtration rate would decrease the speed of urine flow in each nephron, so that the almost normally functioning tubules (transport mechanisms) would reabsorb more Na and Cl and water. But if we assume that the filtered load for each remaining nephron increases with progressive renal arteriolosclerosis, we would have to abandon this hypothesis.

Without intending to predict the nature of antinatriuresis in heart failure, it could be claimed that hypertensives with low salt excretion are those suffering from latent or obvious heart failure. Our negative results with regard to right heart failure do not rule out latent failure of the left heart.

A new distribution of the intrarenal blood flow, i.e. a change of the medullary blood flow due to arteriolar spasms or arteriolosclerosis could represent a factor inducing antinatriuresis.

An increase in aldosterone secretion due to heart failure or as a compensatory phenomenon following the hypernatriuretic phase can be discussed. Our data concerning aldosteronuria and natriuresis are probably not decisive, since aldosteronuria and the secretory rate of this hormone do not have to parallel each other. There are no data available for the assumption that a natriuretic hormone, which could be secreted in excess during the natriuretic phase of hypertension, is secreted at a lower rate in the course of the antinatriuretic phase.

We may assume that either the renal arterial blood pressure itself or the consequent elevation of the intrarenal pressure represents the crucial factor in the promotion of hypernatriuresis. This would become obvious under special circumstances (oral or parenteral loads with water or salt or osmotic diuresis) only. However, we feel that the changed tubular behaviour with respect to sodium, chloride, and water reabsorption is already present under basal conditions, but has to be elicited by procedures promoting diuresis. Later on we shall mention the bulk of evidence in favour of the view that the arterial blood pressure in the kidney is of great importance for the regulation of sodium chloride and water excretion.

6. Specificity of hypernatriuresis

As we have already mentioned, it is important to know to what extent hypernatriuresis is a specific feature of essential hypertension. If it is specific, hypernatriuresis represents the only clinically detectable disorder of salt and water metabolism in human hypertension and, therefore, is of pathogenetic interest. In approaching this problem, we first compared natriuresis in 4 patients with essential hypertension and 2 patients with arteriosclerotic hypertension. We presume that the two forms of hypertension are not identical nosologically, although considerable overlapping of the two hypertensive states may sometimes render differentiation quite difficult or impossible. The differentiation in arteriosclerotic and essential hypertension was based on clinical grounds and on the test of Conway (5), performed by Dr. A. Schmid. As can be seen from Table 2, the tubular rejection of sodium is similarly increased in essential and arteriosclerotic hypertensives (3.2—6% instead of 1.7 $\pm$ 0.4% in normal individuals).

The same is true of renal hypertension. We had the opportunity to follow two patients with comparable hypertension and glomerular filtration rate; one, K. W., was suffering from chronic glomerulonephritis (diagnosis was proved at autopsy) and the other was affected with nephrosclerosis. Both patients showed an almost identical tubular rejection of sodium under isotonic and hypertonic saline infusion (11, 12).

7. Effect of hypotensive therapy on natriuresis

On the assumption that arterial pressure plays an important part in renal handling of sodium, chloride, and water excretion, one

Table 2. *Arterial blood pressure, renal hemodynamics, urine flow and sodium clearance under isotonic NaCl infusion in normotensives and patients with arteriosclerotic or essential hypertension*

Groups	No.	Initials Age	Art. blood pressure syst. diast. mean BP mm Hg		C_{In}	C_{PAH} ml/min/1.73	FF	Total renal resist. dynes/sec/ cm^{-5}	V/min	C_{Na} ml/min/1.73	$\dfrac{C_{na}\,100}{C_{In}}$ %
Normotensives	1—5	Mean standard deviation	115/65	90 ±5.1	94 ±18.5	577 ±62	0.166 ±0.040	6490 ±2906	1.39 ±0.74	1.6 ±0.2	1.7 ±0.4
Arteriosclerotic *hypertension*	6 7	S. L.* 43 B. B.* 72	170/113 220/75	142 148	104 117	520 518	0.200 0.226	12200 11450	4.44 6.25	3.3 3.7	3.2 3.2
Essential *hypertension*	8 9 10 11	H. E.* 49 W. L. 26 J. M. 31 F. A.* 63	161/93 160/120 177/122 196/115	127 140 146 156	84 138 97 95	385 575 507 448	0.212 0.240 0.192 0.212	13650 11000 11180 12300	5.92 3.78 6.17 7.09	3.3 5.0 4.6 5.7	3.9 3.5 4.7 6.0

Note: With respect to urine flow, Na-clearance, or tubular rejection of Na no differentiation between essential and arteriosclerotic hypertension is possible.

In the case of the patients marked with * a test described by Conway (5) to measure the vascular reactivity was performed by Dr. A. Schmid.

would expect a decrease in diuresis and sodium clearance or tubular rejection of sodium under the influence of an effective hypotensive therapy. This antinatriuresis should occur irrespectively of the therapeutic measure applied. As a matter of fact, we found, parallel to the hypotensive effect, an average fall in sodium clearance and diuresis in the patients treated for 4 weeks with reserpine, mecamylamine and chlorothiazide. The antinatriuresis occurring during prolonged chlorothiazide therapy may very well represent a compensatory phenomenon following exaggerated natriuresis due to the initial natriuretic effect of the drug. On the other hand, hydralazine appeared to promote diuresis and natriuresis after this lapse of time. Among the hypotensive agents studied (reserpine, hydralazine, mecamylamine and chlorothiazide), hydralazine was the only one to increase the average glomerular filtration rate $(+2.1\%)$, whereas the renal plasma flow was unchanged after a 4-week period of treatment (Table 3).

In a 16-year-old girl with unilateral kidney disease (pyelonephritic atrophic cirrhosis) and extreme arterial hypertension, we found a prompt decrease in the tubular rejection of sodium following nephrectomy and the significant drop in arterial blood pressure (Table 4).

Table 3. *Mean change in percent of the mean arterial blood pressure, glomerular filtration rate (C_{In}), renal plasma flow (C_{PAH}), urine flow, clearances of Na, Cl, and K and tubular rejection of Na following 4 weeks' hypotensive therapy (with chlorothiazide, mecamylamine, hydralazine, and reserpine)*

Drug	Mean art. BP. %	C_{In} %	C_{PAH} %	Urine flow per min %	C_{Na} %	C_{Cl} %	C_K %	$\dfrac{C_{Na}\,100}{C_{In}}$ %
1. *Chlorothiazide* (10 cases)	—10.0	— 4.9	0	— 4.2	—23.8	—16.3	+26.8	—19.7
2. *Mecamylamine* (10 cases)	—6.3 recumbent	—13.6	—9.7	—23.1	—34.2	—24.0	— 6.1	—1.9
3. *Hydralazine* (10 cases)	—5.1	+ 2.1	—2.1	+20.3	+25.0	+19.1	— 2.2	+20.7
4. *Reserpine* (10 cases)	—2.9	— 3.7	—6.5	—17.3	—10.8	—11.3	+17.9	— 4.5

Table 4. *Arterial blood pressure, glomerular filtration rate (C_{In}), renal plasma flow (C_{PAH}), filtration fraction (FF), and tubular rejection of Na $\dfrac{(C_{Na}\,100)}{C_{In}}$ prior to and following nephrectomy in patient Z. M. (16 years old)*

Date	Art. blood pressure mm Hg	C_{In} ml/min	C_{PAH} ml/min	FF	$\dfrac{C_{Na}\,100}{C_{In}}$ %
8. 5. 1959 prior to nephrectomy .	205/135	100	350	0.286	5.30
3. 7. 1959 6 weeks following nephrectomy	140/100	93	406	0.228	2.14
Normal					1.70 ± 0.40

In a 56-year-old male undergoing Peet's sympathectomy, a marked reduction in diuresis, sodium clearance, and tubular rejection of sodium paralleled the drop in mean arterial blood pressure.

It thus follows that any kind of hypotensive measure (drug therapy, nephrectomy, or sympathectomy) tends to reduce diuresis and natriuresis. Treatment with hydralazine represents so far the only exception to this rule.

What are, in sum, the arguments in favour of our assumption that the hypernatriuresis observed in hypertensives is merely a consequence of the elevated arterial blood pressure and not the expression of a primary disorder of salt and water metabolism ?

A number of experimental studies have shown that diuresis and natriuresis correlate well with the perfusion pressure in the kidney (*22, 23, 24*).

Various experimental forms of hypertension (endocrine, salt, renal) are accompanied by an increase in diuresis and natriuresis as soon as the animals are loaded with salt or fluid.

In patients with hypertension of any origin there appears to be a significant correlation between natriuresis and height of the arterial blood pressure, as long as renal plasma flow and glomerular filtration rate are not considerably reduced (filtrate below 70ml/min). This explains the correlation observed between natriuresis and renal resistance up to a value of 18,000 dynes/sec/cm^{-5}.

Patients with hypertension of various origin (essential, renal, endocrine) exhibit the same behaviour with regard to natriuresis.

Labile hypertensives in a phase of normotension behave like normotensives (*8*).

In hypertensive patients with unilateral obstruction of the renal artery, natriuresis is diminished on the side affected (*3*, *14*).

Possible extrarenal factors which could be responsible for the phenomenon described, such as increased extracellular fluid volume, exchangeable sodium, aldosterone, and hemodynamic influences, did not correlate with natriuresis.

With the exception of hydralazine, any therapeutic measure which lowers the blood pressure will be followed by a decrease in sodium clearance.

Although our studies impose the assumption that the hypernatriuresis which can be observed in hypertensives under special conditions represents a blood-pressure dependent phenomenon of renal function, we still have to consider the possibility that a primary, not yet detectable, disorder of salt and water distribution in the tissue (vessel walls) could be the cause of an altered vasoreaction to various pressor stimuli.

Summary

Despite the established data concerning exaggerated natriuresis in essential hypertension, we still do not know what the intimate nature of this disturbance is. The arterial blood pressure seems to exert a direct effect on tubular function. The fact that exaggerated natriuresis parallels blood pressure also in arteriosclerotic hypertension and in patients with renal and endocrine hypertension and that hypernatriuresis may disappear with successful hypotensive therapy of any type (with the exception of hydralazine), suggests that increased natriuresis in hypertension is a passive, blood-pressure dependent phenomenon. We have no reason to consider it as the manifestation of a primary disorder of salt and water metabolism which could be related to the genesis of hypertension. Other factors possibly responsible for the changed renal handling of sodium chloride and water, such as extracellular fluid volume, aldosterone, and extrarenal hemodynamic changes, were not found to correlate with natriuresis.

Résumé

Malgré l'existence bien établie d'une natriurèse exagérée dans l'hypertension, nous ne connaissons pas encore la nature intime de ce trouble. La pression artérielle semble exercer un effet direct sur la fonction tubulaire. Le fait que la natriurèse exagérée est parallèle à la tension artérielle aussi bien dans l'hypertension artérioscléreuse que chez les malades atteints d'hypertension rénale et endocrinienne, et que cette hypernatriurèse peut disparaître lors d'un traitement hypotenseur de quelque type qu'il soit (sauf l'hydralazine) suggère que cette augmentation de la natriurèse dans l'hypertension est un phénomène passif dépendant de la tension artérielle. Nous n'avons aucune raison de le considérer comme une manifestation d'un désordre primaire du métabolisme de l'eau et des électrolytes qui pourrait conditionner le développement de l'hypertension. Nous n'avons pas décelé d'autres facteurs qui pourraient être responsables d'une élimination anormale de l'eau et du NaCl par le rein, tels que par exemple le volume du liquide extra-cellulaire, d'aldostérone et des changements hémodynamiques extra-rénaux.

References

1. Baldwin, D. S., A. W. Biggs, W. Goldring, W. H. Hulet, and H. Chasis: Amer. J. Med. **24**, 893 (1958).
2. Birchall, R., S. W. Tuthill, W. S. Jacobs, W. J. Trautman, and T. Findley: Circulation (U.S.A.) **7**, 258 (1953).
3. Birchall, R., H. M. Batson, and C. B. Moore: Amer. Heart J. **56**, 616 (1958).
4. Brodsky, W. A., and H. N. Graubarth: J. Laborat. Clin. Med. (U.S.A.) **41**, 43 (1953).
5. Conway, J.: Circulation (U.S.A.) **17**, 807 (1958).
6. Cottier, P. T., J. M. Weller, and S. W. Hoobler: Cardiologia (Switz.) **31**, 278 (1957).
7. Cottier, P. T., J. M. Weller, and S. W. Hoobler: Circulation (U.S.A.) **17**, 750 (1958).
8. Cottier, P. T., J. M. Weller, and S. W. Hoobler: Circulation (U.S.A.) **18**, 196 (1958).
9. Cottier, P. T., A. F. Muller, and A. Schmid: Schweiz. med. Wschr. **89**, 376 (1959).
10. Cottier, P. T., A. Schmid, and A. F. Muller: 3rd World Congress of Cardiology, Brussels. Commun. 598, 1958. Abstract.
11. Cottier, P.: Cardiologia (Switz.) **35**, 410 (1959).
12. Cottier, P.: Helv. med. Acta, Suppl. 39 (1960).
13. Cottier, P., H. J. Schafroth, and A. Basevi: Non-published data.
14. Dustan, H. P.: Personal communication.
15. Farnsworth, E. B., and M. H. Barker: Proc. Soc. Exper. Biol. (U.S.A.) **52**, 74 (1943).
16. Farnsworth, E. B.: J. Clin. Invest. (U.S.A.) **25**, 897 (1946).
17. Green, D. M., H. G. Wedell, M. H. Wald, and B. Learned: Circulation (U.S.A.) **6**, 919 (1952).
18. Green, D. M., and E. J. Ellis: Circulation (U.S.A.) **10**, 536 (1954).
19. Peyer, M.: Thesis. Berne 1958.
20. Reubi, F.: 3rd Internat. Congress Clin. Biol.: Presses Acad. Europ. Brussels 376 (1958).
21. Reubi, F.: Schweiz. med. Wschr. **15**, 385 (1956).
22. Selkurt, E. E., P. W. Hall, and M. P. Spencer: Amer. J. Physiol. **159**, 369 (1949).
23. Selkurt, E. E.: Circulation (U.S.A.) **4**, 541 (1951).
24. Shipley, R. E., and R. S. Study: Amer. J. Physiol. **167**, 676 (1951).
25. Taquini, A. C., S. A. Plesch, T. A. Capris, and B. N. Badano: Acta cardiol. (Belg.) **11**, 109 (1956).

Discussion

REUBI: At the beginning of this session, I should like to read a few lines taken from the "Ciba Foundation Symposium on Hypertension", which was published in 1954. In his closing remarks, Dr. PICKERING made the following statement: "Then there are the corticosteroids, and here the discussion is so recent that I have not had time to think very much about them. But it is quite clear that all the time the methods of assay of these substances are improving and that one substance after another is being identified. In the next few years we shall get a clearer conception as to what part, if any, which corticosteroid, if any, plays in the development of hypertension. There has also been the question of alteration in electrolytes and extracellular fluid volume. Perhaps at a subsequent meeting we may have a clearer answer to this problem".

I hope that we shall be able now to bring a new answer to these problems. We had yesterday two very interesting papers, and I think it would be very nice if we could succeed in correlating intake and excretion of salt, but I do not know if we shall be able to do so. Let us discuss first Dr. DAHL's paper. I personally have been impressed by the data he has presented. I must say, however, that these data would be even more impressive if the different groups of patients could be taken among the same population. If you have to compare Eskimos, Japanese, and Americans, it is quite conceivable that racial and geographical factors may play a rôle, more than salt intake itself. I have been quite struck by Dr. DAHL's last slide, representing a chart of Japan. I think the same chart has been shown in Prague by Dr. SCHROEDER, who found a very good correlation between the composition of drinking water and the existence of cardiovascular disease. Now in Japan, Dr. DAHL also found a good correlation between salt intake and hypertension, and I think that is one point which should be discussed. I still believe there must be something in Dr. DAHL's views. We all know that in chronic pyelonephritis, for instance, a small amount of salt may raise the blood pressure. If one patient takes 2 or 3 grams a day, he may have a normal blood pressure, and if the same patient takes 6 or 10 grams of sodium chloride his blood pressure may rise markedly. It may well be that the salt intake is at least one contributory or environmental factor in essential hypertension. Now, there is one more point which should be made clear: is the salt appetite inherited or not? I do not know whether this problem has been investigated. It is quite conceivable that some people eat more salt just because they like it, and therefore develop hypertension rather than other subjects. A last point should perhaps also be discussed: is the increase in salt intake a consequence of the increased excretion as shown by Dr. COTTIER?

SCHROEDER: May I show two slides?

I would like to emphasize Dr. DAHL's point on the geographical variations of death rates from vascular lesions affecting the central nervous system in Japan. This slide was taken from ISSHIKI and the data are based on 350,000 applicants for life insurance, grouped according to the prefecture in which they resided. The upper curve shows the mean systolic pressure of persons aged 50 to 65, the middle the incidence of hypertension, and the lower the death rate from cerebral vascular disease, mainly cerebral hemorrhage. The different prefectures are arranged geographically from north-east to west. The curves are identical and show high incidences in the north-eastern part of Japan. The data have been analyzed and the differences are considered to be significant, with a doubling of the death rate in the highest as compared to the lowest area.

I have no fault to find with Dr. DAHL's excellent data, but I think we must be careful in drawing conclusions. KOBAYASHI has found a correlation with the death rate from strokes in the different prefectures and the sulfate/ bicarbonate ratio of river water. This next slide shows the distribution of cadmium in the intestines of a widely eaten fish in the rivers of Japan, and again shows an apparent cluster of high values in the north-eastern prefectures, with low values in the west. Cadmium accumulates in the human kidney with age. So there may be other factors associated with salt, but not dependent upon salt, which affect the death rate.

A third point: Would Dr. COTTIER show us his data on the actual increase in sodium excretion in resting hypertensives so that we may compare them with Dr. DAHL's data? If hypertensive people excrete more salt than normotensives, obviously they must eat more salt in order to remain in sodium balance. If this increment is fairly large, approaching Dr. DAHL's figures for Americans, then Dr. DAHL may be showing us a result of hypertension and not a cause.

If the increment is small, then there may be something in Dr. DAHL's hypothesis.

HOOBLER: In regard to Dr. DAHL's report, I think the theory of chronic salt over-ingestion is an appealing one, but I believe we should not be led to false conclusions by an attractive theory alone. Let us reconsider some lines of evidence which Dr. DAHL has proposed. First: the evidence for the production of experimental hypertension by salt over-feeding. This is a difficult type of hypertension to produce, as manifested by the substantial number of rats which he has admitted do not respond to the regimen — I believe a failure rate of 20—30%. In the experiments conducted by Dr. WELLER at the University of Michigan, he was not able to make rats hypertensive after several years of salt feeding. I do not deny that it is possible to produce such hypertension, but I only wish to point out that it is difficult and that such difficulties do not make the theory very attractive. Furthermore, salt feeding in experimental hypertension of other varieties has often been reported not to aggravate the condition.

Now, with respect to the allegedly increased salt appetite of hypertensive persons as reported by Dr. DAHL, you have already heard that MIALL & OLDHAM found contrary results, but these may be disposed of by the infrequency of true hypertension in their studies. In a very careful study conducted under the direction of Dr. WELLER at Michigan, questioning of hypertensive and normotensive subjects revealed no difference in salt habits between the two. I believe that a study by Dr. RODBARD at Buffalo was also inconclusive. If we wish to correlate salt intake and hypertension, we should measure the salt output in the urine and, so far as I know, no study has shown significant difference between normotensives and hypertensives in this regard.

Dr. DAHL has quite wisely stressed that high salt intake might bring out hypertension in the individual genetically predisposed to hypertension. This would account for the observations made by MOSER and myself in various partly inbred family groups in the Bahamas who all have a high salt intake and output but who have varying prevalence rates of hypertension. As for Dr. DAHL's studies in Japan and elsewhere, I would gather that there is a high variability in salt output within each group, shedding some doubt on the validity of the mean values; and all groups studied had an excess salt intake by his criteria. Therefore racial and other factors, which a high salt intake might permit to operate, may account for the apparent frequency of hypertension. What we need are figures for an area with a high genetic or racial predisposition and a low salt output (perhaps less than 5 grams per day ?). I suggest some Carribean islands (possibly Dr. CORCORAN's data on St. Kitt's would be helpful), but would warn against primitive areas with high infective disease rates, since such concurrent diseases may reduce the prevalence of hypertension.

In conclusion then, I submit that the interesting hypothesis of Dr. DAHL, while deceptively simple in appearance, remains entirely unproven.

DAHL: Dr. HOOBLER raised many questions which are important. I hope that I was able to write them down as fast as he brought them up.

He suggests that since we have studied several population groups which appear to have differences in prevalence of hypertension, such differences may be due largely to racial factors rather than variations in salt intake. I agree that the relative importance of these two variables would be clearer if the studies could be made on a genetically homogeneous population among which certain segments had a high, and others a low, salt intake. I have not been able to find such an ideal situation. I had hoped to be able to find an isolated group in Japan with a low salt consumption, but inquiries among many Japanese friends failed to reveal such a population. Therefore as a substitute for the more ideal situation we have studied groups in which average salt intakes vary markedly. Communities have been sought, but thus far have not been found, in which salt consumption was low and the prevalence of hypertension high, or in which salt consumption was high but the prevalence of hypertension was low. I am afraid I cannot say much about Dr. SCHROEDER's thesis relative to the correlation of cadmium intake with the prevalence of hypertension in the Japanese. I would only say, I think — and no doubt from a biased position — that there is much more evidence for sodium being involved than there is for cadmium, but I am prepared to be shown my error.

Whether or not an enhanced salt appetite is inherited in hypertensives I cannot say. We explored the sensitivity to salt-taste in both hypertensives and non-hypertensives before and after salt restriction and could find no differences. Nonetheless, it is possible that there could be subtle differences which would result in the development of greater appetites in certain individuals than in others. In our considerable experience with prolonged and drastic salt restriction, however, we have found no evidence which indicates that hypertensives have more or less distress than do non-hypertensives from eliminating salt as a condiment. Whether a high salt intake is the cause or consequence of this disease is a question which has been raised by many people quite deservedly, and there is no unequivocal answer. If it were a consequence, one might reasonably expect more distress following dietary salt restriction in hypertensives than normotensives: this is not the case. Hypertensives do not lose more salt in the urine when salt is restricted in the diet, so that they do not have a greater need for replacement. Finally, the fact that hypertension can be produced experimentally by excess salt feeding indicates that in animals at least the salt is causal to, and not in consequence of, the disease.

The production of experimental hypertension in rats by salt feeding is an accomplished fact. I have been using this technique in one fashion or another since 1951, and at the present moment have 5 or 6 colonies of salt-fed rats with hypertension. Failure to produce it, in these animals at least, suggests to me that it has not been continued over a long enough period or that insufficient salt is being ingested.

TAQUINI: May I ask a question? Did the rats develop changes in the vessels of the kidney?

DAHL: No.

HOOBLER: Is the incidence of hypertension in salt-fed rats 100%?

DAHL: No. I said 80%. Indeed, I think it is important from the standpoint of the theory that not all rats should develop hypertension from excess salt feeding. The entire concept of LD_{50} is based on the variability in response of different organisms to the same stimulus. I am unaware of any disease-inciting agent which always produces the disease, even in genetically homogeneous populations.

Dr. **HOOBLER** has suggested that the average intakes which I have shown in my graphs and tables may not give a true indication of the usual salt intake, by virtue of the effect of a few very high or low values on the arithmetical average. I do not believe this is the case. In our Brookhaven series, the mean and median values were almost identical. In northern Japan, among the approximately 300 people studied by FUKUDA, there was none eating less than 5 g a day, and only 10 people were eating less than 10 g a day. Actually, there were about 250 of these 300 adults who were consuming in excess of 20 g a day. This is, in my experience, a high salt intake. Among the few Eskimos that we have studied, we have only one — a female in her first trimester of pregnancy — who was eating 10 g of salt; 16 of the remaining 20 Eskimos were on intakes of from 1 to 5 g a day. Among the Marshallese, the median may be slightly lower than the average of 7 g a day, although the data on these people are becoming increasingly beclouded by their consumption of "C" rations, which contain 2% added NaCl. Our data suggest that the usual salt consumption of a northern Jaganese farmer is much greater than the usual salt consumption of an Alaskan Eskimo, and that both of these differ significantly from the usual consumption of Brookhaven male employees.

Now as to the poisoning level being above 5 g a day: I think you are referring to a paper of ours which appeared in *Nature* a few years ago, aren't you? In that paper, I predicted that in areas where the *sodium* intake was above 5 g a day, hypertension would be common and that in areas where it was less than 2 g a day, hypertension would be uncommon. In terms of sodium chloride, 5 g of sodium would be equivalent to about 12.5 g, and 2 g of sodium to about 5 g. I would hate to have my name associated with a fixed number like 5 g — of anything — whereby 4.9 would be a "good" number and 5.1 would be a "bad" number. If there is a poisoning level, and I do happen to regard salt as one of the chronic poisons, I think the effects of this level will be modified by both genetic and environmental factors — potassium intake for instance.

The implication that we have not previously considered the interaction of genetic susceptibility and salt is not correct. In our first paper on this subject in 1954, we suggested that tissue susceptibility to the effects of salt might be inherited. I have discussed this at some length in the paper presented at this Symposium, because it was apparent that some people failed to appreciate our interest in the possible interaction between genetic susceptibility and salt.

MACH: Dr. DAHL, what do you think about the proportion between sodium and potassium? For instance in the KEMPNER diet, we have a low sodium and a high potassium and also a low protein content. I think the proportion between sodium and potassium is important.

DAHL: With regard to the possible importance of potassium to sodium ratios in the diet, I think there is evidence which suggests that this may be significant. Low sodium diets are ordinarily high potassium diets as well. Several years ago, we fed large amounts of additional potassium to some half a dozen patients on low sodium diets in an effort to see whether further lowering of blood pressure would result. It did not. However, I was not convinced that potassium played no rôle. As many of you know, MENEELY and his group were able to modify the toxic effects of salt ingestion in rats very strikingly by feeding added potassium chloride. During the past year, we have been studying patients with a whole body counter using the isotope Na^{22} which permits long-term observation by virtue of a physical half-life of 2.6 years. We have found the biological half-life of sodium can be markedly decreased by dietary increments of various potassium salts.

HOOD: If in a case of hypertension you hydrate intensely, you can demonstrate not only a flow-dependent natriuresis as shown by many people, but also a parallel increase in the excretion of chloride, ammonia, phosphate, bicarbonate, and total osmolarity, while potassium on the whole remains unchanged. Acute reduction of blood pressure induces a parallel decrease in the excretion of the same ions, while again potassium remains wholly or relatively unchanged. This is based upon the findings in about 25 cases. As to the possible mechanism involved, we have made the observation that in those cases where intense peroral hydration produced distress and vomiting and a small but probably significant decrease in filtration rate, the excretion of ions went down even if the urine volume increased somewhat.

Naturally, we are thinking in terms of mechanical factors as the explanation and particularly in terms of the markedly increased display in glomerular activity in hypertension demonstrated in 1943 by HOMER SMITH, who showed that the hypertensive kidney began to spill glucose at lower plasma levels than the normal kidney.

REUBI: I am not sure that Dr. HOOD's remark applies to Dr. COTTIER's findings. If you give a ganglionic blocking agent, you decrease the glomerular filtration rate abruptly, and not only the blood pressure. The second point is that I do not see how you could correlate the hypernatriuresis observed in hypertensive patients with the degree of dispersion in glomerular-tubular activity. The existence of two different nephron populations with respect to glucose reabsorption has been observed in many renal diseases without hypertension.

HOOD: During heavy hydration we observed a simultaneous and parallel increase in the excretion of the ions measured at an unchanged or increased filtration rate. In the graph illustrating the effect of a ganglionic blocking agent I especially pointed out the right part of the graph, where the inulin and PAH clearances after the initial depression had regained values slightly above the basal levels. The excretion of all the measured ions, with the exception of potassium and to some extent of phosphate, was still very strikingly depressed and to a parallel extent.

FREIS: It is interesting that exaggerated natriuresis in hypertensive patients is not dependent upon sodium loading alone, as it has been observed following infusion of mannitol or 5% glucose in distilled water after the oral ingestion of water or beer. BALDWIN has further observed that the normotensive subject could be made to respond with a natriuresis if the hypertonic saline infusion were prolonged to several hours. It has also been observed in normal individuals that a massive oral water load can induce a delayed natriuresis and that cortisone pretreatment will induce exaggerated natriuresis in the normotensive. These observations suggest that the normotensive requires greater filling of his plasma and/or total extracellular fluid space to elicit the natriuretic response. The evidence presented by Dr. COTTIER and also by others indicates that the extracellular fluid volume is normal in uncomplicated hypertension. Finally, BALDWIN showed that exaggerated natriuresis following salt load can be abolished in hypertensive patients by pretreatment with a low sodium diet, which incidentally reduces plasma volume.

These various observations suggest that the phenomenon of exaggerated natriuresis in hypertensive patients might in some way be dependent upon a disturbance in the relationship between the blood volume and the vascular capacity. Since the blood volume is normal in hypertension, this hypothesis would necessitate that the vascular capacity is relatively reduced in hypertension. I realize that this is purely speculative and do not wish to imply that the mechanism of exaggerated natriuresis is due to stimulation of "volume receptors" concerned with aldosterone secretion, since we know that sodium conservation by the kidney begins almost immediately after reduction of blood volume or blood pressure. The finding that antihypertensive agents abolish exaggerated natriuresis in hypertensive patients does not rule out the concept of a disturbance in vascular capacity, since some antihypertensive agents, particularly the ganglion blocking drugs, increase peripheral vascular capacity.

TAQUINI: Some years ago, we made a study similar to Dr. COTTIER's and we arrived at similar conclusions with respect to the excretion of water and electrolytes in hypertensives. In the last year we have been interested in the hemodynamic renal excretory changes produced after tilting. We have studied a group of hypertensives in the supine position after two hours' equilibration and in the semivertical position after 30 minutes. Cardiac output, renal blood flow, glomerular filtration rate, and excretion of water and electrolytes were determined. In keeping with what is known to occur, renal blood flow was found to be below normal in the severe cases. Irrespective of what happened to cardiac output, tilting brought about a further decrease in the great majority of the cases.

Change from recumbency to the semivertical position elicited in hypertensives the usual response of fall in sodium excretion. Since in some patients there was also a decrease in glomerular filtration, the fall in sodium excretion could be the result of the filtered load. Nevertheless, the glomerular filtration rate often did not drop upon tilting, or, if it did so, it later returned to, or exceeded initial levels. It may thus be concluded that the fall in sodium excretion was due to increased tubular reabsorption. In accordance with Dr. COTTIER's results, we attempted to correlate the fall in sodium excretion with the renal resistance. The fall in sodium excretion could not be correlated with renal resistance, either with initial values or with subsequent changes.

The drop in sodium excretion attending the fall in renal blood flow with lowered or unchanged glomerular filtration rate has been ascribed to "skimming" of plasma consequent to an increase in the filtered fraction. This supposed mechanism does not seem to operate in hypertensives during tilting, as no relationship could be found between changes in the filtered fraction and the decrease in sodium excretion.

HOOBLER: Before the impression is started that Dr. COTTIER's hyper-excretion of salt is related to a volume receptor or to a hypothetical endocrine secretion, I would like to recall that the perfusion pressure of the kidney is a most direct determinant of renal sodium and water elimination, and this factor should be excluded in comparing hypertensive and normal subjects. The HOWARD test shows that local perfusion pressure determines water and sodium output in the one kidney with a decreased perfusion pressure. In Dr. COTTIER's studies, minor changes in blood pressure, hardly enough to change body fluid volume, altered the sodium and water excretion. Thus, while it is true that volume receptors and endocrine states may also affect the renal handling of sodium and water in a similar direction to that seen in hypertension, the direct effect of perfusion pressure on renal function must always be taken into consideration.

With respect to Dr. COTTIER's suggestion of a slightly higher level of serum sodium after infusions into patients with mild elevation of blood pressure, I must say that further studies undertaken at Michigan by Dr. WELLER with the strictest control of the determinations has yielded no evidence whatsoever of an increased serum sodium level in the hypertensive subject. I wish to put this on record, since less careful studies reported at the Michigan Symposium, published in the journal Circulation, tended to suggest a difference in serum sodium levels in hypertension and in normotension.

PLATT: It may be of interest to recall that VERNEY & WINTON showed about 1929 that salt excretion changed with a change in perfusion pressure in experiments with heart-lung-kidney preparations.

BROD: I have been very interested in Dr. COTTIER's data. They seem to prove that the disturbances of salt metabolism are a secondary consequence of hypertension and not an event connected with the pathogenesis of the disease. In attempting to interpret this phenomenon, it would seem to me that the hypertensive subject responds to an expansion of his extracellular fluid volume with greater readiness than a normal person. In this connection, I would like to ask Dr. COTTIER how he explains the difference between his findings of a normal extracellular fluid volume and those of COVIAN and BRAUN-MÉNÉNDEZ and JAROŠOVÁ et al., who reported increased extracellular fluid volumes in this disease. A second possibility emerges from the analysis of our haemodynamic data mentioned yesterday, suggesting in the hypertensive subjects a shift of blood into the central vascular bed where the hypothetic volume receptors are supposed to be located.

HILDEN: The reason for the hypernatriuresis being less pronounced in hypertensives with decreased kidney function is not clear. However, these patients have to be compared — I think — with normotensives having a similar degree of reduction in kidney function.

As to the increased excretion of sodium after loading in hypertensives, I find this very difficult to explain. However, even the normal response to sodium loading is far from clear. I think it will be necessary to get a better understanding of the normal response before we try to explain what happens in the hypertensives. It may be that in hypertensives we are dealing with a change in the proportion between proximal and distal tubular sodium reabsorption. In this respect it would be interesting to know how patients with primary hyperaldosteronism react to sodium loading.

SCHROEDER: I would like to ask Dr. COTTIER to give us the actual figures on the elevated sodium excretion of moderate hypertensive patients as compared to normal controls, so that we can compare them with the figures of Dr. DAHL. It is most important to decide whether hypertensive patients eat more salt than normotensives because they are losing salt via their kidneys, or whether they ate more salt prior to hypertension as Dr. DAHL suggested, and continue to do so. Has Dr. COTTIER any ideas on this subject? If elevations of urinary sodium chloride are great enough to approach those reported by Dr. DAHL, perhaps we may come closer to an agreement as to whether salt loss or excretion is the cause or the effect of hypertension. Of course, continued salt loss is incompatible with health unless conserving mechanisms come into play or more salt is eaten.

COTTIER: You don't mind if I begin with Dr. SCHROEDER's question. We studied the basal urinary excretion of Na in normotensives and hypertensives in Dr. HOOBLER's laboratory in Ann Arbor (U.S.A.) and in Berne (Switzerland). We found the following differences between normotensives and the group with moderately severe hypertension ("high salt excretors").

	Ann Arbor (U.S.A.)	*Berne (Switzerland)*
Normotensives:	6.2 mEq/hr (10 indiv.)	4.8 mEq/hr (10 indiv.)
Moderately severe hypertensives:	7.9 mEq/hr (14 indiv.)	7.8 mEq/hr (13 indiv.)
Difference:	1.7 mEq/hr	3.0 mEq/hr

If you calculate these differences for 24 hours, which is not suitable because only the 12 hour-night urine was collected, it would mean that the hypertensives in Ann Arbor excreted 938 mg of Na and the ones in Berne 1656 mg of Na in excess of the normotensives. In view of the small number of patients studied we cannot attach any statistical significance to these findings. But it appears as if there is a higher excretion of Na in the group with moderately severe hypertension than in normotensives already under basal conditions. If no differentiation of the various grades of hypertensive disease were made we could not find such a difference in basal sodium excretion. Comparative studies with a pool of patients with hypertension of various degree are therefore not an adequate procedure.

I was interested to hear that Dr. HOOD also found an increased excretion of bicarbonate and ammonia in hypertensives under diuretic conditions. It is tempting, I agree, to assume that a higher speed of urine flow in the tubules could partially account for this excretory pattern. Whether a non-measurable increase of glomerular filtration rate, which could induce marked natriuresis as long as tubular transport remains unchanged, is responsible for the hypernatriuresis or whether it is really an increase in tubular rejection, is very difficult to decide, since we do not have at our disposal a more accurate method for measuring the glomerular filtration rate than the inulin clearance.

Dr. FREIS, I know that BALDWIN and co-workers (Am. J. Med. **24**, 893, 1958) were able to induce hypernatriuresis in normotensives when prolonging the fluid load. There is no doubt that one can increase natriuresis by expanding the extracellular fluid volume. But it is interesting to note that hypertensives excrete more Na than normotensives in a similar state of hydration. The data of BALDWIN do not justify the assumption that the extracellular fluid volume or its change must therefore be the adequate stimulus inducing hypernatriuresis in hypertensives. We could not find any correlation between inulin-space and natriuresis in normotensives and hypertensives. We would then have to assume that the volume receptors are more susceptible in hypertensives than in normotensives, a possibility which we could not prove to be of importance.

There is no doubt that various measures like the administration of cortical steroids or dietary factors may influence natriuresis. But the fact that they alter natriuresis does not permit us to assume that they are of primary importance with respect to the pathogenesis of the hypernatriuresis in hypertensives. They may very well represent conditional or permissive factors.

Dr. FREIS mentioned reduced vascular capacity as a disorder that is possibly also responsible for hypernatriuresis. I, too, find this idea rather intriguing. One could imagine that in hypertension there is a rearrangement of the hemodynamics insofar as the arterial blood volume is excessively elevated with regard to the reduced arterial capacity. In heart failure, which leads to antinatriuresis, the venous system is overfilled and there may be a relative arterial hypovolemia. I would then suggest that one should look within the kidneys for the postulated volume receptors or baroreceptors regulating natriuresis following hemodynamic changes. Otherwise it is hardly understandable why the perfused isolated and denervated kidney responds so promptly with hypernatriuresis as soon as the perfusion pressure is augmented.

Dr. HILDEN wanted to know how the normal individual excretes the sodium load. In our groups of normotensives and hypertensives we could find no difference in the increase of the plasma concentration of Na, nor could we on the whole detect any measurable increase of the glomerular filtration rate when changing from the isotonic saline infusion to the hypertonic (2.5%) solution. Thus it appears that the increment of filtered load does not differ measurably in the various groups, and yet the sodium clearance rises more markedly in the group with moderately severe hypertension.

If tubular rejection of Na $\left(\dfrac{C_{Na}\ 100}{C_{In}} \right)$ reaches values as high as 15% (Normal 1—2%), this would certainly seem to suggest that decreased tubular reabsorption is responsible for the hypernatriuresis, at least under load conditions. It apparently needs a certain lapse of time until elevation of blood pressure induces hypernatriuresis. In the course of our clearance studies on normotensives, who showed a slight but definite increase of arterial blood pressure due to emotion, we found a natriuresis within the normal range.

Patients with CONN's syndrome also exhibit a hypernatriuretic response when loaded with NaCl or mannitol, as DUSTAN, CORCORAN and PAGE (J. Clin. Invest. **35**, 1357, 1956) have shown. One may wonder whether hypertensive hypernatriuresis and diuresis may be one factor preventing edema formation in primary aldosteronism accompanied by arterial hypertension.

Adrenocortical function and renal pressor mechanisms in experimental hypertension

By

F. GROSS

There is a lot of evidence — admittedly in part contradictory and confusing — that the adrenal cortex is involved in the pathogenesis of experimental as well as of various forms of clinical hypertension. We are, however, far from understanding how and where the cortical hormones interfere with the mechanisms leading eventually to the development of chronic high blood pressure. The main reasons for our lack of knowledge are the inadequacy of the methods available for assessing the functions of the adrenal cortex, the generally short observation periods, which in extreme cases may consist of only a single determination of adrenal hormone excretion, and the wide range of physiological variations in the activity of the adrenal cortex which effaces the border-line between the normal and the pathological state. Another reason why most of the efforts based on animal experiments have so far failed to elucidate the connection between the adrenal cortex and high blood pressure is the fact that the rat is much too obliging an animal for this purpose. This is exemplified not only by its ready development of hypertension in the absence of the adrenals, but also by the way in which it reacts to overdosage of adrenal hormones with chronic elevation of blood pressure. Hence we have to be most reserved in drawing general conclusions from experiments in the rat and to be cautious in assuming that mechanisms or changes demonstrable in this animal are of comparable importance or indeed involved at all in the human disease. In view of the fact that most of our experimental work to which I would like to refer was done in the rat, I have to be careful not to fall into this trap myself.

Since we have recently dealt with the subject of the adrenal cortex in hypertension (*15*), on this occasion reference will be made only to investigations on:

1) the importance of corticoids in salt-dependent forms of experimental hypertension, and

2) the variations of renin and other enzymes in these forms of hypertension and in relation to adrenocortical function.

I. Adrenal cortical hormones in salt-dependent forms of hypertension

In the rat, administration of excess cortexone and salt leads to chronic elevation of blood pressure, particularly if the animal is unilaterally nephrectomised (*44*). Aldosterone, too, may produce hypertension, but it has to be given in relatively higher amounts to obtain a comparable increase in blood pressure, and it does not simultaneously produce the severe renal lesions observed under the influence of cortexone (*27*). The hypertensive effect of very small doses of aldosterone reported by one group of investigators (*16*, *32*) could not be confirmed by others (*13*, *14*, *15*). Cortexone or aldosterone hypertension occurs only if large quantities of salt are taken up simultaneously (*18*). Under the influence of cortexone, a rat of 150—200 g body weight drinks about 100 ml of 1% saline per day, which is equivalent to 0.4 g of sodium per animal or 2—2.5 g per kg body weight. This type of hypertension is fairly specific for the rat, as neither the rabbit, the cat nor the dog react to cortexone or aldosterone and salt overdosage by developing chronic elevation of blood pressure. In this respect, the human being shows

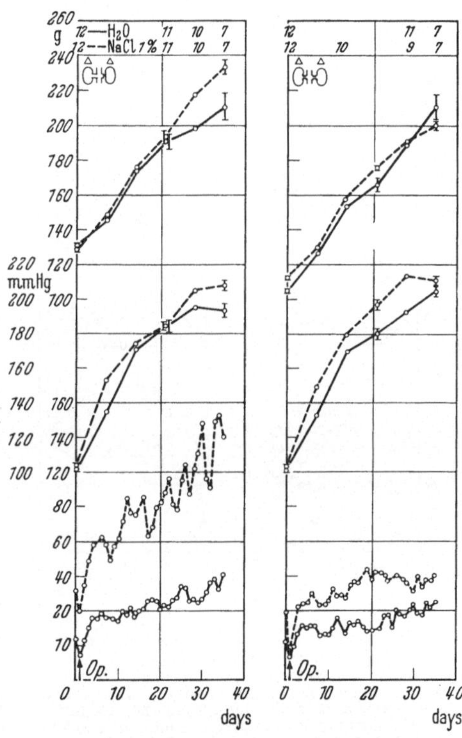

Fig. 1. Weight gain, development of hypertension and fluid intake after unilateral (left) and bilateral clamping of the renal arteries. Solid lines: groups having water to drink. Broken lines: groups with 1% saline as drinking fluid. From top to bottom: body weight in g, blood pressure in mm Hg, fluid uptake in g

some similarity to the rat in that he becomes hypertensive when given high doses of cortexone, provided there is no salt restriction. So far, it is not clear what dose of aldosterone has to be

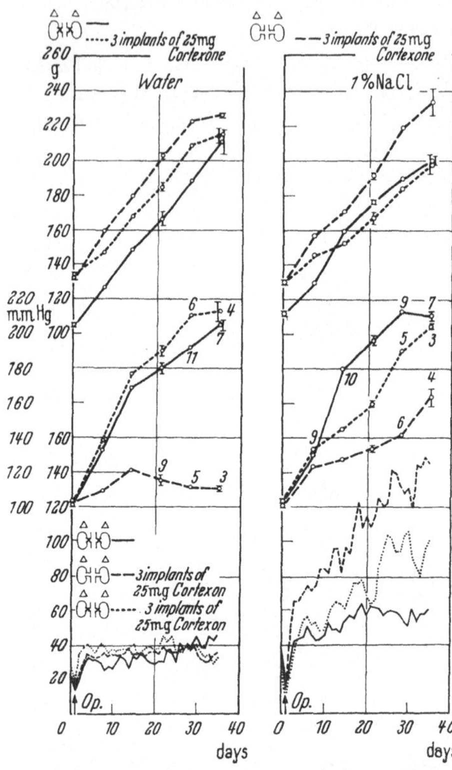

Fig. 2. Body weight, blood pressure, and fluid intake following: a) bilateral clamping of renal arteries (solid lines), b) implantation of 3 pellets of 25 mg cortexone-acetate each (broken lines), and c) combined treatment (dotted lines). Left side: water as drinking fluid. Right side: 1% saline as drinking fluid. From top to bottom: body weight in g, blood pressure in mm Hg, fluid uptake in g. Figures on blood pressure curves indicate the number of animals. Decreasing numbers are due to testing the kidneys for renin content at various stages of the experiment

administered in order to obtain a comparable hypertensive effect in man, but from observations in patients with primary hyperaldosteronism it is likely that chronic elevation of blood pressure may be induced by large amounts of aldosterone.

Another salt-dependent form of hypertension produced so far only in the rat is adrenal regeneration hypertension, which, in addition to 1% saline, requires unilateral nephrectomy as a prerequisite for its development (47, 48). It was impossible to elicit by these measures a comparable elevation of blood pressure in the dog (17).

Renal hypertension in the rat does not depend on excess sodium uptake as do the forms due to hormone overdosage or altered adrenal cortical function, and whether the animals have water or 1% saline as drinking fluid is only of secondary importance as regards the height of blood pressure (Fig. 1). Unilateral or bilateral clamping of the renal arteries and simultaneous overdosage with cortexone may be followed by a more rapid increase in blood pressure, leading occasionally to somewhat higher levels than clamping alone, but combined measures may also result in lower values than simple clamping. This occurs in spite of the lower sodium uptake by animals with both kidneys clamped compared with the same treatment and cortexone in addition. These rats, however, drink less saline than animals implanted with cortexone tablets only (Fig. 2). Sodium depletion, on the other hand, in spite of leading to hypertrophy of the adrenal zona glomerulosa (*8*), prevents the rise in blood pressure. From our experiments on the influence of salt overdosage on the development of renal hypertension in rats we may conclude that unilateral or bilateral clamping of the renal artery is so strong a pathogenic stimulus for the production of hypertension that it can be enhanced only slightly, if at all, by simultaneous loading with salt.

II. Influence of adrenal function on experimental hypertension

While overdosage with cortexone — or aldosterone — and salt leads to hypertension, regardless of the presence or absence of the adrenals, endogenous secretion of cortical hormones is of importance in *renal* hypertension. In adrenalectomised rats, unilateral or bilateral clamping of the renal arteries may also lead to an elevation of blood pressure if sufficient cortexone or aldosterone is given to prevent severe adrenal insufficiency. With water as drinking fluid, in the animal with a unilateral clamp, the threshold dosage is 0.1 mg of cortexone acetate daily, injected in oily solution. In contrast, if d, 1-aldosterone is given either in the relatively high dose of 0.1 mg daily or only 0.02 mg, the animals survive well, but blood pressure cannot be maintained at the pre-adrenalectomy level and comes down more or less slowly toward normal values (Fig. 3). In the adrenalectomised and simultaneously unilaterally nephrectomised animal bearing a clip on the remaining renal artery and given water to drink, 0.1 mg of cortexone daily is a sufficiently high dose to establish as marked a degree of hypertension as in the animal with intact adrenals (*36*). If 1% saline is provided instead of water, together with a daily dose of 0.025 mg of cortexone, which is insufficient to maintain the adrenalectomised animal given water, blood pressure will not reach values as high as with 0.1 mg daily, although definite hypertension does develop (*36*). If only 0.33% saline is given to drink, this dose of cortexone is not completely adequate to maintain life, but in the surviving animals (50%), a moderate degree of hypertension develops. It is even possible to produce a mild degree of renal hypertension in the adrenalectomised rat by giving nothing but 1% saline to substitute for adrenal hormones (*11, 12*). Furthermore, established hypertension may be maintained by 1% saline, although sodium consumption may actually fall as a consequence of the removal of the adrenals (Fig. 4). Hence we may state that, at least in the rat, renal hypertension may develop or be maintained after adrenalectomy either by the administration of salt

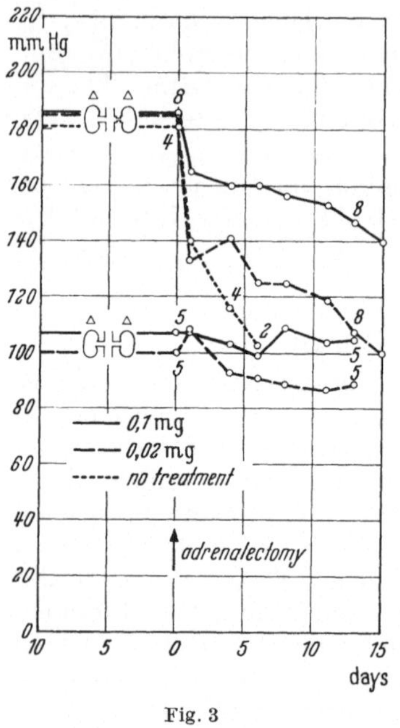

Fig. 3

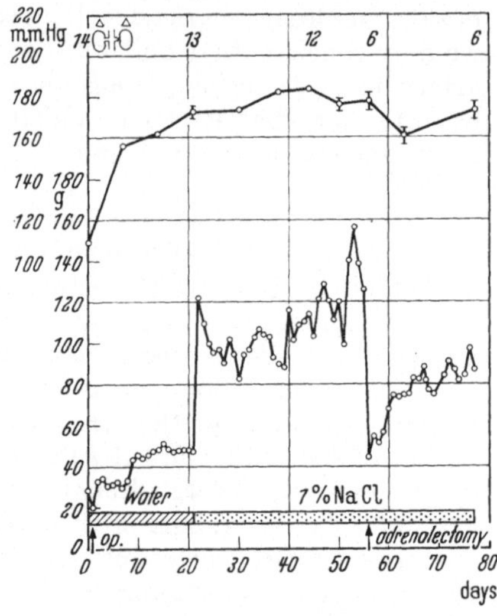

Fig. 4

Fig. 3. Hypertension induced by unilateral clamping of renal artery. Animals were adrenalectomized after established hypertension and subsequently given daily injections of d,l-aldosterone (0.1 mg and 0.02 mg). Aldosterone, even in relatively high doses, cannot prevent blood pressure decrease

Fig. 4. Hypertension induced by unilateral clamping of renal artery. During the first 3 weeks, water was given as drinking fluid, then 1% saline. Animals were adrenalectomized after 56 days and given no maintenance treatment. Upper curve: blood pressure in mm Hg. Lower curve: fluid uptake in g. Decrease in number of animals (figures at top) is due to testing the renin content of the kidneys

alone or by an amount of a salt-retaining corticoid in a dosage which, according to present knowledge of the rate of secretion of aldosterone by the rat adrenal (*45, 46*), is not extraordinarily high and certainly far below the dosage range necessary to produce corticoid hypertension. On the other hand, in animals with functioning adrenals, after clamping one or both renal arteries, the endogenous cortical hormone production is sufficient to achieve as high a pressure as overdosage with cortexone or aldosterone, but without the excessive salt load which is a prerequisite for that type of corticoid hypertension.

The maintenance or the development of renal hypertension in the adrenalectomised animal treated either with small doses of corticoids or only with saline might be compared with the situation in adrenal regeneration hypertension, in which an elevated salt intake together with a low secretory rate of adrenal hormones (2, 48), in addition to some renal manipulation, result in an increase of blood pressure. In renal hypertension in the rat, the adrenal factor may be completely absent; however, as kidney function may be more profoundly disturbed than in adrenal regeneration hypertension and — as a result of adrenalectomy — salt intake is also substantially elevated, the effect on the blood pressure is the same.

However, when the two forms of hypertension were combined by placing a clip on the artery of the remaining kidney of unilaterally nephrectomised animals with regenerating adrenal remnants, the resulting hypertension was not definitely more severe than in animals with simple renal hypertension (Fig. 5).

The fact that renal hypertension may develop in the rat in the absence of the adrenals does not mean that cortical hormones are not involved in the pathogenesis of hypertension in other species in which it is not possible to replace vital adrenal cortical function by giving only saline. It merely enables one to conclude that, if adrenal cortical hormones are of importance, these are the sodium retaining hormones which in the rat may be replaced by a dietary supplement of salt.

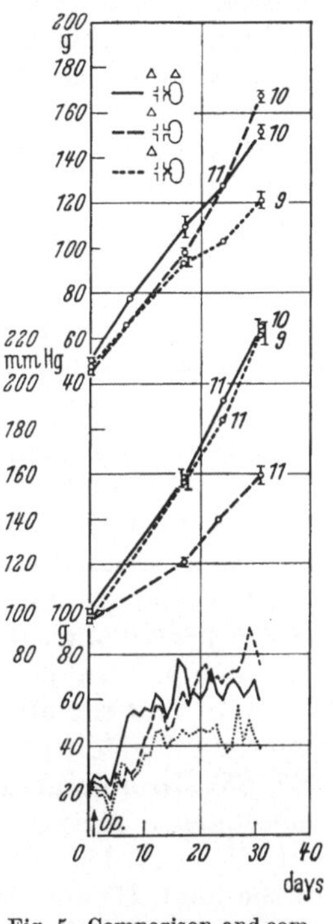

Fig. 5. Comparison and combination of renal and adrenal regeneration hypertension in the rat. Solid lines: clamping of renal artery and contralateral nephrectomy. Broken lines: regeneration period following adrenal enucleation Dotted lines: combined clamping and adrenal regeneration. All animals received 1% saline as drinking fluid. From top to bottom: body weight in g, blood pressure in mm Hg, fluid uptake in g

III. Renal pressor mechanism

Renal pressor mechanism as it is understood to-day means the renin-angiotensin system, which is chemically only clearly defined on the side of the reaction product but is still obscure for the enzyme and for the substrate. Thus, when considering the hypertensive principle(s) found in the kidney, we have to realise that our understanding and the interpretation of results is restricted not only by the incomplete chemical characterisation of these substances, but also by the inadequacy of the methods for their biological evaluation. In subsequently discussing variations in the renin concentration of the kidneys, we are aware of the fact that the content of a secretory product in a gland does not permit direct conclusions as to the rate and regulation of the secretion of this substance and does not tell us anything about its metabolism. Thus, we have to be careful when interpreting the results obtained in this way.

1. Renin content of the kidneys

a) *Overdosage with sodium-retaining corticoids.* When we consider the variations which the concentration of pressor material in the kidneys undergoes under different experimental conditions, we have to bear in mind that what we at present define as renin is a constituent of the normal kidney. There is much evidence that this substance "originates in cells in, or close to, the glomerula" (*3, 4, 39*) and that the granules demonstrable by special staining techniques in the juxtaglomerular cells of the vas afferens are the morphological substrate of renin (*6, 7, 40, 41, 42, 54*). We demonstrated formerly that the amount of renin extractable from the kidneys is inversely related to the salt or, more precisely, to the sodium intake (*25, 28*). In animals receiving an overdose of cortexone, renin in consequence disappears from the kidneys within 2—3 weeks, but only if either 1% saline or sufficient salt is given simultaneously in the food. If, however, a sodium-poor diet is given and water is provided as drinking fluid, the renin content remains unaffected by cortexone. The reduction in renin concentration is a reversible process, since it reappears in the kidneys after interruption of cortexone administration and the replacement of saline by water as drinking fluid (*28*). Overdosage with aldosterone leads to the same result, and a large intake of salt alone will also cause a reduction in renin levels, although it takes longer to achieve as profound a fall as is obtained by the simultaneous administration of a salt-retaining corticoid (*28*). The disappearance of renin from the kidney is accompanied by increased sensitivity of the animal to injected renin or freshly prepared kidney extract, reaching almost the same degree as in the nephrectomised rat (*22*).

Overdosage with cortisol or related corticoids, which also leads to hypertension in the rat, is not accompanied by a diminution of renin in the kidneys, regardless of whether water or saline is given as drinking fluid.

b) *Adrenal insufficiency.* Adrenalectomy resulting in sodium loss is accompanied by an increase of renin concentration in the extracts prepared from the kidneys (*26*). Simultaneously, a decreased sensitivity to injected renin may be observed in these animals, but if the kidneys are removed, the adrenalectomised animal also responds with a prolonged hypertensive reaction to injected renin, reaching approximately the intensity seen in the nephrectomised animal having normal adrenal function (*26*).

c) *Adrenal regeneration hypertension.* In adrenal regeneration hypertension, a decrease of renal pressor substances occurs, comparable to that found in cortexone-induced hypertension (Fig. 6). There is no evidence for increased secretion of either aldosterone or corticosterone by the regenerating adrenal, but, on the contrary, a transient stage of adrenal insufficiency is present for 1—2 weeks after the operation (*17, 34, 35*). As neither unilateral nephrectomy and administration of 1 % saline nor this procedure combined with adrenalectomy lead to hypertension or disappearance

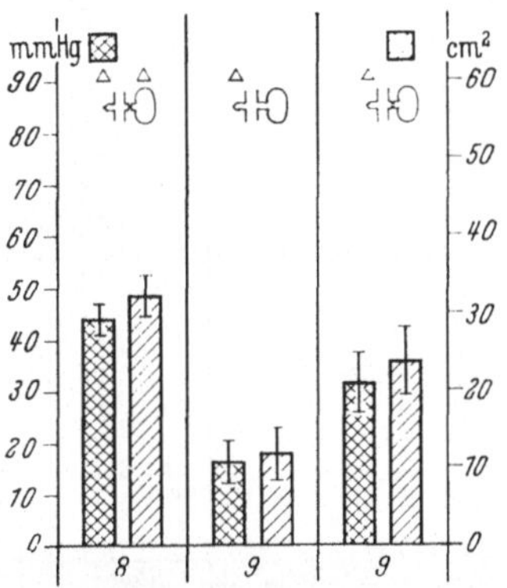

Fig. 6. Comparison of renin content of kidneys following: clamping of renal artery and contralateral nephrectomy (left compartment), adrenal regeneration (centre compartment), combined clamping and adrenal regeneration (right compartment). Left ordinate: maximum pressure response of the nephrectomized test animal. Right ordinate: area in cm² under 30′ of pressure curve in nephrectomized test animals. (Same animals as in Fig. 5)

of renin from the kidney, the special situation provoked either by relative adrenal insufficiency (*34*) or by the process of regeneration must be held responsible for the development of hypertension. It might be that during the phase of partial adrenal insufficiency, the rats drink more saline, to which they are simultaneously more sensitive owing both to the inadequate secretion of corticosterone and to the unilateral nephrectomy, and that it is in fact a relative excess of salt which is a prerequisite for the development of elevated blood pressure. The observation that the renin content of the kidney is diminished in this form of hypertension and that saline and unilateral nephrectomy are necessary for the manifestation of high blood pressure puts adrenal regeneration hypertension in the same category as cortexone or aldosterone hypertension, although these forms differ in principle as regards the levels of sodium-retaining steroids circulating in the body.

d) *Renal hypertension*. In rats with experimental renal hypertension due either to unilateral clamping of the renal artery or to encapsulation of one kidney, the renin in the clamped kidney is

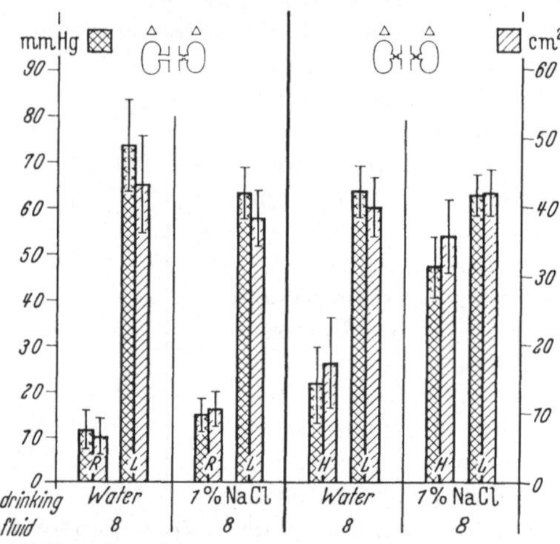

Fig. 7. Pressor activity in kidneys after unilateral (left side of figure) or bilateral clamping of the renal artery with water or 1% saline as drinking fluid. Left columns and ordinate: maximum pressure response. Right columns and ordinate: area under first 30′ of the pressure curve in the nephrectomized test animal. R: right kidney. L: left kidney. H: heavier kidney. L: lighter kidney. (Same animals as in Fig. 1)

normal or elevated, while that of the contralateral kidney is markedly diminished or disappears completely (*19*). This pattern of renin distribution occurs no matter whether water or 1% saline is given as drinking fluid (Fig. 7). Thus, as regards the renin content, the non-clamped kidney is comparable to the kidney in hypertension depending on excess salt. Hence it is not surprising that, after removal of the clamped kidney, the animal shows the same increased sensitivity to injected renin as the rat overdosed with cortexone and salt (*21*), while the presence of the renin-containing clamped kidney prevents an enhanced reaction to exogenous renin.

If both renal arteries or that of the remaining kidney after unilateral nephrectomy are clamped, a certain diminution of the renin content may occur if 1% saline is given as drinking fluid. In the unilaterally nephrectomised animal given water, no definite difference in renin concentration as compared with the animal having clips on both kidney arteries can be observed.

By clamping both renal arteries it is impossible to obtain an absolutely identical degree of diminution in blood supply to each kidney, and slight differences in flow between the two sides are unavoidable. We found that the content of renin was always somewhat more diminished in the heavier kidney than in the lighter one, indicating that the kidney with the lesser reduction in flow

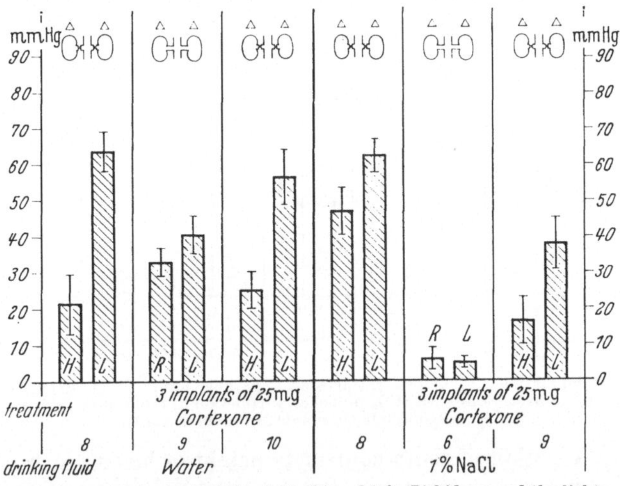

Fig. 8. Pressor material, content of the right (R) and left (L) kidney and the lighter (L) and heavier (H) kidney in rats having either bilateral clamping of renal arteries, treatment with cortexone or both procedures together. Left side: water as drinking fluid. Right side: 1% saline. Ordinate: maximum pressure response of the test animal to kidney extract. (Same animals as in Fig. 2)

contains less renin than the other one (Fig. 8). This is comparable to the situation in the animal with unilateral clamping, in which the difference between the two kidneys is at a maximum.

2. Importance of sodium ion

In order to find out whether sodium or chloride is the ion responsible for the disappearance of renin, experiments were performed with various other salts, such as sodium bicarbonate or ammonium chloride, given together with an overdosage of cortexone. It turned out that 1.4% sodium bicarbonate solution influenced the content of renin in the same way as 1% saline, although the animals drank less of the bicarbonate solution, with the consequence that the intake of sodium ion was smaller and therefore the degree of hypertension was less pronounced (Fig. 9). Ammonium chloride had no influence at all, either on the renin content of the kidney extracts or on the blood pressure. From these results we may conclude that loading with sodium and consequently — as we shall see later — retention of this ion are the factors responsible for the disappearance of renin from the kidney.

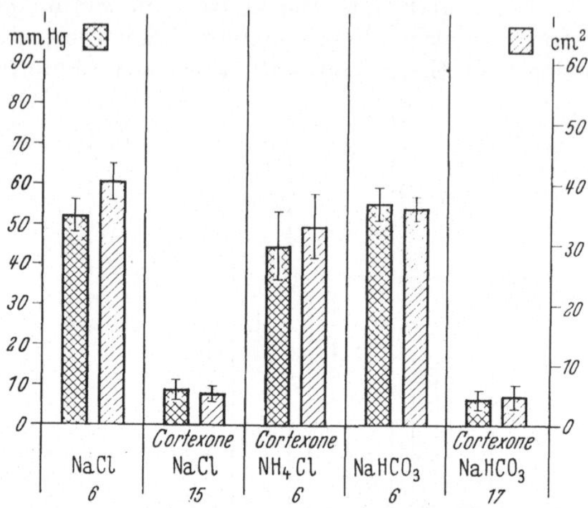

Fig. 9. Pressor activity of kidney extracts after various forms of treatment. Cortexone together with either NaCl or NaHCO₃ provokes a reduction of renin in the kidneys. Figures at bottom indicate number of animals tested

3. Relation of renin content to height of blood pressure

The diminution of the renin concentration in the kidney can, but need not necessarily, go parallel with the development of hypertension. Overdosage with cortexone and salt causes disappearance of renin from the kidneys in all animal species investigated — mouse, rat, rabbit, cat, dog — whether or not hypertension occurs, and the rat and the rabbit show this same response to high doses of aldosterone (23, 27). In rats with unilaterally clamped kidneys, we often observed a diminution of the renin content in the unclamped kidney when there was only a slight or equivocal elevation of blood pressure. If, however, clamping was too strong and consequently marked atrophy or even necrosis of the corresponding kidney developed, no change in the renin concentration in the untouched kidney occurred. This lack of correlation between the renin concentration in the kidney and the height of blood pressure argues against the assumption (52, 55) that the uneven distribution of renin observed during unilateral renal clamping is due to different arterial pressures acting on the kidneys. It also seems unlikely that changes in systemic blood pressure are directly responsible for variations in renin content. On the other hand, the incomplete disappearance of renin from the kidneys of rats overdosed with cortexone and salt and simultaneously bearing renal artery clamps may indicate that intrarenal blood pressure might be related to the renin concentration.

IV. Variations in other enzymatic activities in the kidney

The disappearance of renin from the kidney is not the only change in enzymatic activity to be observed under the conditions

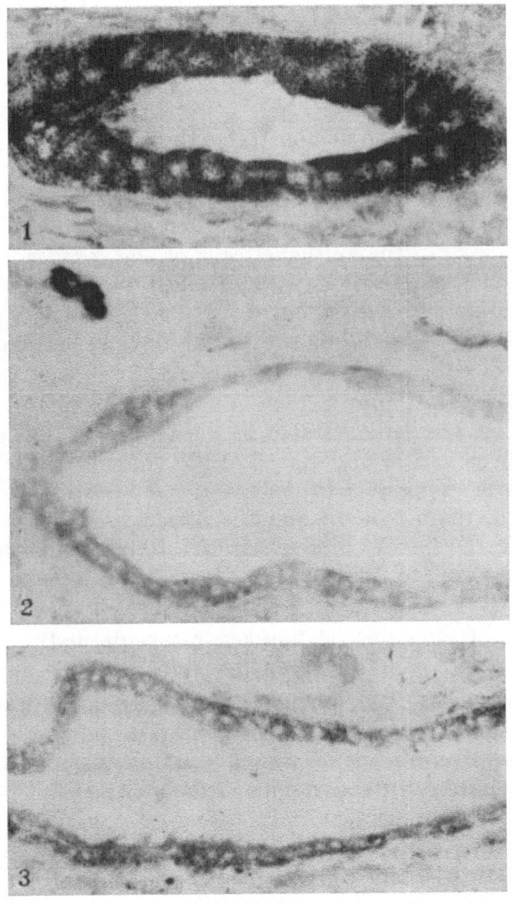

Fig. 10. Activity of glucose-6-phosphate dehydrogenase in the epithelial cells of ducts of the submaxillary gland of intact rat (1, above). The activity in animals with cortexone overdosage (2, middle) is diminished in the same way as in animals with renal hypertension (3, lower). Simultaneously, flattening of the epithelium and widening of the lumen occurs

of sodium retention. We found, in collaboration with HESS (*29*), that the activity of glucose-6-phosphate dehydrogenase in the cells of the macula densa is markedly decreased in animals with cortexone and salt overdosage and is above normal in adrenal insufficiency. In addition, HESS and PEARSE (*30*) demonstrated that, in renal hypertension with unilateral clamping of the renal artery, the glucose-6-phosphate dehydrogenase in the clamped kidney is about normal or slightly elevated, while it almost. disappears from the contralateral kidney. Under various conditions, therefore, this enzyme shows the same changes as the concentration of renin. A decrease in the phosphatase concentration in the unclamped kidney has been reported by PASQUALINO and BOURNE (*37*).

A recent observation demonstrates that changes comparable to those which occur in the kidney are also detectable in other organs. We found that not only in cortexone overdosage, but also in renal hypertension, the glucose-6-phosphate dehydrogenase is diminished in the same way in the epithelial cells of the salivary ducts as in the macula densa cells (Fig. 10). In addition, the salivary ducts show dilatation and flattening of the epithelium comparable to that seen in the distal tubules of the kidneys in cortexone hypertension (*20*).

After adrenalectomy, a high glucose-6-phosphate dehydrogenase activity was demonstrable in the duct cells, but no definite increase such as had been detected in the macula densa cells (*29*). Although it is impossible to discern the connection between the fluctuation in renin content and the activity of this key enzyme concerned in the hexose monophosphate oxidative pathway, it is tempting to correlate them.

V. Possible relation between renin and the adrenal cortex

It was formerly shown by DEANE and MASSON (*5*) that injection of renin in the rat leads to morphological alterations in the cells of the glomerular zone of the adrenal cortex, which may be related to increased activity. Recently, it was demonstrated in the rat that 2 days after clamping one renal artery, the width of the zona glomerulosa increases (*37*). It may therefore be supposed that renin stimulates the zona glomerulosa either directly or indirectly to produce more aldosterone, which leads to an increased tubular reabsorption of sodium. As a consequence of the resulting sodium retention, aldosterone output would be reduced, while on the other hand, under the conditions of sodium depletion, secretion increases. In the adrenalectomised animal which loses sodium, renin is secreted in abundance, but there is no adrenal cortex present to respond with the appropriate production of aldosterone necessary to maintain sodium balance (Fig. 11).

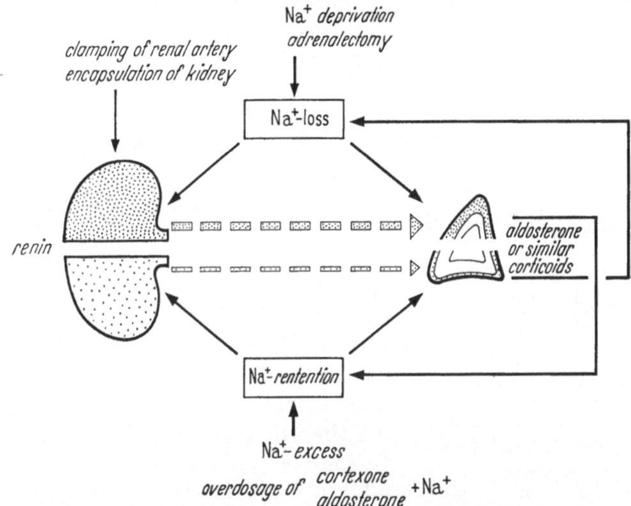

Fig. 11. Hypothetic relationship between secretory activity of the kidney and the adrenals in the regulation of sodium metabolism. Intensity of the shading of the kidney (on left) and adrenal cortex (on right) indicates the content of renin or aldosterone. Intensity of shaded arrows from kidney to adrenal represents relative intensity of renin stimulation of the cortex. The secretion of aldosterone or similar corticoids in large quantity from the strongly stimulated cortex leads to Na retention, while reduced secretion from the weakly stimulated cortex leads to Na⁺ loss. The subsequent action of Na⁺ retention to reduce renin secretion is blocked in the clamped kidney

Clamping one renal artery stimulates the production of renin in that kidney, and consequently the zona glomerulosa of the adrenal cortex reacts with an augmented aldosterone output. It is, however, only the contralateral kidney which corresponds in the appropriate manner with a diminution of renin secretion, while the clamped kidney continues to pour out renin, in this way continuously stimulating the zona glomerulosa to secrete aldosterone in amounts inappropriate to the existing condition. Thus, the clip would initiate a vicious circle which, if maintained over a prolonged period, will finally lead to a manifest pathological condition, the main expression of which is high blood pressure. In such a case, the rate of aldosterone secretion need not necessarily increase beyond the normal range, but the ability to adjust adrenal function to the prevailing conditions is lost.

We have to admit that this hypothesis is far from being established, but in addition to the observations already mentioned we would like to discuss a few other results which support this concept, as well as others which do not.

a) *Rapid variations of renin concentration in the kidney.* In order to investigate if immediate reactions of renin concentration to changes in salt balance may occur, we performed short-term experiments. By continuous infusion of 0.9% saline at 4 ml per hour into a tail vein of the rat for 6—16 hrs it was possible to reduce the renin content of the kidney by about 30%, while infusion of the same amount of an isotonic sucrose solution was without effect on the renin concentration (Fig. 12). This demonstrates that an acute salt load causes the renin concentration of the kidney to decline, but it has so far been impossible to obtain a more marked reduction, even by increasing the salt concentration up to 2%(*1*). In spite of the fact that our assay method for renin is crude and only semi-quantitative, we may nevertheless conclude that under suitable experimental conditions a prompt reduction of the renin content and probably also of its secretion can be obtained. This is consistent with the view that this substance exerts a regulatory function not necessarily concerned with blood pressure. More definite proof for this interpretation requires a method by which it is possible to follow the secretion of renin continuously.

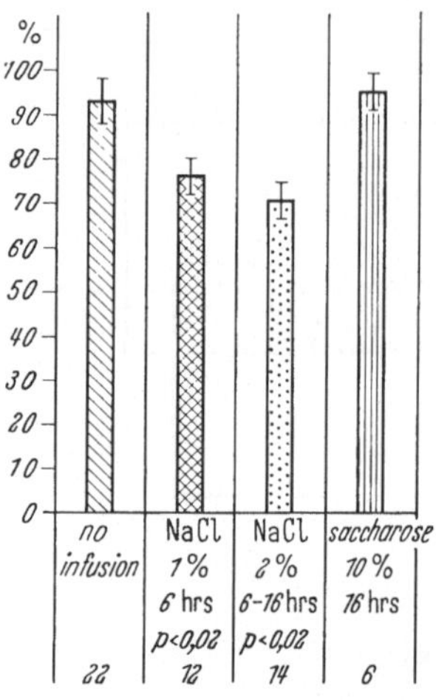

Fig. 12. Influence of saline and sucrose infusions in unanaesthetized animals on renin content of the kidneys. Ordinate: hypertensive activity liberated from rat plasma by renal extracts expressed as percent of standard dose of synthetic angiotensin (0.08 γ). Figures at bottom indicate number of animals tested

If the adrenals are removed from rats with hypertension due to unilateral clamping of the renal artery, blood pressure usually comes down to normal within 3—6 days, coincident with the development of severe adrenal insufficiency (*43*). At this time, the difference in renin content of the clamped and unclamped kidney is definitely less marked than in the non-adrenalectomised clamped animals. In animals in which adrenal insufficiency is prevented by small doses of aldosterone, as the blood pressure falls the difference in renin concentration between the clamped and unclamped kidney becomes less prominent owing to the fact that the renin content of the unclamped kidney increases (*43, 22*).

b) *Sodium retention in experimental hypertension.* Various investigators have shown that in cortexone and aldosterone hypertension there is an increase in sodium concentration, especially in the skeletal muscle, but also in the aortic wall, in which potassium concentration also rises simultaneously (*24, 33, 50, 53*). In renal hypertension, similar but not as pronounced electrolyte changes were found in the aorta (*49*). If we assume that sodium retention is a common pathogenic mechanism for the forms of experimental hypertension discussed, the question arises how we may reconcile the relatively small quantities of sodium taken up by animals developing renal hypertension with the large amounts consumed in corticoid-salt hypertension. In either case, the elevation of sodium concentration in various tissues does not differ very much (*49, 50*). On the other hand, no marked endogenous overproduction of adrenal hormones is necessary in order to elicit renal hypertension in the rat, but even a decreased secretion rate of the adrenal cortex, such as occurs after adrenal enucleation, permits chronic elevation of blood pressure as does salt alone, which, in the absence of cortical hormones, may also be an adequate stimulus (*11, 12*). This complicated picture reflects the fact that the rat, which has the ability to take up and to eliminate salt in large quantities, shows some peculiarities as regards regulation of blood pressure not present in other species, at least not to such a marked degree.

c) *Arguments against renin-aldosterone relation.* One finding which is inconsistent with the pathogenic rôle of a hypothetical renin-aldosterone system is the prompt fall of high blood pressure to normal levels after removal of the clamped kidney (*9*). If the renin, secreted by this kidney, acted through stimulation of aldosterone secretion, one would not expect a more rapid fall of blood pressure after taking the kidney out than after removal of the adrenals. The prompt decrease of blood pressure after eliminating the clamped kidney argues very much in favour of the view that a substance produced by the kidney participates in the pathogenesis of this stage of hypertension (*10*).

The fact that hypertension may also develop in the absence of kidneys does not in our opinion necessarily eliminate the kidney as a pathogenic factor but demonstrates only that the reaction of the organism to different noxious stimuli may be similar.

Another strong argument against the importance of sodium retention in the pathogenesis of renal hypertension is its resistance

to saluretic substances. While hydrochlorothiazide or similar
diuretics not only delay the development of cortexone-salt hypertension, but also diminish its intensity, renal hypertension is not
influenced at all. Although we can assume that hydrochlorothiazide
prevents the retention of sodium, there is neither a delay in the
appearance of hypertension nor a reduction in that already existing.
This is true for the rat. Similar experiments in other animal species
capable of developing renal hypertension have not yet come to our
knowledge.

VI. Physiological significance of renin

If we try to bring the various data available to-day into agreement
with the hypothesis just outlined, we become aware of discrepancies
and gaps in our knowledge, especially as regards how the many
observations might be related or connected with each other. The
possible rôle which renin might play in the pathogenesis of hypertension has hitherto been sought mainly on the basis of the direct
effects exercised on blood pressure either by renin itself or by angiotensin. Although, since the investigations of PICKERING and his
group (*31*), renin has been known to influence kidney function,
these results have always been overshadowed by the direct effect
of the substance on blood pressure. However, the lack of evidence
for the direct involvement of renin in the maintenance of hypertension, the failure to demonstrate a continuous overproduction of
it in experimental renal as well as in human hypertension (*38*), and
various other discrepancies have steadily increased doubts about
the part this substance may play in the pathogenesis of hypertension.

The parallel changes in glucose-6-phosphate dehydrogenase
activity in the macula densa cells and the salivary duct epithelium,
as well as similar morphological changes in these two duct systems
in various forms of experimental hypertension, demonstrate that
two different organs involved in sodium transfer react in the same
way under conditions which may fundamentally influence sodium
metabolism. If we compare the disappearance of renin and of
glucose-6-phosphate dehydrogenase in the contralateral kidney
with that occurring with overdosage of salt-retaining hormones
and conclude that the untouched kidney reacts in a normal and
appropriate manner to a pathogenic process elicited and maintained
by the clamped kidney, we may now add that other organs involved
in sodium metabolism also reflect what are perhaps compensatory
efforts to counteract a situation which otherwise will finally result
in irreversible pathological changes.

In view of the new findings which relate renin in some way to sodium metabolism, its position in the pathogenesis of hypertension needs reconsideration, and it cannot be excluded that a new interpretation of various long-standing observations will become necessary.

Conclusions

Experimental renal hypertension in the rat develops and can be maintained in the absence of the adrenals if one of the following treatments is given:

a) threshold doses of cortexone or aldosterone together with water as drinking fluid,

b) sub-threshold doses of cortexone together with 1% saline, or

c) 1% saline alone.

Combination of clamping one or both renal arteries together with either 1% saline or additional cortexone does not substantially increase the degree of hypertension nor does adrenal regeneration.

Overdosage with either cortexone or aldosterone and with salt leads to the disappearance of renin from the kidneys and glucose-6-phosphate dehydrogenase from the macula densa. The same reaction occurs in the contralateral kidney after clamping one renal artery. Glucose-6-phosphate dehydrogenase in the epithelial cells of the salivary ducts behaves in a similar way to that in the macula densa cells, indicating that both structures are influenced similarly by changes in sodium balance.

By variations in sodium uptake, the content of renin in the kidney is changed in the same direction as the secretion of aldosterone. There is an inverse relationship between the renin concentration in the kidney and the sodium content of the organism.

It is suggested that renin is involved in the pathogenesis of experimental hypertension not on the basis of its direct activity on blood pressure, but because it is involved in sodium metabolism. Much, however, remains to be done in order to prove this hypothesis.

Résumé

L'hypertension rénale expérimentale chez le rat se manifeste ou peut être maintenue en l'absence de surrénales si on administre un des traitements suivants:

a) Doses suffisantes de cortexone ou d'aldostérone en même temps que l'absorption d'eau comme boisson.

b) Doses subliminaires de cortexone concurremment à une solution salée à 1%.

c) Solution salée à 1% administrée seule.

La combinaison du clampage de l'une ou des deux artères rénales avec soit une solution salée à 1% soit de desoxycorticosterone en complément n'augmente pas sensiblement le degré de l'hypertension et ne stimule pas la régénération surrénalienne.

Un surdosage de cortexone ou d'aldostérone ou de sel conduit à la disparition de la rénine du parenchyme rénal et de la déshydrogénase glucose-6-phosphorique de la macula densa. La même réaction apparaît dans le rein contra-latéral après clampage d'une artère rénale. La déshydrogénase glucose-6-phosphorique contenue dans les cellules épithéliales des canaux salivaires se comporte de la même façon que celle se trouvant dans les cellules de la macula densa, ce qui indique que les deux éléments sont influencés de la même façon par les variations de l'équilibre du sodium.

Lorsqu'on fait varier la quantité de sodium ingérée, le taux de rénine dans le rein varie dans le même sens que la sécrétion de l'aldostérone, soit en raison inverse de la concentration de rénine dans le rein par rapport au taux de sodium dans l'organisme.

Ceci laisse supposer que la rénine est impliquée dans la pathogénie de l'hypertension expérimentale, non par une action directe sur la pression sanguine, mais par l'intermédiaire du métabolisme du sodium. Cette hypothèse reste cependant à démontrer.

I have to thank Dr. G. T. BASSIL for his help in preparing the English version of the text and Mr. R. DOEBELIN for technical assistance in the animal experiments.

References

1. BERSET, J.: Thesis, Berne, 1960.
2. BROGI, M. P., and C. PELLEGRINO: J. Physiol. (G. B.) **146**, 165 (1959).
3. COOK, W. F., and G. W. PICKERING: J. Physiol. (G. B.) **143**, 78 (1958).
4. COOK, W., D. B. GORDON, and W. S. PEART: J. Physiol. (G. B.) **135**, 46 P, 1957.
5. DEANE, H. W., and G. M. C. MASSON: J. Clin. Endocr. (U.S.A.) **11**, 193 (1951).
6. DUNIHUE, F. W.: Amer. J. Path. **23**, 906 (1947).
7. DUNIHUE, F. W.: Anat. Rec. (U.S.A.) **103**, 442 (1949).
8. EISENSTEIN, A. B.: Proc. Soc. Exper. Biol. Med. (U.S.A.) **101**, 850 (1959).
9. FLOYER, M. A.: Clin. Sc. (G. B.) **10**, 405 (1951).
10. FLOYER, M. A.: Clin. Sc. (G. B.) **14**, 163 (1955).
11. FREGLY, M. J.: Amer. J. Physiol. **191**, 542 (1957).
12. FREGLY, M. J.: Endocrinology (U.S.A.) **66**, 240 (1960).
13. FREGLY, M. J., and V. M. AREAN: Acta physiol. pharmacol. Neerl. 8, 162 (1959).
14. GAUNT, R., G. J. ULSAMER, and J. J. CHART: Arch. internat. pharmacodyn. thérap. (Belg.) **110**, 114 (1957).
15. GAUNT, R., F. GROSS, A. A. RENZI, and J. J. CHART: The adrenal cortex in hypertension (with particular reference to adrenal regeneration hypertension). Hypertension. Philadelphia 1959, p. 219.
16. GORNALL, A. G., H. M. GRUNDY, and C. J. KOLADICH: Canad. J. Biochem. Physiol. **38**, 43 (1960).
17. GROLLMAN, A.: The pathogenesis of "adrenal regeneration" hypertension. Endocrinology (U.S.A.) **63**, 460 (1958).
18. GROSS, F.: Naunyn-Schmiedebergs Arch. exper. Path. (G.) **232**, 161 (1957).
19. GROSS, F.: Klin. Wschr. (G.) **36**, 693 (1958).
20. GROSS, F., and R. HESS: Histochemical changes in the kidneys and in the salivary glands of rats with experimental hypertension. (In press).
21. GROSS, F., and P. LICHTLEN: Naunyn-Schmiedebergs Arch. exper. Path. (G.) **233**, 323 (1958).

22. Gross, F., and P. Lichtlen: Proc. Soc. Exper. Biol. Med. (U.S.A.) **98**, 341 (1958).
23. Gross, F., und H. Schmidt: Naunyn-Schmiedebergs Arch. exper. Path. (G.) **232**, 408 (1958).
24. Gross, F., und H. Schmidt: Naunyn-Schmiedebergs Arch. exper. Path. (G.) **233**, 311 (1958).
25. Gross, F., und F. Sulser: Naunyn-Schmiedebergs Arch. exper. Path. (G.) **229**, 374 (1956).
26. Gross, F., und F. Sulser: Naunyn-Schmiedebergs Arch. exper. Path. (G.) **230**, 274 (1957).
27. Gross, F., P. Loustalot, and R. Meier: Acta endocr. (Den.) **26**, 417 (1957).
28. Gross, F., P. Loustalot und F. Sulser: Naunyn-Schmiedebergs Arch. exper. Path. (G.) **229**, 381 (1956).
29. Hess, R., and F. Gross: Amer. J. Physiol. **197**, 869 (1959).
30. Hess, R., and A. G. E. Pearse: Brit. J. Exper. Path. **40**, 243 (1959).
31. Hughes-Jones, N. C., G. W. Pickering, P. H. Sanderson, H. Scarborough, and J. Vandenbroucke: J. Physiol. (G. B.) **109**, 288 (1949).
32. Kumar, D., A. E. D. Hall, R. Nakashima, and A. G. Gornall: Canad. J. Biochem. Physiol. **35**, 113 (1957).
33. Laramore, D. C., and A. Grollman: Amer. J. Physiol. **161**, 278 (1950).
34. Masson, G. M. C., and A. C. Corcoran: Arch. internat. pharmacodyn. thérap. (Belg.) **114**, 322 (1958).
35. Masson, G. M. C., S. B. Koritz, and F. G. Peron: Endocrinology (U.S.A.) **62**, 229 (1958).
36. Meier, R., und F. Gross: In press.
37. Pasqualino, A., and G. H. Bourne: Nature (G. B.) **182**, 1426 (1958).
38. Peart, W. S.: Brit. Med. J. **1959/II**, 1353.
39. Peart, W. S., D. B. Gordon, W. F. Cook, and G. W. Pickering: Circulation (U.S.A.) **14**, 981 (1956).
40. Pitcock, J. A., and P. M. Hartroft: Amer. J. Path. **34**, 863 (1958).
41. Pitcock, J. A., and P. M. Hartroft: Fed. Proc. (U.S.A.) **18**, 500 (1959).
42. Pitcock, J. A., P. M. Hartroft, and L. N. Newmark: Proc. Soc. Exper. Biol. Med. (U.S.A.) **100**, 868 (1959).
43. Rondell, P.: Personal communication.
44. Selye, H., C. E. Hall, and E. M. Rowley: Canad. Med. Ass. J. **49**, 88 (1943).
45. Singer, B.: J. Endocr. (G. B.) **19**, 310 (1959).
46. Singer, B., and M. P. Stack-Dunne: J. Endocr. (G. B.) **12**, 130 (1955).
47. Skelton, F. R.: Proc. Soc. Exper. Biol. Med. (U.S.A.) **90**, 342 (1955).
48. Skelton, F. R.: Physiol. Rev. (U.S.A.) **39**, 162 (1959).
49. Tobian, L.: Circulation Res. (U.S.A.) **4**, 671 (1956).
50. Tobian, L.: J. Clin. Invest. (U.S.A.) **35**, 740 (1956).
51. Tobian, L.: J. Laborat. Clin. Med. (U.S.A.) **54**, 951 (1959).
52. Tobian, L.: Ann. Int. Med. (U.S.A.) **52**, 395 (1960).
53. Tobian, L., and P. D. Redleaf: Amer. J. Physiol. **189**, 451 (1957).
54. Tobian, L., J. Janacek, and A. Tomboulian: Proc. Soc. Exper. Biol. Med. (U.S.A.) **100**, 94 (1959).
55. Tobian, L., A. Tomboulian, and J. Janacek: J. Clin. Invest. (U.S.A.) **38**, 605 (1959).

Possible relationship between salt metabolism and the angiotensin system

By

W. S. PEART

The mechanisms by which the kidney can very rapidly alter its output of water and electrolyte under physiological and pathological conditions are imperfectly understood. In relation to hypertension interesting variations are the increased excretion of water and sodium, especially in relation to appropriate loading (FARNSWORTH and BARKER 1943, BRODSKY and GRAUBARTH 1953, COTTIER, WELLER and HOOBLER 1958, SAPIRSTEIN 1958) and the osmotic diuresis probably precipitated by emotion (MILES and DE WARDENER 1953). We are still in the descriptive phases of these phenomena, and the actions of vasopressin and the steroids are perhaps best understood but they do not, nevertheless, explain the best known differences from normal of the kidney in hypertension.

The functions of renin and angiotensin in relation to hypertension are still in considerable doubt, but the observations which I now wish to report may throw a new light both on the kidney in hypertension and on the functions of angiotensin. This would be a relief to me, since it seems the fate of most substances in the body

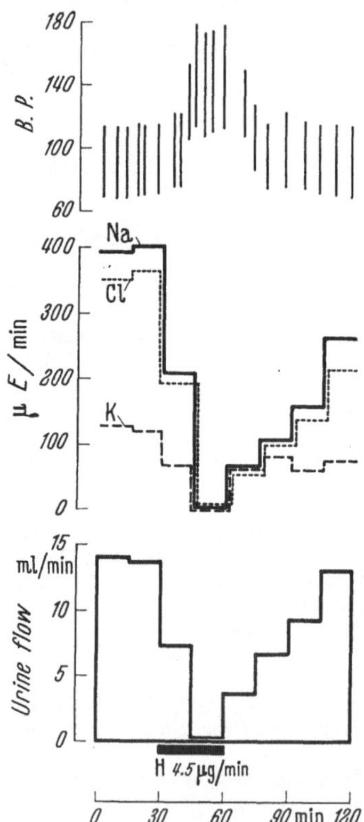

Fig. 1. Effect of infusion of angiotensin (H. 4.5 µg/min) on urine flow and electrolyte excretion in a normal man

which are discovered to have a marked effect on smooth muscle to languish henceforth with an undiscovered function. Histamine and 5-HT come readily to mind. Angiotensin has a similarly profound effect on smooth muscle. The actions of the enzyme renin injected into the blood stream are almost purely exerted by its product

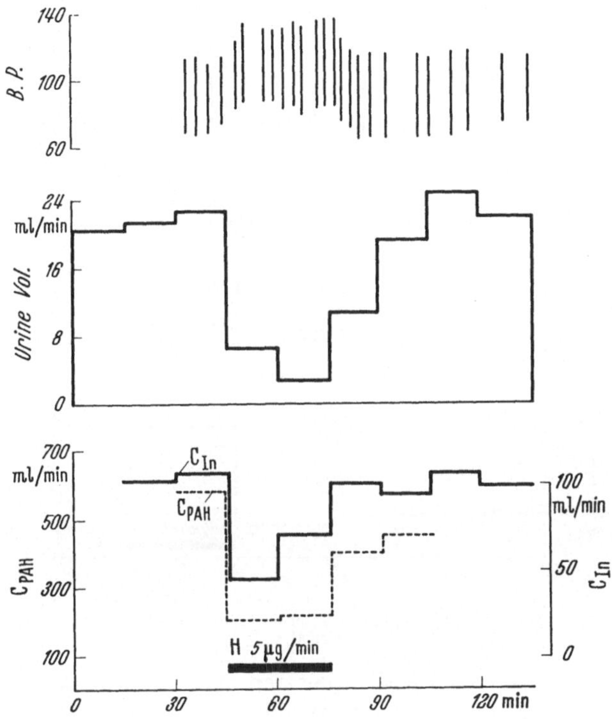

Fig. 2. As in Fig. 1 to show reduction of inulin clearance (C_{In}) and PAH-clearance (C_{PAH})

angiotensin. The use of pure angiotensin removes the doubt as to the effects of impure renin preparations previously used, and in the experiments now described the synthetic valine$_5$-octapeptide (CIBA) has been used (Asparagine-Arginine-Valine-Tyrosine-Valine-Histidine-Proline-Phenylalanine).

Our first observations (PICKERING, SANDERSON and PEART) on normal human subjects showed that in doses up to 5 µg per minute an anti-diuresis was produced (PEART 1959). These are the same as the observations of BOCK and his colleagues (BOCK et al. 1958, BOCK and KRECKE 1958). Fig. 1 illustrates the effect, and it can be seen to be accompanied by a similar reduction in electrolyte excretion. This also occurs at low urine flows. It is a consistent effect and is accompanied by a profound fall in the inulin and PAH clearances as shown in Fig. 2. The implication of this is presumably of very great vasoconstriction in the renal arterioles, and the effect

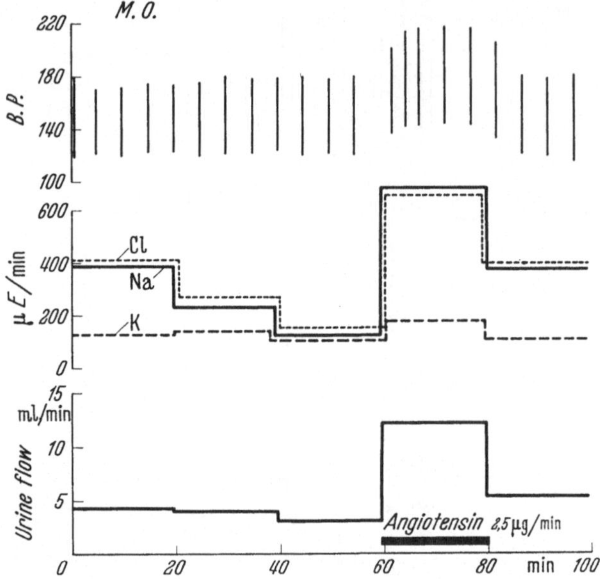

Fig. 3. Effect of an infuson of angiotensin (2.5 µg/min) on the urine flow and electrolyte excretion in a patient with severe renal hypertension. Both factors rise in contrast with the normal

is much greater than with other reported vasoconstrictors; for example, noradrenaline in comparable pressor doses has a rather variable and not great effect on inulin clearance, though some on PAH clearance (Barnett et al. 1950). That this effect is due to vasoconstriction of greater degree in the kidney than elsewhere is suggested by the effects of very small doses insufficient to raise the general blood pressure. The anti-diuresis and decrease in electrolyte excretion can be achieved in this way. These results, like the subsequent one to be reported, were obtained by Dr. J. J. Brown in my department. Whether any physiological renal response could be expected by supposing the release of angiotensin either generally or locally within the kidney is not clear, but one can reflect that vasopressin may not be the only antidiuretic hormone. From a pathological point of view the nearest analogy to this situation is acute glomerulonephritis, where the glomerular filtration rate and tubular function are cut down markedly. In addition to the anatomical damage it is possible that local release of renin and subsequently of angiotensin within the kidney could play a part — in much the way that bradykinin has been shown to cause vasodilatation in the salivary glands by release of the formative enzyme

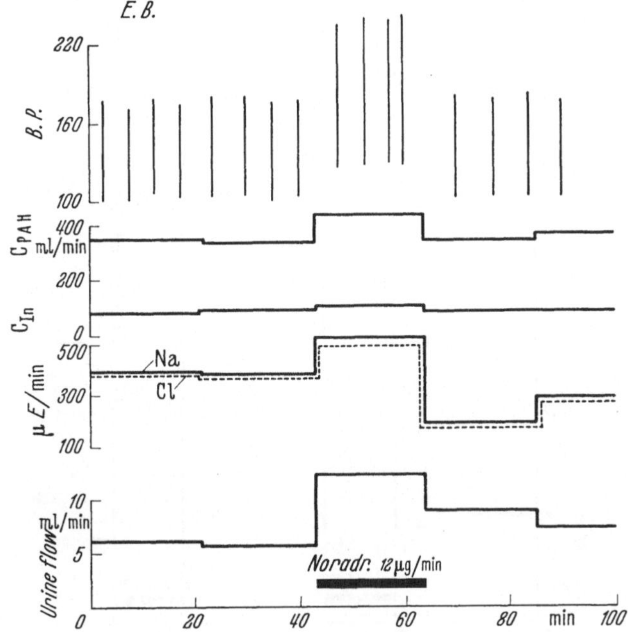

Fig. 4. Effect on renal function of an infusion of noradrenaline in a patient with high blood pressure

into extracellular fluid (HILTON and LEWIS 1957). As we know that renin is formed very close to the glomerulus this needs very careful consideration.

I had considered that the study of the renal effects of angiotensin in patients with hypertension would give a clear indication of the possibility of its presence in the circulation, since its normal effect was to cause an anti-diuresis. The opposite effects in such patients therefore came as a surprise. Diuresis is the usual response and this is illustrated in Fig. 3. It can be seen that the diuresis is osmotic, and sodium and chloride are the main ions affected. This gives another aspect to the hypertensive kidney, and the type of patient studied is shown in Table 1. It can be seen that there is no relation to the type of hypertension, and out of these patients only two did not show diuresis; one had coarctation of the aorta, the other had essential hypertension. The diuretic response is present at both high and low urine flows and at varying levels of blood

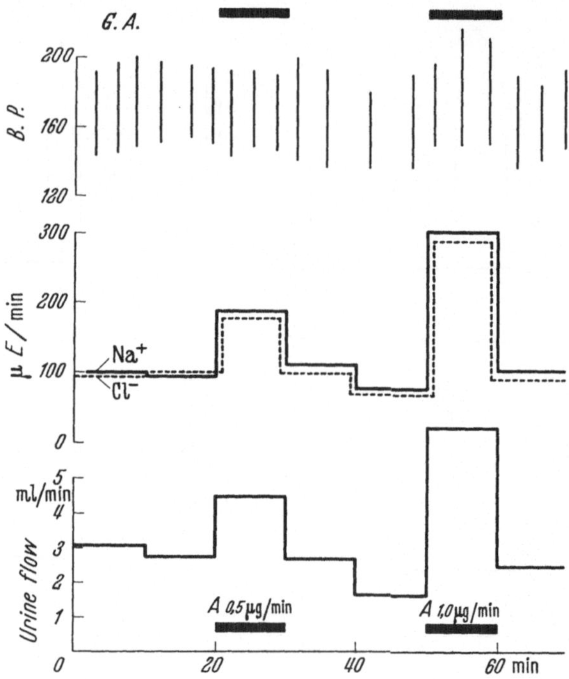

Fig. 5. Effect on renal function of a small infusion of angiotensin insufficient to raise the blood pressure in a patient with high blood pressure

Table 1. *Type of patient who received infusions of angiotensin*

	No.	B.P.
Renal Art. Stenosis	7	160/110—250/150
Essential	6	160/100—240/150
Bilat. Pyelonephritis	3	190/120—240/140
Unil. Tub. Pyelonephritis	1	190/120
Unil. Pyelonephritis	1	220/120
Coarctation	1	200/110
Cushing's Syndrome	1	190/120
	20	

pressure. Most of the patients studied, however, had very high blood pressure. The detailed study of renal function shows somewhat variable effects, and in Table 2 some typical results are given. It can be seen that it is possible to have both a slight decrease or increase in the inulin clearance but that the PAH clearance almost always drops, though not always to a very great degree. Only in one patient have we seen a large increase in the inulin clearance. We can therefore assume that the diuresis is not due to a large increase in the filtered load.

Table 2. *Effects on renal function of angiotensin infusions in patients with high blood pressure*

Name	B.P.	% Change				
		Urine vol.	$U_{Na}V$	$U_K V$	C_{In}	C_{PAH}
E. B.	200/110	+150	+150	+100	+22	+ 3
F. C.	180/120	+ 38	+ 53	— 20	+17	—10
P. F.	226/120	+ 31	+100	— 26	+ 6	—18
A. T.	210/124	+ 21	+ 52	+ 7	—13	—30

We next investigated the basis for this remarkable change. The change in blood pressure itself might clearly play a big part. It has been shown in the dog that changes in the renal artery pressure itself will cause changes in the sodium and water excretion, and that increases in pressure increase both water and sodium output and vice versa (WHITE 1950). We have shown that noradrenaline, in raising the blood pressure, may have a similar effect to angiotensin but to a lesser degree. Fig. 4 illustrates this. However, I think that a local effect on the kidney is the dominant one, and Fig. 5 shows the effect of a small angiotensin infusion into a patient with essential hypertension. No change in blood pressure occurred but an osmotic diuresis followed. Further evidence against the change of blood pressure being the main factor is obtained when the effects of lowering blood pressure are studied. The blood pressure of some of these patients has been lowered acutely by ganglion blocking drugs. However, these changes are reversible and can thus be shown to be due to some effect of hypertension on the kidney.

Fig. 6 shows the typical diuretic response in a patient with hypertension due to renal artery stenosis. After he was operated on and some months had elapsed with his blood pressure lowered to normal levels the observations were repeated, and Fig. 7 shows that he had returned to the normal anti-diuretic pattern. We have shown this successfully in three patients with renal artery stenosis

and one who had a nephrectomy for tuberculosis. This change is
not peculiar, however, to patients treated surgically; this is illustrated
by the progress of a patient successfully treated with ganglion
blocking drugs. Initially he had the typical diuretic response, but
over the months this gradually changed until anti-diuresis appeared.

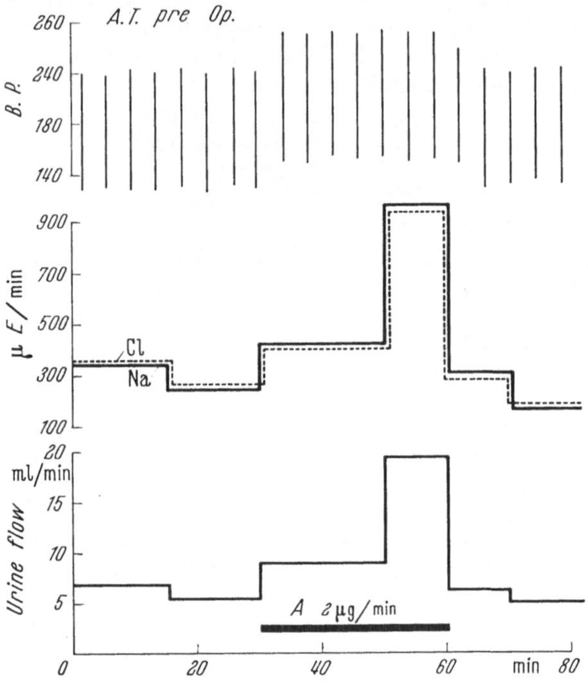

Fig. 6. Usual diuretic response to angiotensin in a patient with hypertension due to renal
artery stenosis

Changes towards the normal response of the kidney to water
and salt loading by successful lowering of the blood pressure have
been shown by THOMPSON et al. (1954) and HOLLANDER, CHOBANI-
AN and BURROWS 1956—1957. The present description of changes
to a vasoconstrictor seems unique, and one looks for a possible
local or general explanation which would fit into the pathological
situation. Except for the osmotic diuresis described by DE WARDE-
NER there is nothing similar, and one wonders what the arrangement
of the circulation of the kidney in hypertension is which brings
about these changes in response to angiotensin. Since there is little
change in the inulin clearance it suggests that there is an equal

effect of the drug on the afferent and efferent arterioles. If this was
a considerable effect one would expect the PAH clearance to drop
uniformly as in the normal subject. This is not our experience, so
it would almost appear that renal arterioles are a little more
resistant than usual to the action of angiotensin. Since the effect

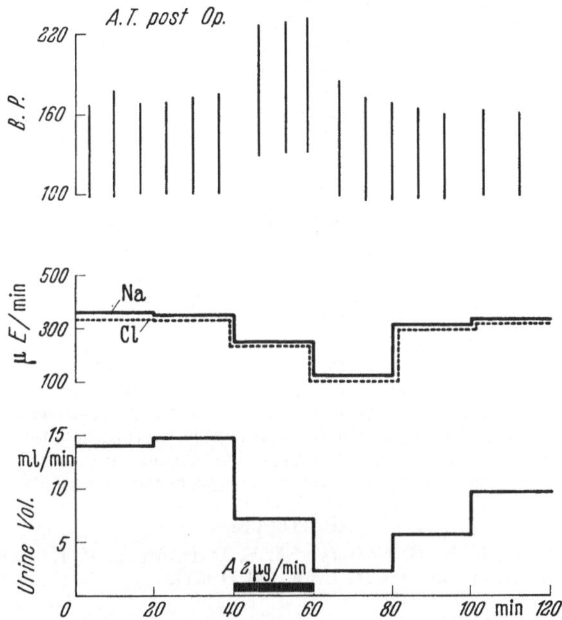

Fig. 7. Return to normal anti-diuresis in response to angiotensin of patient in Fig. 6, after
lowering blood pressure to normal by disobliteration of renal artery five months before

of angiotensin can be obtained in a patient with hypertension
without a change in the blood pressure, it will have to be considered
as a possible local hormonal substance which can cause changes
in electrolyte and water excretion by direct tubular action, though
it cannot at present explain the response of the kidney in hypertension to water and salt loading. Perhaps therefore we should change
our emphasis and look at renin and angiotensin apart from their
pressor effects and towards the direct renal effects. Certainly, if
released into the circulation, renin and therefore angiotensin would
have marked effects on water and electrolyte excretion in the normal and hypertensive subject. The most stimulating point to me
is the possibility of the altered vascular response in the kidney to
angiotensin. This may show that there is a change in blood vessel

walls peculiar to hypertension, or that we have to consider regional blood flow in the kidney more carefully, especially in relation to these altered responses.

Summary

The effects of synthetic val_5-angiotensin on the excretion of water and salt have been studied in normal and hypertensive subjects. In the normal a reduction in excretion of water and electrolytes has been consistently found. In patients with severe hypertension the contrary surprising observation was made that diuresis of water and of electrolytes occurred in most cases. That this was probably due to the effect of the raised blood pressure itself was shown in patients who had their blood pressure returned to normal either by renal artery reconstruction or by drugs, when a slow return to the antidiuretic pattern of response was observed. The possible implications of these observations have been discussed.

Résumé

L'action du produit synthétique «val_5-angiotensine» sur l'élimination de l'eau et du sel a été étudiée chez l'individu normal et chez l'hypertendu. Chez le sujet sain, une réduction de l'excrétion de l'eau et des électrolytes a été démontrée. Chez les malades atteints d'hypertension, on a observé au contraire que l'élimination de l'eau et des électrolytes par les urines était augmentée dans de nombreux cas. Ceci est probablement pour une part en rapport avec le niveau de la tension artérielle, mais aussi avec un effet local sur le rein lui-même. Une baisse de tension transitoire reste sans influence sur le type de réponse des hypertendus. Par contre, un traitement hypotenseur prolongé provoque un lent retour au type de réaction antidiurétique normal. Les implications possibles concernant ces observations ont été discutées.

References

BARNETT, A. J., R. B. BLACKET, A. E. DEPOORTER, P. H. SANDERSON, and G. M. WILSON: Clin. Sc. (G.B.) **9**, 151 (1951).

BOCK, K. D., H. DENGLER, H. J. KRECKE, and G. REICHEL: Klin. Wschr. (G.) **1958/II**, 808.

BOCK, K. D., and H. I. KRECKE: Klin. Wschr. (G.) **1958/II**, 69.

BRODSKY, W. A., and H. N. GRAUBARTH: J. Laborat. Clin. Med. (U.S.A.) **41**, 43 (1953).

COTTIER, P. T., J. M. WELLER, and S. W. HOOBLER: Circulation (U.S.A.) **17**, 750 (1958).

FARNSWORTH, E. B., and M. H. BARKER: Proc. Soc. Exper. Biol. Med. (U.S.A.) **52**, 74 (1943).

HILTON, S. M., and G. P. LEWIS: Brit. Med. Bull. **13**, 189 (1957).

HOLLANDER, W., A. V. CHOBANIAN, and B. A. BURROWS: Proc. N. England Cardiovas. Soc. **15**, 19 (1956/57).

MILES, B. E., and H. E. DE WARDENER: Lancet (G. B.) **1953/II**, 539.

PEART, W. S.: Brit. Med. J. **1959/II**, 1353 and 1421.

SAPIRSTEIN, L. A.: In Hypertension, Vol. 6, p. 28 (1958). Proceedings of the Council for High Blood Pressure Research. Amer. Heart. Ass., Nov. 1957.

THOMPSON, J. E., T. F. SILVA, D. KINSEY, and R. H. SMITHWICK: Circulation (U.S.A.) **10**, 912 (1954).

WHITE, H. L.: Renal function: Transactions of the Second Conference. Ed.: STANLEY E. BRADLEY, p. 127, New York: Josiah Macy Jr. Foundation 1950.

Discussion

WILSON: First of all I want to thank Dr. GROSS for what seems to me an exceptionally helpful piece of work. I found it a little difficult to follow the individual steps in his idea of the vicious circle, but in particular I should like to know how it fits in with three well-established experimental findings. First, when in the rat one kidney is removed and the artery in the remaining kidney is clipped, hypertension is produced. After 8 months of chronic hypertension, removal of the clip from the renal artery produces a prompt fall in blood pressure within less than 12 hours in some animals. I would like Dr. GROSS to tell us how this is explained on his hypothesis. This is the first problem I have. Second, in the last experiment we now take out that kidney and we see the gradual production of renoprival hypertension over 3—4 days. If, on the other hand, instead of removing the clip, we excise the clipped kidney, we do not get a prompt fall in blood pressure with a delayed rise; instead, we get a continuation of the hypertension. This has always seemed to me one of the most important facts in renal hypertension, because this fall and subsequent rise should occur if we are dealing with an exclusively renal factor in renal hypertension, i.e. the same kind of extrarenal factor, whatever it is, must be present in renal as in renoprival hypertension. This is the second thing I would like Dr. GROSS to explain on his hypothesis. The third experimental observation is the production of renal hypertension in an animal in which the kidney is not excreting externally. If one kidney is removed, hypertension due to clipping the artery of the remaining kidney persists after uretero-caval anastomosis, but when you take off the clip, the blood pressure returns to normal. I would like Dr. GROSS to explain, if he can, this occurrence on the basis of the renin-aldosterone hypothesis. I am sure Dr. GROLLMAN will have a great deal to say about this, because it was largely his work which stimulated Dr. FLOYER in our laboratory to do these experiments relating renal to renoprival hypertension.

GROSS: I cannot answer all your questions, but I will try to give a few additional explanations. I omitted in my lecture one part of my manuscript which is entitled "arguments against renin-aldosterone relation". Here, I reported findings which are inconsistent with the pathogenic rôle of a hypothetical renin-aldosterone system. One is the prompt fall of high blood pressure to normal levels after removal of the clamped kidney, as Dr. WILSON and his collaborators, especially Dr. FLOYER, demonstrated years ago. If we assume that the adrenal cortex or aldosterone is responsible for the maintenance of elevated blood pressure in renal hypertension, we cannot explain the discrepancy that blood pressure comes down after removal of the clamped kidney within 8—12 hours, but much more slowly when the adrenals are removed. Adrenalectomy is followed by blood pressure decrease only after 3-4-5 days, in contrast to the rapid normalisation after removal of the clamped kidney. There is much evidence that a substance produced by the kidney, not considered so far here, is involved in the pathogenesis of experimental renal hypertension, but this remains one of the problems which needs further work.

Now, to turn to renoprival hypertension, I think the fact that hypertension may develop in the absence of the kidneys does not necessarily eliminate the kidney as a pathogenic factor in other forms but demonstrates only that the reaction of the organism to different noxious stimuli might be similar. I don't know if Dr. GROLLMAN will agree with this, but renoprival hypertension was for me always something different from the other types of experimental hypertension. The fact that hypertension may develop in the absence of the adrenals is also no argument against the pathogenetic rôle of these glands responsible for the development of special forms of hypertension.

I have one question, too. In your second slide, Dr. WILSON, I saw that you maintained your animals by peritoneal dialysis and I would like to ask you and also Dr. GROLLMAN if there is no possibility that a certain retention of sodium occurs. Did you ever do tissue analysis in these animals besides determination of plasma concentration?

WILSON: Doesn't your hypothesis depend on the ability of the kidney to vary body sodium by changes in excretion? In the rat with uretero-caval anastomosis, there is no possibility of external excretion. If changes in body sodium or water are responsible for the production or abolition of hypertension in this experiment, it must be some redistribution within the body not involving external excretion?

GROSS: Yes, I have to add here that aldosterone is a hormone which not only has an influence on kidney function, but also has extrarenal effects.

GROLLMAN: The disturbances in electrolyte and water metabolism in hypertension have directed attention to the adrenal cortex as a possible mediator or as primarily responsible for such disturbances. However, attempts to incriminate the adrenal cortex as an etiologic agent in essential hypertension have not succeeded. Dogs maintained in electrolyte balance by peritoneal lavage develop hypertension following bilateral adrenalectomy and nephrectomy without the administration of adrenal cortical hormone. Adrenalectomized rats, likewise, ingesting 2% saline, as Dr. GROSS has indicated, also develop hypertension. The so-called adrenal regeneration hypertension of the rat is also not attributable to the production of abnormal or excessive hormone by the regenerating tissue. It must be concluded accordingly that the adrenal plays only a permissive rôle in the pathogenesis of hypertension and that it is not primarily responsible for the electrolyte disturbances observed in this disease. However, the adrenal may influence the level of the blood pressure

1. by its effects on electrolyte-water metabolism;
2. by direct effects on the renal vasculature; and as shown by Dr. GROSS
3. by its effects on the angiotensin mechanism.

With reference to Dr. WILSON's remark, the fact that elevations in blood pressure occur following removal of renal tissue need not indicate that such elevations are induced by extra-renal factors. One would not deny that the diabetes mellitus induced by pancreatectomy is of pancreatic origin. One can only conclude that the elevation in blood pressure is not a consequence of the liberation of a pressor factor by the kidney.

PEART: I would just like to come back to Dr. GROLLMAN's thesis. It seems to me very difficult when one considers branch stenosis in renal arteries with very small portions of the kidney responsible for the high blood pressure. You could argue your way out of it by saying something is wrong with that part of the kidney which influences the metabolism of the other 7/8 or 3/4 of the kidney substance. But it seems to me that the most intriguing thing in the experimental situation still remains the renal artery clip both in man and in the rat, and particularly the branch stenosis. It leads me at any rate to take the simpler view that something is actually coming out of the kidney to directly cause hypertension rather than that you have to explain it away by something coming out which then influences the whole metabolism of all renal tissue so that you in fact get hypertension.

GROLLMAN: I would not deny that under certain circumstances, such as in so-called "unilateral renal disease" or its experimental analogues, one is dealing with hypertension secondary to the elaboration by the kidney of a pressor agent. We should not insist, however, on attributing all hypertension — and particularly the most prevalent "essential" hypertension — to this exceptional and unique form of blood-pressure elevation.

PEART: I was not talking about essential hypertension; it was just because of the fact that the kidney had been implicated in your statement.

WILSON: But does not Dr. GROSS's work provide a possible clue to the hitherto insoluble problem of how an abnormal kidney can influence the opposite normal kidney so that it cannot maintain the blood pressure normal? I think his hypothesis might also fit in with our view that renal hypertension, after the early stages, involves an extra-renal as well as a renal factor.

PICKERING: I want to say a few words about an old observation that we made 20 years ago which suggests in my mind very strongly that renin and presumably hypertensin (angiotensin) may function as a local hormone in the kidney. This was made in the rabbit. When you inject renin intravenously in the rabbit, the blood pressure goes up and reaches its peak in about 2 minutes, and in about half an hour the whole thing is over. Now, during the first 15 minutes, the urine flow goes down, and this is associated with a decrease in both inulin and diodone clearance and a slight increase in the filtration fraction. I think one can explain that as a vascular effect on the kidney. But this phase is succeeded by a phase of the most intense diuresis. The urine flow rises to levels which are very much higher than you can get by giving the animal water. And this urine is very odd, because its sodium and chloride contents are just a little bit higher than those of plasma; at least they tend to be so. So that if you start with a urine which contains very little salt, the salt content rises, and if you feed your animals on hypertonic saline so that you start with a very high salt content of the urine, the sodium and chloride content of the urine falls during the diuresis so that the content of the urine approximates to the level which WALKER and his colleagues found in proximal tubular urine in the rat. Now, in this phase, the sodium and chloride content changes as I have mentioned, but there is not much change in the excretion of potassium or of the other anions. This diuresis cannot be explained on an osmotic basis. Not only that, but the inulin and diodone clearances have now returned to more or less normal levels. We wondered if this was due to a change in the kind of nephrons being perfused by the blood, and so we injected Berlin blue into the aorta at the height of the diuresis and then clamped the kidney, cut it out, froze it, and cut sections from it, but there did not seem to be any change in the distribution of blood. And so I think the only reasonable conclusion was that this was an effect on the tubule. I have always thought that it was on the distal tubules, because there is close similarity between the urine at the height of the diuresis and the proximal tubular fluid. Now, that observation so far is peculiar to the rabbit, and I don't know its counterpart in man. But at any rate, in the rabbit it did suggest that there was a local hormone action.

BROD: I would like to discuss the first paper. I have been especially intrigued by your comparison of the osmotic effect of angiotensin on the kidney in hypertensives with the effect DE WARDENER and MILES noticed in some subjects after emotion. I have always been wondering about the reason for this osmotic diuresis. Now, under emotion, you can get either a vasoconstriction in the kidneys accompanied by a fall of urine and sodium output, or you can get an increased ADH output accompanied again by a drop in urine flow. The osmotic diuresis occurring especially in hypertensive subjects under emotion is obviously due to something overcoming these two physiologically occurring mechanisms. We have been studying very closely the effect of acute emotional stress on haemodynamics and we did not find any qualitative difference in the normotensive and hypertensive subjects. But there were quantitative differences. Under acute emotional stress in hypertensive subjects, the blood pressure rose to a higher level. Now, if this were connected with your osmotic effect on the kidneys, there should be perhaps an increase in renal blood flow due to a higher perfusing pressure. But it is not so. These patients have a higher degree of renal vasoconstriction, so that actually they have a lesser blood flow to the kidneys. In addition to this effect on blood pressure, there is a greater shift of blood from the viscera (where a higher degree of vasoconstriction occurred), to the central vascular bed, because these subjects do not have a similarly higher degree of vasodilatation in the muscle. I wonder whether really your effect could not be accounted for by some changes in the central vascular bed, where volume-receptors are supposed to be localized. I also wanted to ask you in what stage of essential hypertension your patients were. We have seen with cold pressor stimuli that in the early stage of hypertension there was a higher degree of renal vasoconstriction than in normal subjects. A paradoxical increase in renal blood flow occurred only in subjects in late stages of hypertension with evidence of nephrosclerosis. This is, I think, similar to what Dr. Hood has also shown to occur after carbon dioxide. And here again I would stress the point that we made several times in Prague, that we should really try to define better the various stages of hypertension with which we are working. We should not throw all essential hypertensives into one and the same bag. And my last point: You have been mentioning that renin might have a direct local effect in the kidneys. Well, I was always intrigued by the question why, if we clamp a renal artery and the clamped kidney is producing more renin, we do not get in this kidney a greater haemodynamic effect and why in fact this kidney is not ischaemic. It has been shown, I think, that a kidney with a clamped renal artery does not necessarily get less blood. On the contrary, there is a vasodilatation, and I always thought that this might be an effect of the fact that an interaction of renin with α_2-globulin takes some time and that probably the blood flow through the kidneys is too short, so that angiotensin is formed somewhere in the postrenal part of the vascular bed and cannot affect renal haemodynamics before reaching the general circulation.

COTTIER: I was impressed by the paper of Dr. PEART. I would like to recall that Dr. K. KIPFER, former associate of Dr. REUBI, started these studies two years ago and that he also found hypernatriuresis in mild hypertensives following infusion of angiotensin. The data were not published. Did you study any labile hypertensives in a normotensive phase? Another question I wanted to ask is whether you did any studies with chronic angiotensin infusion in normal subjects, and after what lapse of time does this phenomenon of hypernatriuresis occur? Then you described one case of unilateral renal artery disease. It would be interesting to know how natriuresis was on the side of the affected renal artery, and it would be a very crucial experiment to find out whether on the affected side there was a lower natriuresis. I think that the idea of the reset of the intrarenal blood flow is very interesting and intriguing; it is conceivable that the medullary blood flow changes. Unfortunately it is difficult to measure, because it is only a very small fraction of the total renal blood flow.

BOCK: May I ask Dr. PEART whether he has done any studies on patients with low blood pressure, for instance on patients in shock?

PEART: (to BOCK) I'd better answer that straight away: the answer is no.

(to COTTIER): We need a lot of patients with hypertension with a lower range of blood pressure before I can answer your question properly. In the patients studied, most had high blood pressure, in fact distinctly high, but two things could be said about them. One is that one of the patients with a renal artery stenosis who had a blood pressure of only 180/100 still had an antidiuresis. The other is that we had ureteric catheters in these patients. It is extremely difficult with catheters in the ureter to get any sort of steady state, unfortunately. We had suggestions that the two kidneys did differ, but I would not commit myself on paper or even in speaking at the moment about that. This is something which must be gone into, because it is an ideal opportunity to see whether the clip in man does protect the kidney from the effects of angiotensin. I hope we will be able to get the answer to that.

REUBI: Dr. GROSS, have you any answer to suggest?

GROSS: No, but I would say one word to Dr. PICKERING. I think it is quite important to bear in mind that renin may have a different action on water and sodium elimination according to the degree of sodium load or the special situation of sodium metabolism. Furthermore, one should not overlook the fact that the reaction to injected renin is probably quite different from the reaction to renin which is produced in the kidney. In my opinion we have in the rat with unilaterally clamped kidney an ideal object by which to examine the function of two kidneys differing in their renin content. We are now doing studies comparing the kidney which contains renin with the kidney depleted of renin. In order to have similar conditions of renal circulation, we remove the clip before we investigate excretory function. Although we are only at the beginning of these experiments, I can say that the renin-containing kidney reabsorbs more sodium than the non-clamped kidney which is free of renin. Whether this has anything to do with what Dr. COTTIER told us about excretion in hypertensives I do not know, but this difference in kidney function will have to be followed up.

PEART: Of course I had better answer Dr. BROD's questions. I think the first thing is that there could be a number of ways in which the effect that we observe could occur. The first I suggested is the vascular one, because it seems that there is such a rapid onset and offset. It would be possible to think of angiotensin competing in some way with steroids at the tubule level and thus affecting function. However, it seems a little unlikely to me in view of this rapidity. I do not associate rapidity of that sort with competition with steroid in the tubule, but I am rather ignorant of this subject and I am not sure whether that could be true. As to the effects on the general distribution of blood, well that may be so, but this is a very quick action and I cannot conceive this as likely. The effects of very small infusions suggest a direct action on the kidney rather than a general redistribution of blood. A further point about the level of pressure: I would point out that in one of the patients with renal artery stenosis his blood pressure dropped to normal levels within 24 hours of having his kidney removed, yet the response to angiotensin on his kidney took months to return to an antidiuretic phase; in other words, time had to elapse before the kidney returned to normal behaviour, and this to me is the most stimulating aspect of the whole investigation.

REUBI: It certainly is, yes.

Adrenocortical function in essential hypertension[1]

By

J. Genest, W. Nowaczynski, E. Koiw, T. Sandor and P. Biron[2]

Introduction

For the last 12 years, our main research work has been devoted to the study of the possible relationship of adrenocortical hormones and arterial hypertension in humans. Much clinical and experimental evidence, some circumstantial and some more direct, favors this approach to the study of the basic mechanism of arterial hypertension in humans. It is not our assignment, nor does time permit us to describe this evidence.

The purpose of this paper is to present: 1) the results obtained from the study of a large urinary steroid spectrum in normal subjects and hypertensive patients; 2) the effects of progesterone administration on blood pressure, sodium and potassium balances of patients with essential and renal hypertension; 3) the effects of valine$_5$-angiotensin II, nor-epinephrine, epinephrine, and neo-synephrine in patients with benign hypertension and in normal male volunteers.

Section I

Study of a large urinary steroid spectrum in normal subjects and hypertensive patients.

Subjects

The normal subjects used as controls were physicians, nurses, technicians and medical students carrying on their usual work. Hypertension was labeled essential when no other cause could be found and in absence of papilledema. It was diagnosed of renal origin when it was clear from the case history that renal disease preceded appearance of hypertension. The presence of papilledema,

[1] Work supported through grants from the Ministries of Health (Federal-Provincial Plan) Ottawa and Quebec, the Life Insurance Medical Research Fund, New York, the National Research Council, Ottawa, Canada, and the CIBA Company, Montreal.

[2] National Research Council Medical Research Fellow, 1958—1961.

usually associated with hematuria and/or diastolic pressure most often above 130 mm Hg, was the main criterion for diagnosis of malignant hypertension.

All hypertensive patients were studied during hospitalisation and none were in congestive heart failure or presented any sign of peripheral edema. There was no dietary restriction of any kind for normal subjects or hypertensive patients, except that about half of patients with malignant hypertension were not permitted to use the salt shaker, but otherwise were given ordinary hospital diets. The number and sex of the subjects and patients studied in each group are indicated in Table 1. The mean age of the group of normal subjects was 15 to 18 years younger than that of the groups of hypertensive patients.

Table 1. *Number and sex of patients studied*

	Aldosterone	Pregnanetriol[1]	Pregnanetriol/ Aldosterone Ratio
Normal subjects . .	23	10	10
	M: 10 W: 13	M: 7 W: 3	M: 7 W: 3
Essential hypertension	46	26	26
	M: 21 W: 25	M: 8 W: 18	M: 8 W: 18
Renal hypertension .	15	8	7
	M: 3 W: 12	M: 1 W: 7	M: 1 W: 6
Malignant hypertension . . .	26	12	11
	M: 15 W: 11	M: 7 W: 5	M: 6 W: 5

A 24 to 72 hr urine collection was made on each patient and immediately placed in a deep-freeze until processed.

Eight steroids were determined in each urine aliquot: cortisone, cortisol and their tetrahydro derivatives, aldosterone, etiocholanolone, pregnanetriol and the tetrahydro derivative of 17-hydroxy, 11-desoxy-corticosterone (Compound "S"), in addition to sodium and sodium/potassium ratio.

Because of the recent observation by PICKETT et al. (*1*) that urinary pregnanetriol is markedly increased during the early phase of the second part of the menstrual cycle, we have eliminated from our series of normal female subjects all pregnanetriol determinations done during the second part of their menstrual cycle. But we have kept all results obtained from hypertensive women without regard to the time of the menstrual cycle during which urine collections were made. This strengthens the significance of

---

[1] EBERLEIN-BONGIOVANNI'S procedure.

the differences obtained between groups of hypertensive patients compared to groups of normal subjects.

Materials and methods

The procedures used for hydrolysis, extraction, purification and determination of the above steroids, as well as the technical details, have been previously described in several publications from our laboratory (*2, 3, 4, 5, 6, 7, 8*). These procedures are essentially based on isolation of the various steroids in a high degree of purity. Identification of the individual steroids is based on chromatographic mobilities on two or three paper systems in comparison to mobilities of standard reference substances, on absorption in ultraviolet light, reaction with blue tetrazolium (*2*) and isonicotinic acid hydrazide (*9*), absorption spectra in concentrated sulfuric acid (*10, 11, 12*), and in 100% phosphoric acid (*13, 14*) and the m-dinitrobenzene reaction (*15*).

In the course of this study, Bongiovanni and Eberlein's procedure (*16*), used for determination of pregnanetriol, was found inaccurate in most cases, because of the presence of at least one or two interfering substances (Δ^5-pregnene-3β, 17α, 20α-triol and a substance already described by us as Compound III [*17*]) in the pregnanetriol fraction eluted from the aluminium oxide column. Modifications of this procedure were made for isolation of pregnanetriol in a highly pure state and free from these two interfering substances (*5*).

Results

I. Aldosterone. All normal subjects and hypertensive patients in whom urinary aldosterone was determined by our physico-chemical method (*4*) are included in these results. This extensive study, being reported elsewhere (*8*) and based on 200 individual determinations in 110 subjects and patients, shows a 2 to 3-fold increase in mean urinary aldosterone excretion of groups of patients with essential, renal and malignant hypertension as compared to that of normal subjects similarly studied (Table 2).

Differences between means of the groups of patients with arterial hypertension and that of normal subjects are statistically significant with "P" values below 0.001 for the groups of essential and malignant hypertension and 0.005 for the group of patients with renal hypertension.

Eighty-three aldosterone determinations were done in the 46 patients with essential hypertension. Thirty-six determinations, or 43%, were above the upper limits of the normal range by our procedure (*2* to 10 μg/day).

Table 2. *Urinary aldosterone excretion* (micrograms/day)

	Normal subjects	Hypertensive patients		
		Essential	Renal	Malignant
No. of determinations	57	83	22	38
No. of patients .	23	46	15	26
Mean excretion and S.E. . . .	4.31±0.37	10.56±0.98	8.53±1.77	12.38±1.73
"t" value		5.1	3.35	5.45
"p"		<0.001	<0.005	<0.001

These results are derived from spot determinations done on hypertensive patients, and a marked overlapping exists between individual values obtained in normal subjects and hypertensive patients. Further studies were undertaken to determine the daily

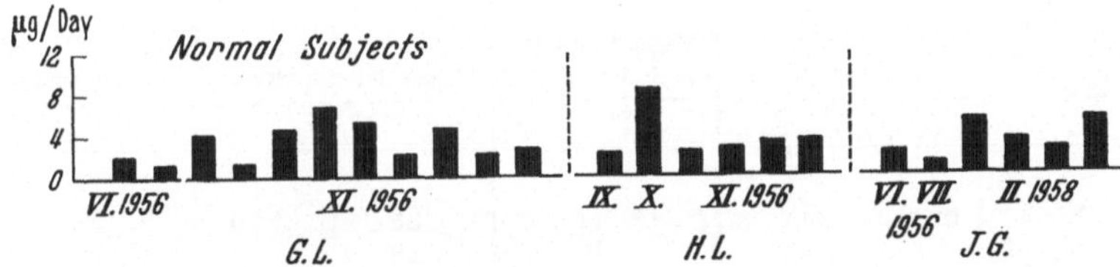

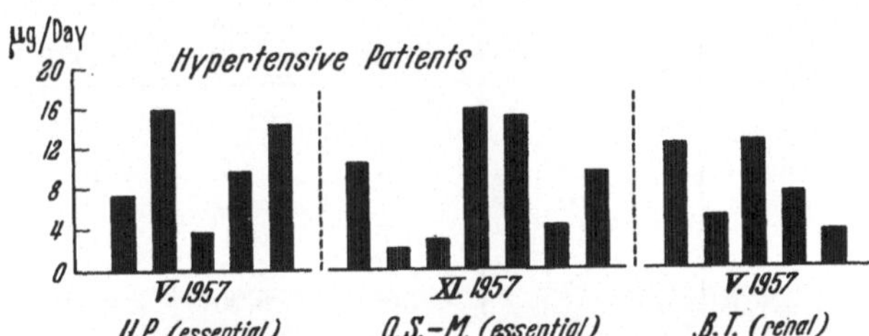

Fig. 1. Dietary sodium intake was not restricted in the normotensive subjects or in the two hypertensive patients B. T. and O. S.-M. Patient U. P. received a diet containing 150 mEq of sodium per day

urinary aldosterone excretion for 5 to 10 consecutive days in several normal subjects and patients with essential or renal hypertension. As shown in Fig. 1, daily urinary aldosterone excretion in normal subjects stays well within normal limits, even when these subjects are carrying on their usual daily work. On the other hand, all hypertensive patients studied but one, and who were asymptomatic and in the early phase of the disease, showed under conditions of hospitalization, a marked fluctuation in daily aldosterone excretion from normal to excessively high levels. A similar fluctuation was also found in one patient with coarctation of the aorta. This confirms our earlier findings (6). These occasionally high levels of urinary aldosterone cannot be explained on the basis of congestive heart failure or edema. No reasons of stress, anxiety, sodium restriction or excessive potassium intake were present, as far as we could determine, to explain these excessive fluctuations, which seemed especially marked in patients with early hypertension.

II. Pregnane-3 α, 17 α, 20 α-triol. Results obtained with Bongiovanni and Eberlein's procedure and with Nowaczynski, Koiw and Genest's procedure (5) are shown in Table 3. Findings with these two methods are similar, although the distribution of individual values obtained with Nowaczynski et al.'s method is not as wide as that found with Bongiovanni and Eberlein's procedure.

Table 3. *Urinary pregnanetriol excretion*

	Normal subjects	Hypertensive patients		
		Essential	Renal	Malignant
I. Bongiovanni-Eberlein's *procedure*				
No. of determinations .	11	33	9	15
No. of patients	10	26	8	12
Mean excretion and S.E.	2105±271	991±119	698±150	770±159
"t" value		4.14	4.06	4.3
"p"		<0.001	<0.001	<0.001
II. Nowaczynski-Koiw *and Genest's procedure*				
No. of determinations .	15	26	6	13
No. of patients	10	21	5	10
Mean excretion	1053	367	162	327
"t" value		4.93	4.0	4.16
"p"		<0.001	<0.001	<0.001

There is a significant decrease in mean pregnanetriol excretion in patients with renal, essential and malignant hypertension as compared to that of normal subjects. The differences between means of groups of patients with hypertension and that of normal subjects are highly significant with "P" values below 0.001.

III. Urinary ratio pregnanetriol/aldosterone. Since the excretion of these two substances varies in opposite directions in hypertensive patients, their ratio may be a more sensitive index of hypertensive cardiovascular disease. Results obtained with aldosterone excretion on the one hand, and pregnanetriol excretion as determined by BONGIOVANNI and EBERLEIN's procedure on the other hand, are shown in Fig. 2. It is obvious that the differences in mean ratio of groups of patients with essential, renal and malignant hypertension as compared to that of normal subjects are statistically

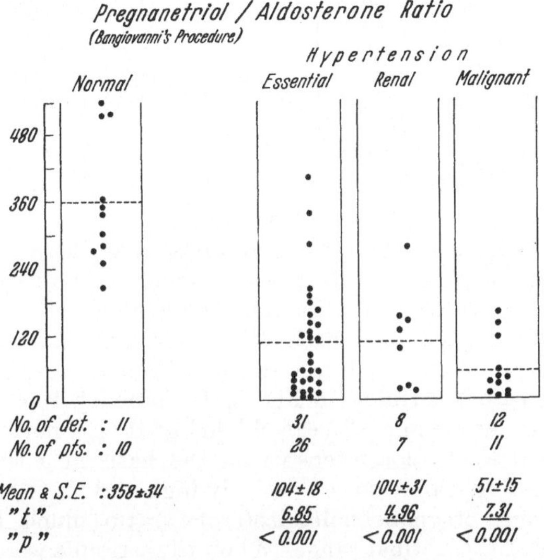

Fig. 2. This ratio appears highly important, as an indication of hypertensive cardio-vascular disease, in the absence of obvious endocrine disorders. Aldosterone and pregnanetriol were determined in the same urine aliquot

significant with "P" values much below 0.001 and "t" values of 6.8, 4.9 and 7.3 respectively for the groups of patients with essential, renal and malignant hypertension.

This ratio in hypertensive patients is lower than the inferior limits of the normal range in 92% of all hypertensive patients studied. Such findings lead us to believe that, in the absence of clear clinical endocrine disorders, a lower ratio of urinary pregnanetriol/aldosterone is suggestive of hypertensive disease (see description of case).

IV. Other corticosteroids. As shown in Table 4, no essential difference is found in mean excretion of cortisone, cortisol and their tetrahydro derivatives, etiocholanolone and the tetrahydro derivative of 17-hydroxy, 11-desoxy-corticosterone in groups of patients with essential, renal and malignant hypertension as compared to that of normal subjects.

Table 4. *Mean values and range of excretion* (μg/day)

	Normal subjects	Hypertension		
		Essential	Renal	Malignant
Cortisone . . .	63	69	91	49
	(10—114)	(11—218)	(16—155)	(11—147)
Tetrahydro	568	542	345	559
cortisone . .	(85—1986)	(119—1401)	(185—700)	(59—1330)
Hydrocortisone	107	131	160	86
	(34—262)	(21—300)	(97—218)	(23—238)
Terahydro	915	1088	751	533
hydrocortisone	(284—2150)	(461—1975)	(90—1920)	(166—1069)
E + THE +	1664	1820	1347	1250
+ F + THF .	(577—2836)	(794—2791)	(509—2577)	(266—2126)

Discussion

These findings establish beyond doubt that there is a disturbance in aldosterone secretion in patients with arterial hypertension of various origins, although they cannot permit any claim that this disturbance is a basic etiological factor in this disease.

It may be of great interest to describe here in detail a most interesting case illustrated in Fig. 3. In January 1959, results of urinary aldosterone in a 23-year-old girl used as a normal control and believed to be normotensive on the basis of a single blood pressure reading, came out excessively high and those of the pregnanetriol and pregnanetriol/aldosterone ratio much below the lower limit of the normal range. When these results were known in March 1959, blood pressure was taken twice a day for two weeks and showed on several occasions systolic readings of 140 and 142 mm Hg and diastolic readings of 90 and 92 mm Hg. Serial daily aldosterone determinations showed marked fluctuations from normal to abnormally high levels, such as those encountered in early asymptomatic hypertension, and the pregnanetriol/aldosterone ratio was much lower than normal. At this point, a family history taken from the patient revealed that one brother and one sister were suffering from hypertension. In September 1959, her blood pressure taken twice a day for a week was found occasionally at 140/110 and 150/100 mm Hg. It is certainly interesting that, without any previous knowledge on our part, this young woman, believed to be normotensive, was found through urinary determinations of aldosterone and pregnanetriol to have fluctuations in blood pressure up to hypertensive levels and to have a family history of hypertension. It appears probable that this girl will develop essential hypertension.

Our findings of the significantly increased mean urinary aldosterone, first reported in 1956 (*18*), in patients with essential, renal and malignant hypertension as compared to normal subjects, and of excessive fluctuations in urinary aldosterone in early asymptomatic hypertension (*6*), have recently been confirmed by TRONCHETTI et al. (*19*), ROMANELLI (*20*) and VENNING (*21*) and their

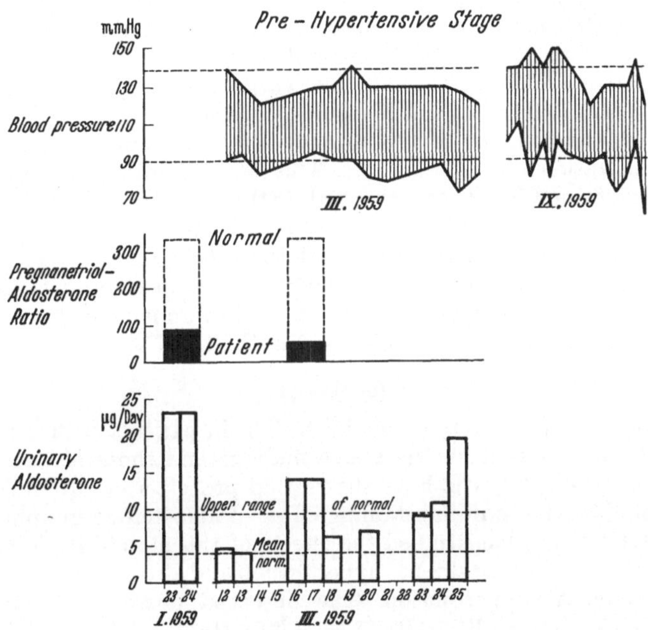

Fig. 3. This subject, apparently in the early or "hyper-reactor" phase of hypertension, shows the same excessive fluctuations in urinary aldosterone as other hypertensive patients

respective groups. LARAGH et al. (*22*) have found significant increases in aldosterone secretion rate in patients with renal and malignant hypertension, but not in those with benign essential hypertension. In view of the excessive fluctuations of aldosterone excretion found in patients with early benign essential hypertension, it is indicated to do repeated studies of aldosterone secretion rate in the same hypertensive patients.

In a recent review of all cases of primary aldosteronism reported in literature up to June 1958 by DELORME and GENEST (*23*), arterial hypertension has been the constant and major finding in this disease. Administration of aldosterone to rats by KUMAR et al. (*24*), GORNALL and co-workers (*25*) and by GROSS et al. (*26, 27*) and in man by August and collaborators (28) has resulted in significant increases of blood pressure.

Our observations tie in with those of: 1) Friedman, who has shown that an increase in blood pressure following administration of various pressor substances to nephrectomized rats and dogs is always accompanied by a parallel shift of sodium into the intra-cellular compartment (29, 30, 31); 2) Tobian, who has found an increase in sodium concentration in arteries and muscles from patients with hypertension as well as in those obtained from animals made hypertensive by various experimental means (32, 40, 41); 3) Deane and Masson (33), who have demonstrated a marked enlargement of the adrenal zona glomerulosa following administration of renin to rats. This latter finding has recently been confirmed by Hartroft et al. (34).

The significance of changes in urinary aldosterone and pregnane-triol is well illustrated by the fact that their ratio is below the lower limit of the normal range in 92% of all hypertensive patients studied (35). The relation between aldosterone and the renal pressor mechanism will be discussed in the third section.

Section II

Effects of progesterone administration in patients with arterial hypertension. Based on the above findings and those of Landau and Lugibihl (36), who have shown that progesterone administration inhibits the sodium-retaining effect of aldosterone in humans, Armstrong (37) has studied the effects of this steroid in rats and dogs with experimental renal hypertension and also in a few patients with essential hypertension. The observed decreases in blood pressure in almost all instances were important.

We have made a similar study in 7 patients, 5 women and 2 men, and the results obtained confirm Armstrong's observations. Six of these patients presented essential hypertension and one had hypertension of renal origin. These patients were studied while in hospital. Five were put under metabolic conditions of fixed sodium and potassium intake before, during and after progesterone administration and two were studied for the effect of progesterone on blood pressure only. Progesterone was given in two divided doses every 12 hrs by deep intramuscular injections. The daily blood pressures are the means of 14 hourly readings in upright and recumbent positions from 8 a. m. to 10 p. m. The figures given in the following table are the averages of the daily blood pressure readings taken during the entire control period and during that of pro-gesterone administration at a given dosage.

Table 5

Patients	Control period (8—15 days)		Progesterone 50—200 mg I-M/day (10—16 days)	
	B.P. Recumbent	B.P. Upright	B.P. Recumbent	P.B. Upright
F. D. Ess. Hypert..	193/110		160/95	134/87
C. L. Ess. Hypert..	182/115	162/110	168/96	145/88
A. L. Ess. Hypert..	174/112	163/106	157/93	141/93
G. G. Ess. Hypert..	158/103	137/103	145/99	124/95
P. B. Ess. Hypert. 1. . . .	188/111	175/115	152/88	137/82
P. B. Ess. Hypert. 2. . . .	196/129	192/127	144/85	137/84
J. Y. Ess. Hypert..	205/106	205/107	187/99	187/99
A. P. Renal Hypert.	213/115	196/107	197/104	167/96

In Table 5 are indicated the overall results obtained in these
seven patients. One patient, P. B., had two courses of progesterone
administration. It can be seen that significant decreases in blood
pressure were obtained in all of the seven patients. In fact, in the

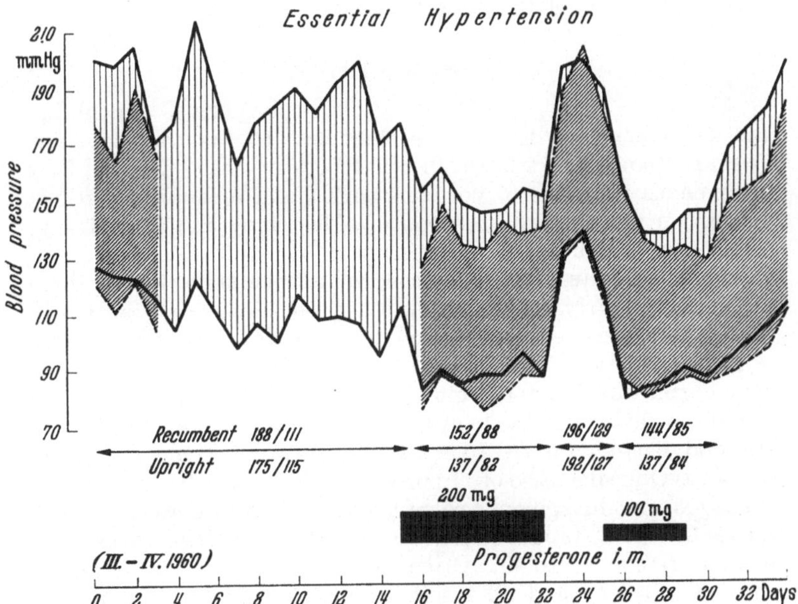

Fig. 4. The hypotensive effects of progesterone in this patient are striking, both at the 100 mg
and 200 mg dosage levels. This 45-year-old patient, P. B., had hypertension known 9 months
previously. Her mother suffered from arterial hypertension. Fundi showed arteriosclerotic
changes without retinopathy. Renal function was fair with urea clearance at 70% of normal,
creatinine clearance of 60 ml/min. Intravenous pyelogram was normal. She complained of
migraine-like attacks which disappeared during the periods of progesterone administration

upright posture, the blood pressure of these seven patients was almost within normal limits.

The effect of progesterone administration on the blood pressure of a patient with essential hypertension is shown in Fig. 4. This patient received two courses of progesterone, one for 7 days at 200 mg/day and the other for 4 days at 100 mg/day. During the interval between these two periods, the patient received placebo injections of isotonic saline. The results of the progesterone administration are striking, with lowering of the blood pressure to normal limits and immediate rise to hypertensive levels following cessation of progesterone and its replacement by placebo injections. Re-administration of progesterone brought blood pressure rapidly down to normal levels.

Such falls in blood pressure are observed without any significant sodium loss during progesterone administration. The metabolic studies done on the five patients show that the decrease in blood pressure is obtained without any negative sodium balance. These studies will be reported in greater detail elsewhere (*38*).

Section III

Effects of valine$_5$-angiotensin II, nor-epinephrine, epinephrine and neo-synephrine infusions in humans. Three years ago, Dr. Joffre Brouillet studied in our laboratory the effects of 8-hr intravenous infusions of nor-epinephrine and epinephrine in 5% glucose on the urinary excretion of aldosterone and 17-hydroxycorticosteroids (measured by Peterson's modification of Silber-Porter's procedure) (*39*). Three normotensive subjects and three patients with early benign essential hypertension were admitted to hospital and received unrestricted diets. On day 1, control infusion of glucose 5% was administered for 8 hrs. On day 2, an 8-hr nor-epinephrine infusion in 5% glucose was given at a rate sufficient to produce a slight increase in systolic (mean: 25; range 12 to 41 mm Hg) and diastolic (mean: 15; range 7 to 24 mm Hg) blood pressure and an average decrease of 11 pulsations per minute (range 5 to 16). On day 3, an 8-hr epinephrine infusion in 5% glucose was given at a rate sufficient to produce an average increase of 29 pulsations per minute (range: 19 to 40). Urines were collected only during the time of infusions, and all results of urinary aldosterone and 17-hydroxycorticosteroids are expressed in micrograms and milligrams/day respectively. The results illustrated in Table 6 indicate that there is essentially no change in urinary aldosterone excretion. There is a very slight, but apparently not significant, rise in

Table 6. *Effects of 8-hour i.v. infusions of nor-epinephrine and epinephrine* (in 5% glucose)

Patients[1]	Age	Diagnosis	Aldosterone[2] (μg/day)			17-Hydroxy-corticosteroids[3] (mg/day)		
			Control glucose 5%	Nor-Epin.	Epin.	Control glucose 5%	Nor-Epin.	Epin.
R. B.	25	Benign Ess. Hypert.	9	3	3	4.3	5.5	6.6
A. C.	18	Benign Ess. Hypert.	3	3	7			
W. C.	41	Benign Ess. Hypert.	8	8	9	6.3	8.0	7.9
C. de B.	18	Normal subject	7	8	11	4.2	5.6	5.2
T. P.	35	Schizophrenia	9	12	4			
A. G.	28	Obesity	5	5		1.6	5.5	

urinary total 17-hydroxycorticosteroids with equal distribution in both free and conjugated fractions.

In October 1959, we reported at the annual meeting of the American Heart Association preliminary experiments showing that urinary aldosterone increased markedly during and following intravenous infusions of valine$_5$-angiotensin II in human volunteers (cited by TOBIAN) (*38*). We have now completed this study in seven healthy male medical students and, in addition to urinary aldosterone, we have determined in four of them the daily excretion of cortisone, cortisol, their tetrahydro-derivatives and the tetrahydro-aldosterone.

These subjects were maintained on a fixed sodium and potassium intake (102 and 90 mEq/day respectively) for a period of 5 to 6 days prior to and during the whole experimental period. Control infusions of glucose 5% were given to 5 subjects. Six experiments were performed with intravenous angiotensin infusions, two with nor-epinephrine and two with neo-synephrine infusions. These pressor substances were diluted in 5% glucose and infused for 7 to 14 hrs at a rate sufficient to maintain a constant elevation of diastolic blood pressure of at least 30 to 40 mm Hg above control levels for the duration of the infusion.

Urines were collected on each day. When infusions were given, they were collected for the period of the infusion and again separately for the rest of the 24-hr period. All experiments were started

---

[1] Unrestricted diet.

[2] NOWACZYNSKI, KOIW and GENEST's procedure.

[3] PETERSON's modification of SILBER-PORTER.

after at least 5 days' equilibration period on a fixed sodium and potassium intake under metabolic balance conditions.

Control infusions of glucose 5% for 8-hr periods did not produce any significant increases in urinary aldosterone during or following the infusions.

The overall effects of the valine[5]-angiotensin II infusions on urinary aldosterone of normal male volunteers are shown in Table 7. In the subjects studied, we observe a 2 to 10-fold increase in urinary aldosterone during and immediately following the angiotensin infusions. This increase can persist for one to two days after the infusions.

Table 7. *Effects of i.v. valine$_5$-angiotensin II infusions in normal male volunteers*[1]

Patients	Dose of Angiotensin	Aldosterone[2] (μg/day)			
		Day 1	Day 2		Day 3
			Angiotension infusion	Post-Angiotensin Infusion	
J. M.	2 mg/14 hrs	14	52	69	68
R. A. 1.	3.1 mg/ 7 hrs	10	14	47	
R. A. 2.	3.4 mg/13 hrs	11	105	98	28
F. M.	1.2 mg/ 8 hrs	19	32	42	23
J.-P. D.	0.9 mg/ 7 hrs	5	36	27	16
H. N.	0.9 mg/12 hrs	23	84	29	25

The results of the daily excretion of urinary cortisol, cortisone and their tetrahydro derivatives are given in Table 8. They show in three subjects a very slight but consistent rise of 20 to 100% in the sum of these steroids above control levels. The slight rise comes mostly from the increase in the values for the tetrahydrocortisone zone, which includes also those of tetrahydro-aldosterone. Subsequent separation of the latter indicates that it accounts for part of this rise and that its urinary levels follow closely those of aldosterone in the patients studied. Only once did the values of the 17-hydroxycorticosteroids rise slightly above the upper limits of the normal range. This order of magnitude of rise, in terms of physiological significance, is small in comparison to that of urinary aldosterone during and following the angiotensin infusion.

In subject R. A., the angiotensin infusion (3.4 mg/13 hrs) was accompanied and followed immediately by a marked sodium retention, a 10-fold increase in urinary aldosterone, and smaller

---

[1] On fixed Na and K intake (102 and 90 mEq/day, respectively).

[2] Nowaczynski, Koiw and Genest's procedure.

Table 8. *Effect of i.v. infusions of angiotensin and nor-epinephrine in normal male subjects*[1]

	Urinary excretion							
	K^2	Na^2	Aldo-sterone[3]	Cortisol[3]	Corti-sone[3]	Tetrahydro-cortisol[3]	Tetrahydro-cortisone[3]	Sum of "F" + "E" THF + THE mg/day
R. A. 22 yr								
Day 1 — Control	84	85	11	70	133	3017	1407	4.6
Day 2 — Angiotensin infusion (3.4 mg/13 hrs)	78	31	105	218	227	2382	6792	9.6
Post-infusion period	46	23	98	444	133	907	2129	3.6
Day 3 — Control	90	108	28	125	153	3744	1815	5.8
Day 4 — Control	75	78	19	180	74	2099	803	3.2
Day 5 — Nor-epinephrine infusions (6.3 mg/7 hrs)	60	230	41	508	511	2348	3259	6.6
Post-infusion period	65	26	26	106	246	990	1445	2.8
J. M. 26 yr								
Day 1 — Control	39	39	14	210	89	1229	790	2.3
Day 2 — Angiotensin infusion (2 mg/13.6 hrs)	81	14	52	248	97	1916	1357	3.6
Post-infusion period	73	12	69	102	137	3752	2358	6.3
Day 3 — Control	48	35	68	193	197	3989	3404	7.8
J. P. D. 21 yr								
Day 1 — Control	67	58	5	107	140	1024	1768	3.0
Day 2 — Angiotensin infusion (0.9 mg/7.3 hrs)	50	6	36	218	249	931	1852	3.2
Post-infusion period	69	31	27	93	85	699	966	1.8
Day 3 — Control	95	39	16	229	197	1954	1162	3.5
H. N. 23 yr								
Day 1 — Control	75	53	23	85	183	2199	1806	4.3
Day 2 — Angiotensin infusion (0.9 mg/12.4 hrs)	70	16	84	137	311	876	3955	5.3
Post-infusion period	44	6	29	117	291	585	1211	2.2
Day 3 — Control	74	88	25	141	239	3317	912	4.6

[1] On a fixed Na and K intake (102 and 90 mEq/day, respectively).
[2] mEq/day.
[3] Micrograms/day.

increases in cortisol, cortisone and tetrahydro-cortisone (including tetrahydro-aldosterone). The sum of these corticosteroids went up from 4.6 to 9.6 mg/day. The nor-epinephrine infusion (6.3 mg/ 7 hrs) provoked a very marked natriuresis and a significant rise in

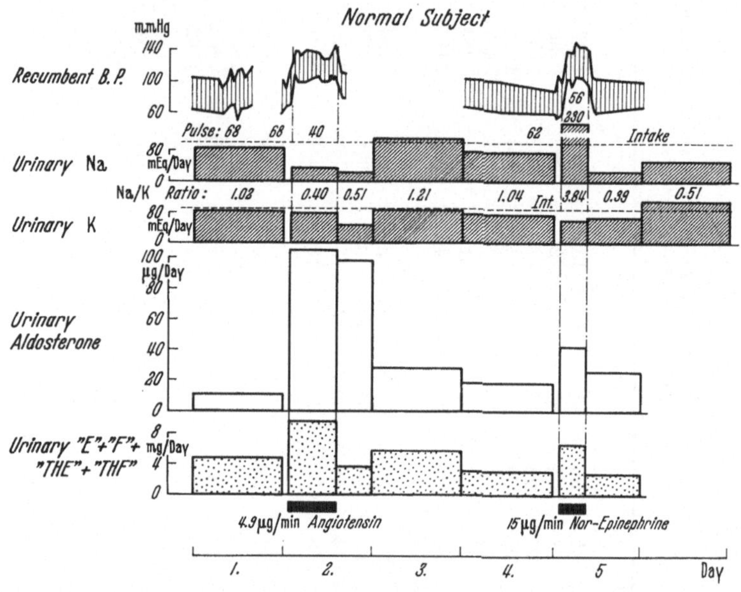

Fig. 5. Note the response in urinary sodium, Na/K ratio, aldosterone and the sum of 17-hydroxycorticosteroids to infusions of angiotensin and nor-epinephrine. Despite similar increases in blood pressure, aldosterone increased only 2-fold during nor-epinephrine infusion in contrast to the 10-fold and more persistent rise produced by angiotensin

aldosterone, cortisol, cortisone and tetrahydro-cortisone. Again, the sum of the 17-hydroxycorticosteroids rose from 3.2 to 6.6 mg/ day. These results are illustrated graphically in Fig. 5.

Another experiment (Fig. 6) was performed on the same subject, who received a control infusion of 5% glucose (8 hrs) and a second infusion of angiotensin (3.1 mg/7 hrs). No change in urinary aldosterone is observed during the glucose infusion, but the angio-tensin administration is accompanied by a marked sodium retention and followed by a large increase in aldosterone.

In subject J. M., the angiotensin infusion (2 mg/14 hrs) (Fig. 7) is accompanied and followed by a severe sodium retention and a very marked increase in urinary aldosterone persisting the day after. The sum of the 17-hydroxycorticosteroids rose progressively from 2.3 to 7.8 mg/day.

A neo-synephrine infusion (40 mg/8 hrs), the results of which are illustrated in Fig. 8, provoked a marked fall in urinary aldosterone with a pronounced natriuresis. This patient also received a nor-epinephrine infusion, but unfortunately an accident happen-

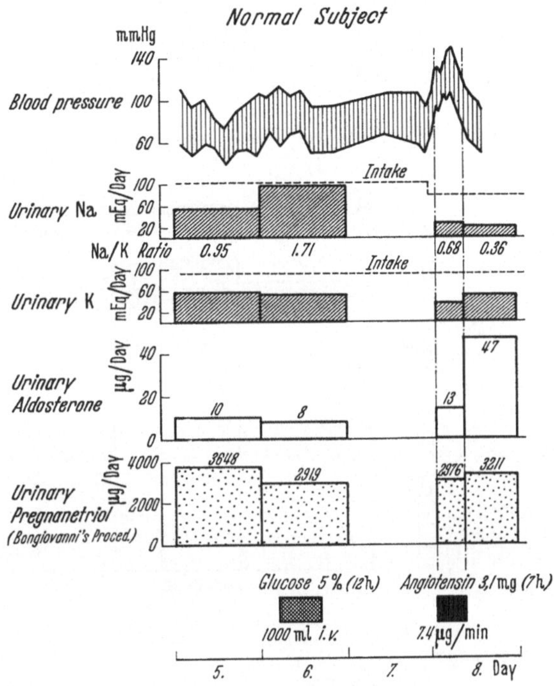

Fig. 6. Same subject as for Fig. 5. No effect of the glucose infusion on aldosterone. But a marked rise occurs immediately following the angiotensin infusion. No change occurs in urinary pregnanetriol

ed during extraction of this urine aliquot and aldosterone determination is not available.

Another subject, a hyper-reactor with blood pressure readings occasionally above 150/90 mm Hg, received a neo-synephrine infusion (48 mg/8 hrs). The urinary aldosterone before, during, immediately after and on the following day was 26, 12, 17 and 12 µg/day, respectively. Sodium excretion went up from a control level of 60 to 274 mEq/day during the neo-synephrine infusion. This patient did not show any change in urinary aldosterone during a control glucose 5% infusion.

These experiments establish that angiotensin has a strong and quite selective trophic effect on aldosterone excretion. Its effect on urinary "glucocorticoids" is very slight and probably not significant. They bring direct evidence of a definite correlation in humans

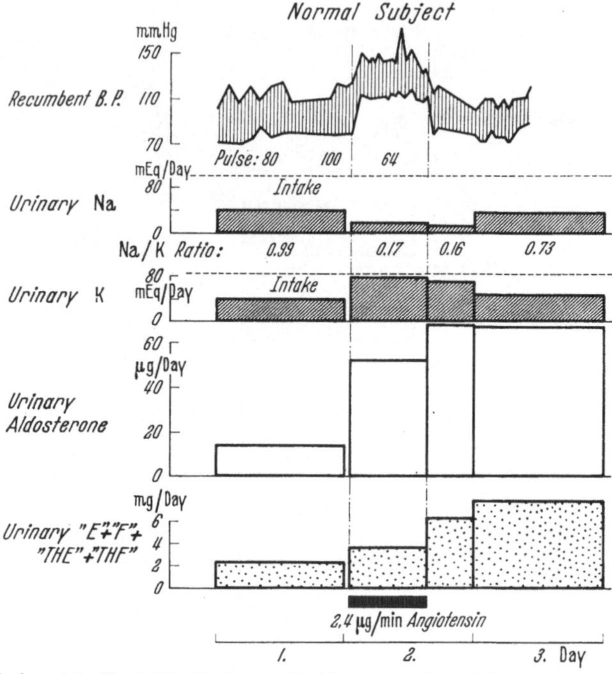

Fig. 7. As for subject R. A. (Fig. 5), it seems that the more prolonged the angiotensin infusion, the more marked and persistent the increase in urinary aldosterone coinciding with a severe sodium retention and a fall of the Na/K ratio

between the adrenal zona glomerulosa and angiotensin. They therefore confirm the experimental data of Tobian (*40*) and Hartroft (*34, 43, 44, 45, 46*) and are quite in accordance with the concept of Gross (*47*). Tobian and Hartroft's groups have demonstrated in rats and dogs a parallel relationship between width of adrenal zona glomerulosa secreting aldosterone and granularity of renal juxta-glomerular cells elaborating renin or a renin-like substance, in response to changes in blood pressure and in sodium or potassium intake. The findings of Deane and Masson (*33*), confirmed recently by Hartroft et al. (*34*), establish that renin administration produces a marked increase in width of the adrenal zona glomerulosa.

The stimulatory effect of angiotensin on aldosterone appears quite marked and specific. Such effect was noted only once (a 2-fold rise) in 7 experiments with nor-epinephrine and not with neo-synephrine. The increase in urinary aldosterone is probably not

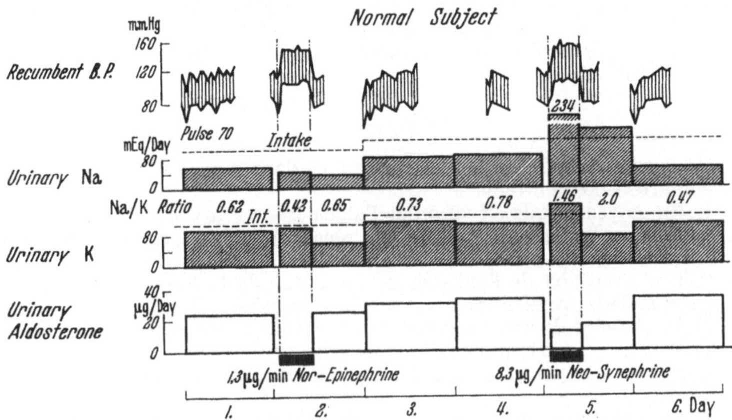

Fig. 8. Note the opposite effect of neo-synephrine infusion on urinary sodium and aldosterone as compared to that of angiotension noted in the previous Fig.

the result of the induced hypertensive state, since it is not encountered with neo-synephrine and nor-epinephrine (with the one exception), although similar increases in blood pressure were achieved. Since some experimental data suggest that hyperfunction of the adrenal zona glomerulosa is accompanied by increased granularity of juxta-glomerular cells and renin content of kidneys, it would be of the utmost interest to determine plasma angiotensin in patients with proven primary hyper-aldosteronism. Studies are actually under way in our laboratory to do simultaneous determinations of blood angiotensin, urinary aldosterone, pregnanetriol and pregnanetriol/aldosterone ratio in hypertensive patients.

Summary

These studies in normal subjects and patients with various types of arterial hypertension show: 1) a mean increase in urinary aldosterone in groups of patients with essential, renal and malignant hypertension as compared to that of normal subjects; 2) an excretion of aldosterone above normal limits in 43% of patients with essential hypertension; 3) an excessive fluctuation in daily urinary aldosterone in patients with arterial hypertension, especially in the early phase of the disease, as compared to normal subjects similarly studied; 4) a mean decrease in urinary pregnanetriol in patients with essential, renal and malignant hypertension as compared to that of normal subjects; 5) a highly significant decrease in pregnanetriol/aldosterone ratio in 92% of all hypertensive patients studied; 6) a significant hypotensive effect of progesterone in 7 patients with arterial hypertension. This effect does not appear to be related to natriuresis; 7) a marked and specific trophic effect of valine$_5$-angiotensin II on urinary aldosterone excretion.

These studies bring definite evidence of abnormalities in adrenal cortical secretion and provide direct evidence of a correlation between the adrenal zona glomerulosa secreting aldosterone, sodium regulation and the renal juxta-glomerular apparatus responsible for the elaboration of renin or of a renin-like substance.

Résumé

Ces études faites chez le sujet normal et dans différents types d'hypertension artérielle montrent:

1. En moyenne, une élévation de l'aldostérone urinaire chez les malades présentant une hypertension essentielle, rénale ou maligne, comparativement aux chiffres des sujets normaux.

2. Une excrétion de l'aldostérone au-dessus de la limite normale chez 43% des malades présentant une hypertension essentielle.

3. De grandes fluctuations dans l'élimination quotidienne d'aldostérone chez les malades avec hypertension essentielle, en particulier au stade précoce de la maladie, comparativement aux sujets normaux étudiés dans les mêmes conditions.

4. En moyenne, une diminution de pregnanetriol urinaire chez les malades présentant une hypertension essentielle, rénale ou maligne, comparativement aux sujets normaux.

5. Une diminution particulièrement significative du rapport pregnanetriol/aldostérone chez 92% de tous les hypertendus étudiés.

6. Un net effet hypotenseur de la progestérone chez 7 hypertendus. Cet effet ne semble pas être en rapport avec la natriurèse.

7. L'accroissement spécifique et prononcé de l'élimination urinaire de l'aldostérone par la valine$_5$-angiotensine II.

Ces études démontrent clairement des troubles de la sécrétion cortico-surrénale et supportent l'existence d'une corrélation entre la zone glomérulaire de la surrénale sécrétant l'aldostérone, la régulation du sodium et le système rénal juxta-glomérulaire, affecté à la formation de la rénine oud'une substance analogue.

Acknowledgements

It is a pleasure to acknowledge the valuable collaboration of Drs. Gilles Pigeon, Jean Davignon, Joffre Brouillet, and Jacques Trudel, Medical Research Fellows of the National Research Council, Ottawa, Canada, and of Dr. Camille Dufault, Research Fellow; of Misses Fernande Salvail, Renée Dansereau, Françoise Vaillancourt and Pierrette Bourque, R. N.; and Mrs. Anne Brossard, Misses Henriette Gilbert and Françoise Martin, dietitians; of Misses Isabelle Morin, Alice Laflamme Pauline Robinson, and Lucienne Monette, medial technologists; of Mr. Roland Paquette, Chief Statistician, Ayerst, McKenna & Harrison, Montreal, for statistical help and advice.

The authors acknowledge with gratitude the generous gifts of d,l-aldosterone, free-alcohol and acetate and of synthetic valine$_5$-angiotensin II from Dr. Franz Gross and Walter Murphy, of the CIBA Company, Basle and

Montreal; of pregnane 3α, 17α, 20α-triol from Dr. ALFRED BONGIOVANNI, Philadelphia, and Dr. NORMAN BRINK, Merck & Company, Rahway; of progesterone from Dr. WALTER MURPHY, CIBA Company, Montreal, and Dr. MICHAEL MIKULASCHEK, Lilly Company, Indianapolis.

References

1. PICKETT, M. T., E. C. KYRIABIDES, M. I. STERN, and L. F. SOMMERVILLE: Lancet (G. B.) **1959/II**, 829.
2. NOWACZYNSKI, W., M. GOLDNER, and J. GENEST: J. Laborat. Clin. Med. (U.S.A.) **45**, 818 (1955).
3. NOWACZYNSKI, W., and E. KOIW: J. Laborat. Clin. Med. (U.S.A.) **49**, 815 (1957).
4. NOWACZYNSKI, W., E. KOIW, and J. GENEST: Canad. J. Biochem. Physiol. **35**, 425 (1957).
5. NOWACZYNSKI, W., E. KOIW, and J. GENEST: J. Clin. Endocr. (U.S.A.) 1960 (in press).
6. GENEST, J., E. KOIW, W. NOWACZYNSKI, and G. LEBOEUF: Proc. Soc. Exper. Biol. Med. (U.S.A.) **97**, 676 (1958).
7. GENEST, J., W. NOWACZYNSKI, E. KOIW, and T. SANDOR: Proc. 4th Intern. Congress of Bioch. Vienna, Sept. 1958. Suppl. Intern. Abstr. Biol. Sci., p. 116.
8. GENEST, J., E. KOIW, W. NOWACZYNSKI, and T. SANDOR: Acta endocr. (Den.) 1960 (in press).
9. WEICHSELBAUM, T. E., and H. W. WARGRAF: J. Clin. Endocr. (U.S.A.) **17**, 959 (1957).
10. ZAFFARONI, A.: J. Amer. Chem. Soc. **72**, 3828 (1950).
11. BERNSTEIN, S., and R. H. LENHARD: J. Org. Chem. (U.S.A.) **19**, 1146 (1954).
12. BERNSTEIN, S., and R. H. LENHARD: J. Org. Chem. (U.S.A.) **19**, 1269 (1954).
13. NOWACZYNSKI, W., and P. STEYERMARK: Arch. Biochem. Physiol. (U.S.A.) **58**, 453 (1955).
14. NOWACZYNSKI, W., and P. STEYERMARK: Canad. J. Biochem. Physiol. **34**, 592 (1956).
15. WILSON, H., and R. FAIRBANKS: Arch. Biochem. Biophys. (U.S.A.) **54**, 440 (1955).
16. BONGIOVANNI, A. M., and W. R. EBERLEIN: Analyt. Chem. (U.S.A.) **30**, 388 (1958).
17. NOWACZYNSKI, W., P. STEYERMARK, E. KOIW, J. GENEST, and R. N. JONES: Canad. J. Biochem. Physiol. **34**, 1023 (1956).
18. GENEST, J., G. LEMIEUX, A. DAVIGNON, E. KOIW, W. NOWACZYNSKI, and P. STEYERMARK: Science (U.S.A.) **123**, 503 (1956).
19. TRONCHETTI, F., G. MUCIO, and R. ROMANELLI: Ann. endocr. (Fr.) **18**, 654 (1957).
20. ROMANELLI, R.: Personal communication, 1960.
21. VENNING, E., I. DYRENFURTH, J. B. DOSSETOR, and J. C. BECK: Paper sent for publication, 1960.
22. LARAGH, J. H., S. ULICK, W. JANUSZEWICZ, Q. B. DEMING, W. G. KELLY, and S. LIEBERMAN: Circulation (U.S.A.) **20**, 725 (1959).
23. DELORME, P., and J. GENEST: Canad. Med. Ass. J. **81**, 893 (1959).
24. KUMAR, D., A. E. D. HALL, R. NAKASHIMA, and A. G. GORNALL: Canad. J. Biochem. Physiol. **35**, 113 (1957).

146   J. Genest, et al.: Adrenocortical function in essential hypertension

25. Gornall, A. G., H. M. Grundy, and C. J. Koladich: Canad. J. Biochem. Physiol. **38**, 43 (1960).
26. Gross, F., P. Loustalot, and R. Meier: Experientia (Switz.) **11**, 67 (1955).
27. Gross, F., P. Loustalot, and R. Meier: Acta endocr. (Den.) **26**, 417 (1957).
28. August, J. T., D. H. Nelson, and G. W. Thorn: J. Clin. Invest. (U.S.A.) **37**, 1549 (1958).
29. Friedman, S. M., M. Nakashima, and C. L. Friedman: Circulation Res. (U.S.A.) **4**, 557 (1956).
30. Friedman, S. M., R. M. Butt, and C. L. Friedman: Amer. J. Physiol. **190**, 507 (1957).
31. Friedman, S. M., C. L. Friedman, and M. Nakashima: Circulation Res. (U.S.A.) **5**, 261 (1957).
32. Tobian, L., and A. Fox: J. Clin. Invest. (U.S.A.) **35**, 297 (1956).
33. Deane, H. W., and G. M. C. Masson: J. Clin. Endocr. (U.S.A.) **11**, 193 (1951).
34. Hartroft, P. M., L. N. Newmark, and J. A. Pitcock: In: Hypertension. Ed.: J. Moyer. Saunders 1959, p. 24.
35. Genest, J., E. Koiw, W. Nowaczynski, and T. Sandor: Abstract. Proc. 32nd Session Amer. Heart Ass. Oct. 1959, Philadelphia. Also published in Circulation (U.S.A.) **20**, 700 (1959).
36. Landau, R. L., and K. Lugibihl: J. Clin. Endocr. (U.S.A.) **18**, 1237 (1958).
37. Armstrong, J. G.: Proc. Soc. Exper. Biol. Med. (U.S.A.) **102**, 452 (1959).
38. Genest, J.: Paper sent for publication.
39. Peterson, R. E., A. Karrer, and S. L. Guerra: Analyt. Chem. (U.S.A.) **29**, 144 (1957).
40. Tobian, L.: Ann. Int. Med. (U.S.A.) **52**, 395 (1960).
41. Tobian, L., and J. Binion: Circulation (U.S.A.) **5**, 754 (1952).
42. Tobian, L., and J. Binion: J. Clin. Invest. (U.S.A.) **37**, 1407 (1954).
43. Hartroft, P. M., and W. S. Hartroft: J. Exper. Med. (U.S.A.) **97**, 415 (1953).
44. Hartroft, P. M., and W. S. Hartroft: J. Exper. Med. (U.S.A.) **102**, 205 (1955).
45. Pitcock, J. A., and P. M. Hartroft: Amer. J. Path. **34**, 863 (1958).
46. Pitcock, J. A., P. M. Hartroft, and L. N. Newmark: Proc. Soc. Exper. Biol. Med. (U.S.A.) **100**, 868 (1959).
47. Gross, F.: Klin. Wschr. (G.) **1958/II**, 693.

The significance of hyperaldosteronuria in hypertension

By

J. WARTER, J. SCHWARTZ and R. BLOCH

In 1913, VAQUEZ referred three hypertensive patients to DELBET for adrenalectomy, which the patients failed to survive. At that time, the aim of adrenalectomy was primarily medullectomy. VAQUEZ had in fact just previously emphasised the atherogenic, in addition to the hypertensive, role of adrenaline. Later, between 1925 and 1930 and as a result of the work of RENÉ LERICHE, adrenalectomy came into its own again at the same time as neurosurgical interventions on the sympathetic system and greater splanchnic nerve were beginning to be performed. However, in those days adrenalectomy was still only unilateral and its effectiveness doubtful.

With the discovery of adrenocortical hormones, the problem took on a new aspect, the role of the catechol amines being henceforth reduced in importance. With the aid of adrenocortical hormones it is easy to reproduce hypertensive disease. Moreover, "metacorticoid" hypertension is bound up with mechanisms involved in hypertension of renal origin. In 1942, GOLDBLATT demonstrated that adrenocortical insufficiency reduces the output of hypertensinogen whereas desoxycorticosterone stimulates it (HELMER, 1951).

After 1945 interest in adrenalectomy for the treatment of arterial hypertension revived; thanks to FONTAINE in France, unilateral adrenalectomy was now superseded by bilateral and subtotal resection of the adrenals. Finally, the failure of extensive thoracolumbar sympathectomies and splanchnicectomies led to the introduction of total adrenalectomy as elaborated by BLAKEMORE in the U.S.A., among others; despite the gravity of this operation, in certain cases it appears to yield more lasting results than even the more radical forms of sympathectomy.

Meanwhile, however, the conception that essential hypertension involved an adrenocortical factor was still based on very tenuous evidence. But in 1955 came CONN's description of primary hyperaldosteronism with arterial hypertension as its major symptom. The occurrence of this hyperaldosteronism was confirmed

10*

Table 1

Case	B.P.	Duration of hypertension	Renal disease	Eyegrounds	Retropneumo-peritoneum	Plasma electro-lytes mg/litre Na+	K+	Sodium intake	Aldosterone (γ/24 h.)
K. Roger 37 years	150/100 to 180/110	1 year	none	normal	normal	3.37	0.201	moderate normal	30 8
B. Gilbert	140/190 to 200/120	2 years	tuberculosis ? Functions normal	normal			0.185	moderate	10 and 7
K. Alice 44 years	260/160 to 300/180		+++	pronounced retinitis		3.15 to 2.59	0.101 to 0.222	moderate	18
E. Emile 57 years	240/150 to 270/170		+++			3.15	0.156	moderate	13
M. François	190/100 to 200/100		none					normal	20
H. Charles 47 years	200/100 to 240/100		+++					normal	16
M. Charles 46 years	250/150 to 310/190		polycystic kidneys		adrenals enlarged			normal	10
R. Joseph 43 years	230/120		none					normal	10
E. Berthe	210/130 to 270/150		none		normal	3.31	0.190	moderate	16 and 6
B. Joseph 56 years	185/110	6 years	none					normal	18

G. Emile 53 years	240/130	6 years	none					moderate	13
B. Pierre 36 years	175/100		none			3.20	0.144	moderate	36.3 and 16
B. Florence 53 years	270/130		lithiasis			3.13 to 2.92	0.203 0.199	moderate	22 and 4
B. Josette 22 years	200/100 to 240/160	7 years	+++		normal	2.99 to 3.24	0.222 to 0.187	moderate	14
D. Marlyse 16 years	170/120 to 220/160	3 years	bifid ureters; functions normal				0.203 to 0.152	normal	1.60 and 6
M. Emile	180/120 to 240/120	10 years	+			3.20	0.117 to 0.184	normal	12
P. Alice 41 years	220/120 to 250/140	6 years	++	vascular sclerosis	normal	3.15 to 3.36	0.119 to 0.163	normal	40.4 and 4
S. Roger 25 years	180/120 to 240/150	2 years	+	pronounced retinitis	normal		0.129 to 0.186	moderate	10
Z. Hélène 47 years	140/80 to 240/110	10 years	none	vascular sclerosis			0.188	moderate	25
W. Eugène 45 years	170/100 to 280/140	1 year	none		right adrenal enlarged	3.22	0.163 to 0.188	moderate	10
B. Dolorès 28 years	145/90 to 240/160	3 years	+	normal	normal	3.24	0.171	moderate	15
H. Alice	210/170	3 years	none	normal	normal	3.02 to 2.99	0.161 to 0.188	normal	20

by analysing the urinary excretion of aldosterone — an analysis which physicochemical techniques were soon to render comparatively easy. In the same year, SKELTON found that by performing nephrectomy and adrenalectomy on one side and a simple adrenal enucleation on the other he could consistently produce permanent hypertension in rats. In this instance, the hypertension is linked up with the process of regeneration of the enucleated adrenal; this type of hypertension is eminently suitable for studying the adrenocortical factors involved.

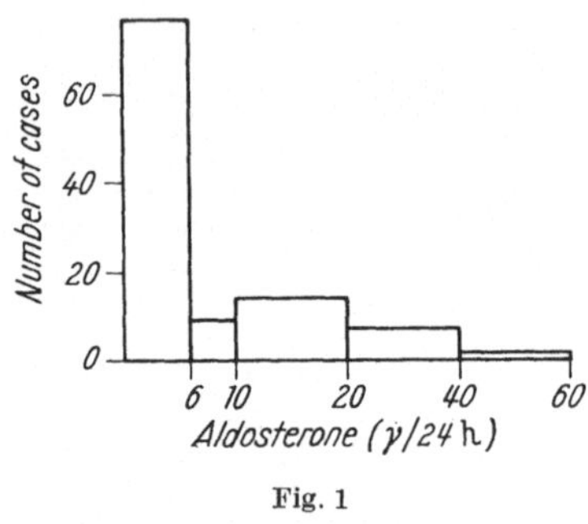

Fig. 1

It is a fact — and one of major significance — that essential hypertension is quite often accompanied by hyperaldosteronuria. As far back as 1956, GENEST stressed the importance of a certain degree of hyperaldosteronuria in essential hypertension. Our own results confirm the frequency of hyperaldosteronuria in hypertensive subjects (Table 1, Fig. 1).

Using the technique of NEHER and WETTSTEIN, we have in fact discovered hyperaldosteronuria in 30 out of 103 patients (6 to 10 γ/24 hrs in 8 cases, and 10 to 60 γ/24 hrs in a further 22).

However, neither the clinical picture (blood pressure, renal exploration) nor the biological data (potassaemia, natraemia, catechol amines, 17-ketosteroids, etc.) revealed any difference between these cases of hypertension and those in which the urinary excretion of aldosterone was normal. In none of the patients with hyperaldosteronuria did the hypertension present any clinical or biochemical signs characteristic of an excess of electrolyte-regulating hormones, although in 5 instances the blood potassium concentration was reduced while the alkali reserve remained normal. Admittedly, 5 of the patients exhibited marked signs of renal disorder (albuminuria, very high diastolic pressure, azotaemia on the upper limits of the normal range), but on the other hand the urinary excretion of aldosterone was normal in other cases of hypertension complicated by similar renal manifestations.

In contrast to COTTIER, we have never encountered hypoaldosteronuria, although it is true that the technique of NEHER and WETTSTEIN makes it difficult to be dogmatic on this point.

Thus, in 29% of our cases, arterial hypertension was associated with manifest hyperaldosteronuria. The latter, however, is not permanent: in the 5 cases in which we were able to keep a check on the urinary aldosterone excretion under the same regimen (though, admittedly, at prolonged intervals), we noted considerable fluctuations (for example, 16 and 6, 36 and 3 γ/24 hrs). Repeated urinanalyses would thus probably reveal a considerably higher incidence of hyperaldosteronuria in the course of hypertension, since in certain cases the hyperaldosteronuria is no doubt intermittent; the same applies to CONN's syndrome.

This hyperaldosteronuria was found on 14 out of 30 occasions in patients subjected to a fairly low-salt diet; their dietary regimen still included a minimum allowance of 80 mEq. of sodium daily; we were able to confirm that with this amount of sodium no rise in the urinary aldosterone concentration occurs in normal subjects at rest. The other patients were kept on a normal diet. The variations in aldosterone excretion in response to sodium restriction in hypertensive patients would appear to call for a careful study, which so far does not seem to have been undertaken.

The hyperaldosteronuria occurring in such cases is a sign of increased aldosterone secretion. We have carried out loading tests

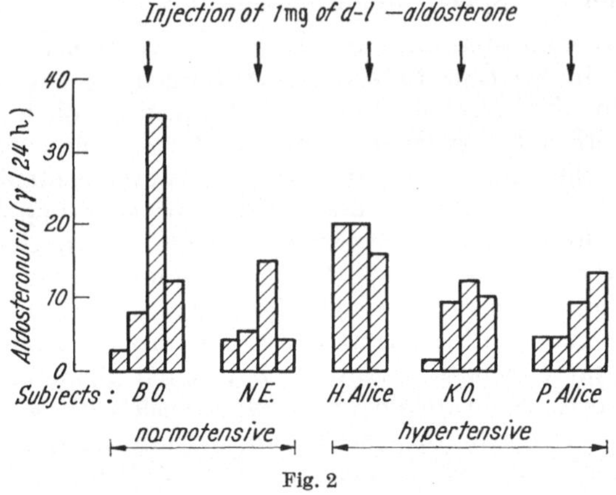

Fig. 2

with DL-aldosterone (a single intramuscular injection of 1,000 γ) and studied the catabolism of this hormone in 5 cases involving normal or hypertensive subjects. In the 24 hrs following the injection, from 1.2 to 2.7% of the injected aldosterone was recovered in the urine of the normal subjects; in the hypertensives the amount recovered was smaller, i. e. 0, 0.8, and 1% in the 3 cases investigated by us (Fig. 2). Our results not only confirm what had already been implied, namely that essential hypertension is frequently associated with hypersecretion of aldosterone, but they also suggest that aldosterone secretion is even greater in these cases than the urinary aldosterone concentration would appear to indicate. These conclusions tie up to some extent with those reached by LARAGH. According to this author, who uses a technique based on isotopic dilution, the patient with benign hypertension has an aldosterone secretion of 175 to 335 γ per day (within normal limits), whereas in the hypertensive with renal or vascular lesions the daily secretion works out at 450 to 1,690 γ; in cases of malignant hypertension, the figure varies between 520 and 2,750 γ. These results, however, conflict with our own as regards one point: according to LARAGH, hyperaldosteronuria is a sign peculiar to severe hypertension.

Routine adrenocortical exploration (17-ketosteroids, formaldehydogenic steroids, dehydro-iso-androsterone), on the other hand, never reveals any significant anomaly. True, the 17-ketosteroid and dehydro-iso-androsterone levels are often subnormal; but the variations in the ratio between aldosterone and dehydro-iso-androsterone are not significant.

The hyperaldosteronism occurring in hypertension must be considered in relation to certain anatomicopathological modifications in the adrenal, consisting frequently of hyperplasia together with subcapsular adenomatous formations composed of fascicular cells. Such changes, which are quite common in the adrenals of elderly subjects, appear to be of some importance in the young hypertensive. Experiments have shown that hypertension of the GOLDBLATT type, like renin administration, produces similar abnormalities in the adrenal cortex. DEANE and MASSON have treated rats with renin and have also provoked renal hypertension in rats: in both instances, they noted glomerular hyperplasia proportional to the degree of hypertension; these structural modifications are invariably encountered in the animals, irrespective of the size of their salt intake. This is a particularly important point, since it is known that in normal animals glomerular hyperplasia develops only when the salt intake is restricted, whereas an excess of salt leads to glomerular hypoplasia.

Though these anatomical changes of the adrenal cortex appear to go hand in hand with hyperaldosteronism, their precise significance is still the subject of controversy.

I. Arterial hypertension with hyperaldosteronism and CONN's syndrome

This hyperaldosteronism certainly seems to contrast readily with the hyperaldosteronism occurring in CONN's syndrome. But, according to CONN himself, experience over the last five years shows that primary hyperaldosteronism appears in its classic guise in less than 30% of cases: only the hypertension is invariable, although it is not always as benign as CONN originally assumed. On the contrary, in certain authenticated cases, it has taken the form of real malignant hypertension with papilloedema and hypertensive retinopathy. The arterial hypertension of CONN's syndrome is not accompanied merely by mild albuminuria, but may well be complicated by severe renal manifestations. The tubular disease associated with potassium depletion is complicated in a certain number of cases by nephro-angiosclerosis and even more often by pyelonephritis. The very frequency with which such renal complications occur suggests that the hypertension in CONN's syndrome may also be bound up with a renal mechanism.

The picture of hypertension provoked by primary aldosteronism is thus liable to afford comparatively few clues. Moreover, the biochemical criteria themselves may also prove unreliable: the blood potassium concentration may remain normal despite repeated determinations, and in certain cases the urinary aldosterone excretion may be within normal limits when measured on successive occasions. Incidentally, the anatomical data are also variable: in 15% of cases of CONN's syndrome, the adrenocortical adenoma is not confined to one adrenal only, and there is thus quite a considerable chance of encountering a case in which the contralateral adrenal is also adenomatous; in 9% of cases, only slight thickening of the adrenal cortex occurs, associated with simple hyperplasia. Finally, in 6% of cases, the appearance of the adrenals remains normal. Even surgical intervention does not always seem to prove decisive: in 25% of cases, the blood pressure shows a marked decline following the operation but fails to revert to normal levels. In 15% of cases, the blood pressure merely drops for a few weeks and then steadily rises again until it reaches the levels recorded prior to surgery.

Though there is still a fundamental difference between primary hyperaldosteronism and the hyperaldosteronism associated with essential hypertension, it cannot be denied that today the outlines of CONN's syndrome have become somewhat indistinct — as witnessed, for example, by the following case. A 44-year-old woman had been admitted to hospital suffering from malignant hypertension; biochemical examination revealed hypopotassaemia (2.5 mEq. per litre) on three successive occasions. Despite the absence of any other humoral disorder, measurement of the urinary aldosterone excretion yielded a figure of 18 γ per 24 hrs. The patient subsequently died suddenly and, when a post-mortem examination was performed, bilateral adenomatous hyperplasia of the adrenals was discovered together with partial stenosis of the right renal artery. In such a case, the clinical and biological data do not enable one to determine the precise nature of the hypertensive disease in question: only an anatomical examination could reveal its renal origin. A number of other observations in cases of primary hyperaldosteronism seem to us to involve similar ambiguity. Conn acknowledges that primary hyperaldosteronism is frequently overlooked; on the other hand, it must now also be recognised that certain of the cases diagnosed as primary hyperaldosteronism are simply cases of essential hypertension with hyperaldosteronuria.

Moreover, it is by no means easy to account for the hypertension occurring in Conn's syndrome. Aldosterone itself has only

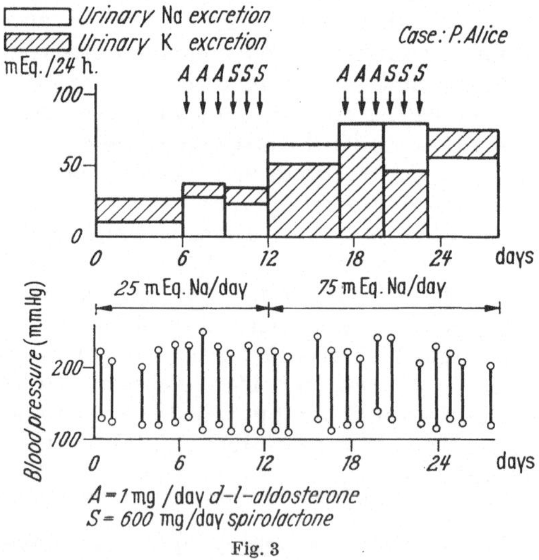

Fig. 3

a mild hypertensive effect. In patients with Addison's disease, treatment with large doses of aldosterone normalises the blood pressure but does not cause hypertension: the effects of aldosterone differ from those of DOCA. In rats sensitised by unilateral nephrectomy, GROSS observed arterial hypertension only when he injected 500 γ of DL-aldosterone daily for 4 weeks by the sub-cutaneous route. GAUNT, on the other hand, noted no signs of hypertension whatever when he administered the same dose (500 γ) to intact rats over a period of 7 months. In man, THORN has shown that a load of aldosterone amounting to 6,000 γ daily for 22 days provokes a rise in blood pressure of only 10 to 22 mm Hg.

It may be that in CONN's syndrome aldosterone provokes hypertension only in the presence of renal lesions, either pre-existing or secondary to the very slow potassium depletion to which aldosterone leads. Another problem is that of the sensitivity of the renal tubule to aldosterone in the hypertensive subject — an aspect which deserves to be studied in greater detail: in one hypertensive patient, administration of 1,000 γ of aldosterone on each of three successive days had no apparent effect on either the blood pressure or the electrolyte balance (Fig. 3).

II. Interpretation of hyperaldosteronuria in essential hypertension

A. The hyperaldosteronuria occurring in essential hypertension is neither constant nor associated with the biochemical manifestations peculiar to CONN's syndrome in its classic form. While it is true that relative hyperaldosteronuria, of the kind suggested by GENEST, may be found — on the basis of an analysis of the ratio between urinary aldosterone and pregnanetriol — in almost every case of essential hypertension, this fact can be variously interpreted: in all deficiency states, the urinary 17-ketosteroid excretion also diminishes, and we have seen that there was no correlation between the dehydro-iso-androsterone and the aldosterone levels in the urine.

But, in fact, this hyperaldosteronism might be bound up with a more complex cortical disorder. Aldosterone is not the only adrenocortical hormone exerting a regulatory action on the electrolytes. Indeed, since the work done by PRADER, a great variety of studies have been devoted to research on a natriuretic factor, though no final conclusions have emerged. In this connection, however, two points should be borne in mind, which emphasise the complexity of the problems involved and the gaps in our knowledge:

Firstly, the corticosteroids such as cortisone and hydrocortisone have a diphasic action on sodium excretion in adrenalectomised animals, i. e. they first cause sodium retention and then sodium diuresis. The intensity and duration of each of the two phases depend, among other things, on the dosage.

Secondly, hardly anything is known about the competitive action of the various steroid hormones. At present we have only a very rough outline of antagonistic hormonal actions and agents. There may even be some doubt as to whether such antagonisms really exist: in normal subjects, for example, we found that an excess of progesterone, administered intravenously, had only a doubtful sodium-excreting effect.

PERERA has suggested that a diminution in glucocorticoid secretion might play a role in the pathogenesis of essential hypertension; but the steroid balances yield no reliable confirmation for such an assumption. COOPER, however, has noted an *in vitro* decrease in corticoidogenesis, which he thinks may be a function of the degree of diastolic hypertension: he suggests that the synthesis of hydrocortisone is more strongly affected than that of corticosterone-type compounds. COOPER concludes that in the course of arterial hypertension, a progressive diminution in 17-hydroxydation occurs.

On the other hand, STURTEVANT has observed that SC-5233 prevents the development of the hypertension associated with adrenocortical regeneration. SC-5233 has an antagonistic action on the mineralocorticoids secreted by the adrenal in process of regeneration, but it may be that its effect on the blood pressure is independent of this action; a "nor-" derivative of SC-5233 endowed with a much more pronounced aldosterone-antagonising action does not display the same hypotensive effect.

The hyperaldosteronism of the hypertensive patient may perhaps be part of a more complex cortical disorder whose importance, however, cannot yet be determined.

B. The variable nature of the hyperaldosteronism and the adrenocortical lesions encountered in the hypertensive contrasts with the consistency of the disorders affecting electrolyte metabolism. Now aldosterone is primarily an electrolyte-regulating hormone. As a factor involved in sodium retention, its secretion depends first and foremost upon variations in the sodium intake and upon the amounts of sodium lost. According to currently accepted theories, sodium influences the secretion of aldosterone by means of alterations in the extra-cellular fluid volumes; and in the hypertensive, the extra-cellular spaces, the volume of blood, and N^{24} and K^{42} spaces are usually normal.

However, two facts seem to have been established with certainty:

1. The frequent incidence of functional disparity between the two kidneys of hypertensive patients. BALDWIN has, in fact, recently shown that, in 80% of hypertensive subjects, comparative exploration of the two kidneys reveals a significant difference in the sodium fraction reabsorbed in the tubule: thus, there is evidence that a renal disorder occurs very early on in the course of hypertension.

2. After infusion of hypertonic solutions, including saline in particular, hypertensives eliminate more sodium than normotensives. This anomaly is encountered in all forms of hypertension, i.e.:

— essential hypertension with or without signs of renal disease,

— hypertension in Cushing's syndrome (here, in response to an excess of hypertonic serum, water diuresis seems to be decidedly greater than sodium diuresis),

— hypertension associated with primary hyperaldosteronism (ORTUZAR), and

— hypertension persisting after bilateral adrenalectomy in a subject receiving 25 mg cortisone daily by mouth and 5 mg DOCA perlingually.

The consistency of these anomalies in the hypertensive and their disappearance in response to effective anti-hypertensive therapy suggests that they play an important role; despite the controversy to which they have given rise, they appear to be bound up with disorders affecting renal haemodynamics: SELKURT observed them in the isolated kidney when he varied the perfusion pressure.

It is only normal that the hyperaldosteronism occasionally noted in hypertensives should be considered in relation to these facts; however, to regard the two as linked by a chain of cause and effect, is — though tempting — no doubt premature.

Summary

Urinary aldosterone levels were measured in 103 hypertensive patients. Hyperaldosteronuria was found in 30 cases; in 8 cases, the aldosterone level was above 6 γ but less than 10 γ/24 hrs; in 22 cases it was above 10 γ/24 hrs, reaching on one occasion 60 γ/24 hrs. Thus, hyperaldosteronuria was present in 29% of these patients suffering from arterial hypertension; but it is not a specific sign for any of the clinical forms of the disease and is never accompanied by the manifestations characteristic of Conn's syndrome. However, in 5 cases, isolated hypopotassaemia was encountered.

Hyperaldosteronuria in hypertensives poses the problem of differential diagnosis as between primary hyperaldosteronism. Certain cases that have been described under Conn's syndrome are simply instances of arterial hypertension with hyperaldosteronuria.

The hyperaldosteronism occurring in hypertension does not appear to be bound up with a more complex pattern of dyscorticism. The alterations seen in the urinary dehydro-iso-androsterone and 17-ketosteroid concentrations are also met with in all chronic affections. It would appear, on the other hand, that this form of hyperaldosteronism can be related to the enhanced sodium excretion typical of all hypertensive patients.

Résumé

Le dosage de l'aldostérone urinaire a été réalisé chez 103 hypertendus: Dans 30 cas, l'aldostéronurie se révèla élevée; dans 8 cas, elle était supérieure à 6 γ, mais inférieure à 10 γ/24 h; dans 22 cas, elle était supérieure à 10 γ/24 h et atteignait une fois 60 γ/24 h. Une hyperaldostéronurie existe donc dans 29% des cas d'hypertension artérielle; elle n'est pourtant spécifique d'aucune de ses formes cliniques, et ne s'accompagne jamais des manifestations propres au syndrome de CONN. Pourtant, dans 5 cas, une hypokaliémie isolée fut notée.

L'hyperaldostéronurie des hypertendus pose un problème de diagnostic différentiel avec l'hyperaldostéronisme primaire. Certains cas décrits sous le nom de syndrome de CONN ne sont que des hypertensions artérielles avec hyperaldostéronurie.

L'hyperaldostéronisme de l'hypertension artérielle ne semble pas lié à un dyscorticisme plus complexe. Les modifications des taux de la déhydro-iso-androstérone et des 17-cétostéroïdes urinaires se retrouvent dans toute affection chronique. Il semble par contre que l'on puisse rapporter cette forme d'hyperaldostéronisme à l'excrétion sodique exagérée propre à tout hypertendu.

Literature

AUGUST, J. I., D. H. NELSON, and G. W. THORN: J. Clin. Invest. (U.S.A.) **37**, 1549 (1958).

BALDWIN, D. S., W. H. HULET, A. W. BIGGS, E. A. GOMBOS, and H. CHASIS: J. Clin. Invest. (U.S.A.) **39**, 395 (1960).

CONN, J. W.: J. Amer. Med. Ass. **172**, 1650 (1960). — COOPER, D. Y., J. C. TOUCHSTONE, and J. M. ROBERTS: J. Clin. Invest. (U.S.A.) **37**, 1524 (1958). — COTTIER, P., A. F. MÜLLER, and A. SCHMID: Schweiz. med. Wschr. **89**, 376 (1959).

DEANE, G. H., and G. M. C. MASSON: J. Clin. Endocr. (U.S.A.) **11**, 143 (1951).

GABE, I., H. I. JORY, L. MULLIGAN, and J. W. WOOLEN: Amer. J. Med. **28**, 311 (1960). — GAUNT, R., G. I. ULSAMEN, and J. J. CHART: Arch. internat. pharmacodyn. thérap. (Belg.) **110**, 114 (1957). — GENEST, J., E. KOIW, W. NOWACZYNSKI, and T. SANDOR: Circulation (U.S.A.) **20**, 700 (1954). — GROSS, F., P. LOUSTALOT, and R. MEIER: Acta endocr. (Den.) **26**, 417 (1957).

HELMER, O. M., and R. S. GRIFFITH: Fed. Proc. (U.S.A.) **10**, 196 (1951). — HOLLANDER, W., and W. E. JUDSON: J. Clin. Invest. (U.S.A.) **36**, 1460 (1957).

LARAGH, J. H., S. ULICK, W. JANUSZEWICZ, Q. B. DEMRIG, W. G. KELLY, and S. LIEBERMAN: Circulation (U.S.A.) **20**, 725 (1959). — LEWIS, H. A., and H. GOLDBLATT: Bull. N. Y. Acad. Med. **18**, 459 (1942).

ORTUZAR, R., R. CROXATTO, P. THOMSEN, and J. GONZALES: J. Laborat. Clin. Med. (U.S.A.) **54**, 712 (1959).

SELKURT, E. E.: Circulation (U.S.A.) **4**, 541 (1951). — STURTEVANT, F. M.: Endocrinology (U.S.A.) **64**, 299 (1959).

WARTER, J., J. SCHWARTZ, and R. BLOCH: Presse méd. (Fr.) **68**, 5 (1960).

Discussion

REUBI: As the data presented by Dr. GENEST have, I think, been questioned by some other authors, I should like to ask Dr. COTTIER and Dr. MULLER to report briefly on their experience in the determination of aldosterone production in hypertensive patients.

MULLER: I wish to congratulate Dr. GENEST on his work. He has given us some convincing arguments in favour of an increased excretion of aldosterone in hypertensive patients. To my mind, however, it is the increased reactivity of aldosterone in the hypertensive subject which is the most important observation. In a preliminary study we were never impressed by particularly high urinary aldosterone excretion values. Recently we have extended our study by determining the secretion rate of aldosterone in four patients, two with essential hypertension and two with malignant hypertension. We used the procedure described by RALPH E. PETERSON. J. H. LARAGH and his collaborators have done a similar study in 23 hypertensive patients. They found normal values in patients with essential hypertension; however, all but one of their subjects with malignant hypertension showed an increased secretion rate. The authors don't mention in their abstract the urinary sodium levels and the urinary excretion values of aldosterone.

The table shows our results. Except for patient R. V. we find normal secretion rates and they correspond rather well with the urinary sodium excretion on the same day (third column). If we take into consideration the urinary sodium of 110 mEq/24 hrs in the first patient, his secretion rate is relatively high. The fourth and fifth columns illustrate the urinary excretion

Table

Name, age, diagnosis	Body weight kg	Aldosterone secretion μg/24 h	Urinary Na excretion mEq/24 h	Aldosterone excretion μg/24 h	Urinary Na excretion mEq/24 h	Na space per l	Na_e per kg body weight
R. V. ♂ 20, Ess. hypert.	53	577	110	5.9	103	16	41
R. M. ♂ 56, Ess. hypert.	86	286	142	6.0	176	18	30
I. J. ♂ 38, Mal. hypert.	56	298	158	6.3	134	16	40
R. L. ♂ 49, Mal. hypert.	78	263	202	12.3	234	23	41

of aldosterone and sodium on the day preceding the measurement of the secretion rates. The correlations between secretion and excretion of aldosterone are not always perfect. We further looked for a correlation between aldosterone and total exchangeable sodium; again it was not possible to find such a correlation and the values are within the normal range[1].

DAHL: Dr. RALPH PETERSON of the New York Hospital has made measurements of aldosterone secretion in a variety of patients. I think it is of interest that the highest values which he has found, about 3000 γ per day, have occurred not in association with primary aldosteronism or a state associated with hypertension, but rather with such states as cirrhosis and heart failure.

PEART: Apart from knowledge about the increased rate of secretion, of course, I'd want to know about blood level, because this might be a more important factor. It is always a worry to me that so much emphasis is placed on urinary excretion, instead of total exchange. I know that blood level measurements are difficult. When one looks at the kidney, that in itself could vary its range of excretion of aldosterone. I think that is something one has to beware of particularly in renal disease. I think urinary figures might vary much in some cases; I think the level in the blood might be more important in looking at this point.

REUBI: Do you think that the blood level would be more important than the total production of endogenous aldosterone, as measured by LARAGH and MULLER?

PEART: Wouldn't it depend really upon the actual facts of a given situation? We have to know about that by giving aldosterone and measuring its blood and urine levels in relation to it effects.

REUBI: Yes, perhaps it might. But of course we have to consider that 99% of aldosterone which has been synthesized in the body is destroyed subsequently, as so little appears in the urine.

MULLER: I agree that it would be very interesting and of great value to know the blood levels of aldosterone. Unfortunately this is technically still very difficult and one needs at least 100 ml of blood for each determination. Maybe one day we will have C^{14} marked aldosterone of high specific activity at our disposal. Then it should be possible to determine the blood levels of aldosterone. Meanwhile we will have to rely on urinary excretion and glandular secretion.

REUBI: Dr. GENEST, I would like to ask you one question: how do you visualise the whole problem? Dr. SCHWARTZ told us that he would interpret the increase in aldosterone production or excretion in hypertensive patients as a secondary phenomenon. What is your own interpretation?

GENEST: May I make a few comments about the main point of disagreement between our results, which have been confirmed by VENNING, ROMANELLI and SCHWARTZ, and those of LARAGH and co-workers. Essentially, our results show an increase in mean urinary aldosterone excretion in groups of patients with essential hypertension, whether of the benign or severe variety as compared to that of normal subjects. Also in these patients, especially in the early phase of the disease, there is an excessive fluctuation in urinary aldosterone from normal to above normal levels for reasons that we cannot account for, on the basis of sodium or potassium intake, stress or anxiety state. LARAGH has recently reported that in malignant and renal hypertensive patients there is an increase in aldosterone secretion rate, whereas in 8 or 10 patients with benign hypertension there is no such increase. There lies the main disagreement between our findings and those of LARAGH. This suggests that it would be necessary to do repeated measurements of aldosterone secretion rate at regular intervals in the same hypertensive

---

[1] Total exchangeable sodium was determined by Dr. R. A. COLLET.

patients in the benign phase of the disease. It might perhaps also suggest that some of the assumptions on which the measurement of secretion rate are based[1] should be re-evaluated. Some of these assumptions are that "the pool of steroid remains constant throughout the period of the study", that "the rate of synthesis of steroid equals the rate of transformation of steroid", that "the mixing of the injected steroid within the pool is homogenous and is rapid compared to its metabolism" and finally that "the rate of metabolism of the steroid is proportional to its concentration" (PETERSON). If one uses the method for aldosterone secretion rate by measuring its labelled tetrahydro derivative in urine, it is not entirely clear to me that the calculation of such secretion rate is entirely valid, if based solely on the matter of isotopic dilution, and can be totally independent of the rate of degradation of aldosterone into its tetrahydro derivative. No one has yet shown that the metabolism of aldosterone is constant in the same individual, in different physiological situations, and in various diseased states, e. g. hypertension. But this point can only be settled when more experience and more data are accumulated. At any rate, in view of our findings of the excessive fluctuation of urinary aldosterone in essential hypertension and especially in the early stage of the disease, it would certainly be necessary to do serial aldosterone secretion rate determinations in such cases.

Now Dr. REUBI asked how I visualize the problem. Working exclusively in the field of human hypertension, it is quite interesting that without consulting with Dr. GROSS, who has been working exclusively in the field of experimental hypertension, we came out with pretty much the same working hypothesis which was described by Dr. GROSS this morning. We have shown that in humans there is a highly specific and important relationship between the renal pressor mechanism and the zona glomerulosa secreting aldosterone. It seems quite unlikely that angiotensin infusion would increase urinary aldosterone by affecting only its renal clearance, because of the very marked increase of aldosterone. The major problem at the present time is to establish if the renal pressor mechanism plays any role at any stage of essential hypertension in humans. For that reason, we have been working for the last two years on a procedure for measuring angiotensin in human blood. We can say that we have at the present time a quite specific and sensitive method for such measurements and I think our method also fits Dr. PEART's criteria of validity.

REUBI: Dr. PEART, are you satisfied with this method?

PEART: Well, I really don't know what it is, so I cannot say.

MULLER: I agree with Dr. GENEST that we have to make certain assumptions in these studies on aldosterone secretion. However, since we are determining the secretion over a relatively long time interval by means of an excreted metabolite in the urine and not by the turnover rate of the free unaltered compound in the blood over a relatively short period, we are dealing with mean values during 24 hrs. It is not possible by these studies to detect rapid changes in the secretion during the day. What we really are determining corresponds to an *average* daily production. Unfortunately these studies cannot be repeated from day to day.

SCHWARTZ: May I ask Dr. GENEST two questions: 1. Did you control the pregnanetriol excretion rate in chronic illness not related to hypertension? 2. What conclusions do you draw from the changes in the pregnanetriol/aldosterone ratio in hypertensive persons?

---

[1] PETERSON, Recent Progress in Hormone Research, Editor G. Pincus, Academic Press (1958).

GENEST: We have not done any serial studies of urinary pregnanetriol or of the urinary ratio of pregnanetriol/aldosterone in non-hypertensive patients. The reason why we determined pregnanetriol, etiocholanolone, and the tetrahydro derivative of 17-hydroxy-cortexone and why we looked for the presence of cortexone and of 17-hydroxy-cortexone, was based on the findings and the beautiful studies of BONGIOVANNI and EBERLEIN in the hypertensive form of adrenal virilizing hyperplasia. The high significance of the mean decrease in urinary pregnanetriol and the even higher significance of the decreased pregnanetriol/aldosterone ratio are not the results of any preconceived idea. We were simply stimulated in doing these studies by the findings of BONGIOVANNI and EBERLEIN. The interpretation of the implications of these data in the pathogenesis of hypertension is certainly not clear. It is only worthwhile to emphasize the relationship of urinary pregnanetriol to 17-hydroxy-progesterone which plays an important role in the biosynthesis of corticosteroids and the fact that progesterone inhibits the sodium-retaining effect of aldosterone and exerts, in high dosage, a significant hypotensive effect. Remember, we do not advocate the treatment of hypertension with high doses of progesterone because of other reasons, but we merely want to emphasize its physiological effect in hypertensive patients.

SCHWARTZ: I would first make one statement: the high dosage of progesterone you need to have an antagonistic action to aldosterone seems to exclude a physiological antagonism between the two hormones. On the other hand, I would ask Dr. GENEST whether he did find a correlation between the pregnanetriol and aldosterone excretion rates.

GENEST: We do not know the secretion of progesterone per day, but it is quite certain that the figures of 100 to 200 mg are quite high and probably do not correspond to the amount secreted per day. We have not made, as I have mentioned, any serial studies of urinary pregnanetriol and of the ratio pregnanetriol/aldosterone in the same normal subject or hypertensive patient. It would certainly be of great interest to do this type of study.

SCHROEDER: I am confused about this important question: Have hypertensive patients increased adrenocortical activity or have they not? Dr. GENEST has found elevated or at least widely fluctuating levels of aldosterone in the urines of early as well as of severely hypertensive persons. Dr. SCHWARTZ indicates that elevated levels are unusual. Dr. WETTSTEIN reported in Prague that they are normal, although they can be elevated in a variety of other conditions. LARAGH and Dr. COTTIER found the same. Are these differences in results due to the use of different normal standards? I would like to ask Dr. SCHWARTZ and Dr. GENEST what their upper limits of normal excretion of aldosterone are. Is there a difference in methodology? Are the patients different in the several series?

REUBI: We know that the normal values for aldosterone excretion and secretion depend on the sodium intake and excretion of sodium in urine, and on the ratio between potassium and sodium as well. I should like to ask whether Dr. GENEST and Dr. SCHWARTZ have been using LUETSCHER'S standards.

GENEST: Our normal values vary between 2 and 10 μg per day for urinary aldosterone. I would like to emphasize that one must not be too absolute or dogmatic about a strict relationship between urinary sodium and urinary aldosterone. In our studies, there is no correlation between the amount of aldosterone in urine and the daily intake of sodium (as measured by the urinary sodium output) with a range of 50 to 250—300 meq per day[1].

---

[1] Proc. Soc. Exper. Biol. Med. **97**, 676 (1958).

This lack of correlation applies also to urinary potassium, to the ratio of sodium/potassium or potassium/sodium. I quite agree that below an intake of 50 meq of sodium per day there is generally an increase in urinary aldosterone, but above this level up to 250—300 meq per day, one must not overemphasize any strict correlation between urinary sodium and aldosterone.

REUBI: Dr. SCHROEDER, are you satisfied?

SCHROEDER: No. When you compare one group with another you must have identical conditions and similar subjects in the two groups. Now, are your conditions and Dr. SCHWARTZ's conditions and LARAGH's conditions identical for comparison? When results of similar experiments are as different as these are, we must look for the explanation.

REUBI: Dr. SCHWARTZ, can you answer this point as far as your own experiments are concerned? What are your normal values of aldosterone excretion in urine?

SCHWARTZ: I never saw at our normal diet and at rest a normal man have a higher level than 6 γ per day.

GROSS: I would add one word. One of the most famous examples of increased aldosterone excretion is normal pregnancy — and we know that in many cases this is not a consequence of increased production of aldosterone, but of a changed metabolism of aldosterone. In normal pregnancy, values up to 40 and 50 γ are found, but the blood pressure remains normal; and in toxaemia of pregnancy, when the blood pressure is elevated, the same values as in normal pregnancy are found. This demonstrates that factors other than those we usually consider may be involved. If the excretion of a hormone is determined, this is comparable to determining the content of a hormone in a gland, which might be influenced by various conditions which we do not know.

It was very striking to me that Dr. GENEST found an inverse ratio between aldosterone and pregnanetriol excretion. In pregnancy aldosterone and *pregnanediol* excretion increase, but in spite of this nothing happens to the blood pressure in normal pregnancy.

Another question: If I am correct, the figures you showed demonstrated that angiotensin led to an increased elimination of aldosterone not only on the day of the infusion, but also on the following day; however, the sodium excretion did not run parallel, as on the day of the infusion sodium elimination was diminished. But on the next day, when aldosterone was still high, sodium had already reverted to nearly normal values. It is most interesting that as a consequence of a rather short infusion of angiotensin you have such a prolonged effect. This only demonstrates that something must happen which is not connected with what we would expect after an infusion of such a rapid-acting substance as angiotensin.

GENEST: The occasional lack of correlation between urinary aldosterone and sodium in some of the patients receiving angiotensin infusion illustrates the point I was making a little earlier. Within a certain range of sodium intake, there is often little correlation between sodium intake and aldosterone excretion. In a population of individual subjects adapted on different sodium intake levels, you have to go to quite extreme ranges of sodium intake (below 50 meq or above 250—300 meq per day) to find a significant correlation.

MULLER: Your urinary aldosterone levels were extremely high with angiotensin. It was surprising to me that the urinary sodium was not always correspondingly low. We have been impressed in our studies by a quite regular correlation between urinary sodium and aldosterone. Naturally the higher the sodium intake, the less the differences in urinary aldosterone. This has as consequence that other influences, such as position, exercise, emotions, etc., play a relatively more important role. However, when we cut down the sodium intake to 30 or even 10 meq per day, the influence of sodium restriction becomes so important that other environmental factors step back.

GENEST: There is some confusion here. If the sodium intake of a given subject or patient is increased from 50 to 200 meq per day or decreased from 200 to 50 meq per day, there will be changes in urinary aldosterone that can be fairly well correlated with the sodium intake. But as in our studies which involve spot determinations of aldosterone in a population of individuals adapted to different salt intakes, we find urinary aldosterone values which have no correlation with the amount of salt ingested within a range of 50 to 250—300 meq per day. But we quite agree that if the same patient is successively put on different salt intakes, his urinary aldosterone will vary inversely.

MULLER: I would like to know in your first slide whether your differences in urinary aldosterone between the normotensive patients and the different forms of hypertensive disease correlate with urinary sodium values.

GENEST: There is no correlation in our hypertensive patients between those who had high urinary aldosterone excretion and their salt intake (as measured by their daily urinary sodium). Like the normal subjects, the hypertensive patients were on an "ad libitum" and unrestricted diet. The upper limit of urinary aldosterone excretion in normal subjects is 10 μg per day by our method. Taking this figure as the dividing line between normal and excessive excretion in our groups of patients with essential hypertension, 8 out of 14 patients with an intake of 50—100 meq of sodium/day (as measured by the daily output in urine), 13 out of 35 patients with an intake of 100—150, and 3 out of 10 with an intake of 150—200, excreted higher amounts of aldosterone than normal. Excessive fluctuation in daily urinary aldosterone occurred whether the patient was on a fixed sodium intake or on "ad libitum" salt intake.

PEART: Just a point about aldosterone. Dr. COTTIER showed that there was a difference in hypertension in the amount of sodium excreted. One would have expected then that there would have been a correlation between the amount of sodium excreted per 24 hrs and the aldosterone secretion if there were a causal relation. Apart from this point I would say that in interpreting the excretion of sodium during infusion of angiotensin, as I tried to show previously, one has to consider the probable direct action on renal function, so that I think you have a rather complicated picture which might not make it so simple to interpret.

To Dr. GENEST: I wonder whether in fact one ought not to look at the effect of angiotensin on excretion during the infusions. Are you absolutely sure the kidney is not excreting aldosterone better under the influence of angiotensin? I think this is very important when one is considering production rates versus clearance rates, and I think it is a point that would have to be answered. The other thing which I wonder: have you got any information about the effects of blood pressure reduction alone on the excretion of aldosterone, because this might be put into the same class as the effect which Dr. COTTIER has found, and HOLLANDER and his colleagues, on the excretion of sodium in the urine of patients with hypertension; it can be reversed by sympathectomy or by ganglion blocking drugs.

GENEST (to PEART): The answer to your first question is that I do not know. But it appears unlikely. The answer to your second question is that this is one thing which has to be done. But you must remember that because of the excessive fluctuation in urinary aldosterone, the amount of work implied in the serial determination of urinary aldosterone when the patients are at high levels of blood pressure and again when the patients' blood pressure has been controlled by surgical or medical means, is quite impressive. To my knowledge it has not been done, at least not by our group, but I certainly agree that it has to be done.

GROSS: We heard this morning from Dr. PEART that angiotensin infusion in normotensive subjects leads to a diminution of sodium excretion and to an antidiuretic effect. This should have the consequence that aldosterone secretion diminishes, and therefore the increase you found is difficult to understand. How long did you infuse?

GENEST: 7 to 14 hrs.

GROSS: This covers almost the whole period of one of your aldosterone determinations. If there is a correlation between sodium and circulating plasma volume, there should be a decrease of aldosterone secretion under this influence. You did not determine the circulating plasma volume?

GENEST: No.

PEART: Wouldn't one have to be rather careful here? The longest period of infusion of angiotensin in the normal subject that we reported is an hour at the present time, and one cannot say what is going to happen to urine flow and electrolyte excretion over 7—14 hrs.

DAHL: I have one question: If excess aldosterone production is primary in this disease, I would expect a correlation between amounts produced and hypertension. However, patients with primary aldosteronism frequently have relatively mild hypertension. And among cirrhotic and certain cardiac patients who may produce extraordinarily large amounts of aldosterone, hypertension is notable by its absence.

REUBI: I wanted to make the same remark as you have done, because I have always been impressed by the fact that patients who are producing the greatest amounts of aldosterone are not hypertensive at all. These are patients with heart failure or liver cirrhosis, and they usually do not have hypertension, so that I wonder whether aldosterone has anything to do with blood pressure. Furthermore, if you give aldosterone up to 6 mg a day to nephrotic patients with oedema, you do not get any elevation of blood pressure. On the other hand, as we learned this afternoon, there is no difference in aldosteronuria between patients with so-called esssntial hypertension and patients with renal hypertension. Unless we assume that essential hypertension is a renal disease — which I do not — we have, therefore, to consider that increased production of aldosterone is only a secondary phenomenon. I do not know whether we all agree with this feeling.

WILSON: It may be that in oedematous states, the volume control mechanism is not responding properly, whereas in hypertension it is a question of redistribution of blood volume. Thus aldosterone is not working under comparable conditions.

REUBI: This would mean that aldosterone has no specific effect on blood pressure, and I think on that we can agree.

WILSON: It might have an effect on blood volume.

REUBI: Perhaps on blood volume, but not on arteriolar tone.

WILSON: We still have to find a mechanism by which redistribution of body water and/or sodium can affect the blood pressure, either through the cardiac output or its effects on arterial tone.

REUBI: Yes.

BROD: We have been working in our laboratory in Prague for many years on haemodynamic adjustments to various emergency states. In still unpublished investigations we found that in heart failure we get the same change of regional haemodynamics as we get under severe muscular stress, under emotion, and also in essential hypertension. The difference of course is that in heart failure this is in response to a failing cardiac output, and hence even if you bring the total peripheral vascular resistance up very high, you will not get a high blood pressure, while in essential hypertension the same thing occurs obviously with a normally functioning heart and therefore you get an increase in blood pressure. Now, in those states where this reaction is mobilised, especially in heart failure, there is a parallel second homeostatic mechanism, obviously involving the adrenal cortex and the secretion of aldosterone. Now, if this is an inherent part of the homeostatic response, it might well be that in essential hypertension we also get this second line mobilised, and this would explain the finding of increased aldosterone secretion; however, the increased aldosterone production (if confirmed) and the increase in blood pressure would be two parallel manifestations of the same homeostatic response without one necessarily being the cause of the other.

GENEST: There has been much emphasis on the high levels of urinary aldosterone in edematous states. But it must be pointed out that in about one third of patients with congestive heart failure and edema, the aldosterone excretion is well within normal limits. Now the way I look at the excessive fluctuation of urinary aldosterone in hypertensive patients is related to the concept of Dr. SYDNEY FRIEDMAN, from Vancouver. Dr. FRIEDMAN has shown that any pressor substance, when injected to nephrectomized rats and dogs, will at the same time increase the rate of transport of sodium from the extracellular to the intracellular space. This correlation is very neat in all cases. Excessive secretion of aldosterone may play the same role in increasing the rate of transfer of sodium to the intracellular space and, in susceptible individuals, increase arteriolar tonicity. The clinical syndrome described by CONN as primary aldosteronism is in favor of that concept and indicates that aldosterone should not be thought of uniquely as a factor concerned in the pathogenesis of edema. Many other factors besides edema play a role in the secretion of aldosterone, blood volume, venous pressure, stresses, anxiety states, exercise, physical activity, and angiotensin, as we have just demonstrated. The highly specific trophic effect of angiotensin on urinary aldosterone and the excessive fluctuation of aldosterone found in hypertensive patients fits in whith the experiments of Dr. GROSS and Dr. FRIEDMAN and their concepts. Our working hypothesis is that either the amount of intracellular sodium, the intracellular sodium/potassium ratio or the rate of transfer of sodium from the extracellular to the intracellular space may basically effect the arteriolar muscle tone and contractility.

REUBI: Dr. GENEST, I forgot something: in your paper you said that you would not believe that a higher pressure is a sufficient reason for the increased excretion of sodium, because using various vasoactive drugs you had obtained for the same blood pressure effect different responses as far as sodium output was concerned. Of course you have to take into account the specific pharmacodynamic effects of the drugs you are using, in addition to their common hypertensive properties.

GENEST: One of the main conclusions of our work is that angiotensin has a marked specific effect on aldosterone whereas other substances like norepinephrine and neo-synephrine, given in amounts sufficient to raise the blood pressure to the same levels as with angiotensin, do not produce the same effect on aldosterone and sodium. In fact, with neo-synephrine there is a markedly increased sodium output, along with a decrease in urinary aldosterone. Epinephrine infusions given at a rate sufficient to increase the pulse rate by an average of 29 pulsations per minute has no effect on urinary aldosterone and 17-hydroxycorticosteroids.

SCHWARTZ: There's just one remark I should like to make. Since this work seems to have a fundamental bearing on the problem of aldosteronism and hypertension, I should like to know whether, in a hypertensive subject, aldosterone hypersecretion following sodium restriction is more marked than in normal subjects.

GENEST: Dr. VENNING kindly permitted me to quote her recent results and the answer is that hypertensive patients submitted to a low sodium diet react in the same way, as far as urinary aldosterone is concerned, as the normal subjects. She has also found that there is no significant difference in urinary aldosterone in response to ACTH stimulation between normotensive subjects and hypertensive patients. Dr. VENNING has also found that the amounts of aldosterone contained in adrenals taken at the autopsy ten to twelve hours after death of two patients with severe hypertension were very high in comparison to the amounts found in normal subjects.

Therapeutic aspects of salt restriction

By

A. Grollman

Salt restriction in the form of a "low-salt" diet has long interested those concerned in the management of hypertension. Although advocated as early as 1905 by Ambard and Beaujard (*2*), it received its greatest impetus from the subsequent studies of Allen and Sherrill (*1*). Although a few authorities, such as Volhard (*41*) utilized salt restriction in the management of their hypertensive patients, this method of therapy was accepted with little enthusiasm or not at all, for a variety of reasons. There was, in the first place, no apparent rationale for a regimen which shared with other forms of dietotherapy a certain stigma of charlatanism. Of more significance in convincing the skeptical of the uselessness of the method was the fact that salt restriction as practised did not lower the blood pressure appreciably nor did the addition of excessive salt load to the hypertensive patient (*31*) or experimental animal tend to elevate it (*16*).

In establishing the validity of the hypertensive rat for the assay of antihypertensive agents, Grollman and Harrison (*18*) noted the capacity of certain synthetic diets to lower the blood pressure to a striking degree. Further investigation revealed that this antihypertensive effect was not a result of the composition of the diets but was related to their sodium content. This led to their application of a low-salt diet to the human and to their advocacy of sodium restriction for the management of the hypertensive patient (*19*).

The effect of sodium depletion in experimental hypertension

The antihypertensive effect of sodium depletion is most readily demonstrable in the rat as shown by Grollman and Harrison (*18*). Diets practically electrolyte-free were prepared by dialyzing the animals' usual food or by mixing naturally occurring food-stuffs which are normally low in sodium content. The effect of adding various salts to such diets demonstrated that deficiency of sodium was responsible for the observed lowering of the blood pressure and that the chloride moiety of the molecule was not related to the effect observed. The addition of sodium chloride to an electrolyte-free diet abolished its hypotensive effect; potassium chloride added to the same diet did not affect its antihypertensive action (*18*).

The administration of single foods such as rice, soya bean, peanut or potato, which are naturally low in sodium content, all resulted in marked reduction in blood pressure which could be counteracted by the addition of 2% sodium chloride. These observations offered a rational explanation and experimental basis for the established effectiveness of the diet in human hypertension, the beneficial effect of which had been attributed by KEMPNER (*27*) to some esoteric property of its protein constituents.

The reduction in blood pressure induced in hypertensive animals by sodium restriction was not encountered in the normotensive animal. The beneficial effect of sodium depletion was also demonstrated by the fact that the survival of hypertensive rats maintained on a low sodium diet was definitely prolonged over control animals suffering from a comparable degree of hypertension maintained on the same diet with added sodium chloride (*18*).

The effects of sodium restriction on the blood pressure have also been investigated in the dog. The results in this species are less dramatic and less rapid in their manifestation, although demonstrable particularly if sodium depletion is accelerated by the administration of such natriuretic agents as the mercurial or benzo-thiadiazine diuretics (*24*).

Effects of sodium restriction in human hypertension

The effectiveness of sodium restriction in the experimental animal suggested its trial in human hypertensive patients (*19*). The numerous subsequent studies on the subject have led to conflicting results (*5, 7, 10, 33*). This is attributable, in part, to the difficulties involved in evaluating the response to any form of therapy of so labile a function as the blood pressure; and, in part, to the poorly controlled sodium intake. Unless the latter is controlled by analysis of the urine one may be grossly deceived as to the actual sodium content of a presumed "salt-free" diet. For example, in a series of 30 hypertensive subjects treated as out-patients, the salt intake as determined by analysis of the urine was less than 1 g in only one patient; the others were ingesting from 5 to 15 g of salt despite the fact that they had been placed on a supposedly salt-free diet (*24*). Conclusions as to the effectiveness of sodium restriction on the blood pressure are of no significance unless the patients are studied on a carefully controlled metabolic ward or under conditions in which the true sodium intake is otherwise measurable.

Few doubt now (*10, 33*) that sodium restriction in man, as in the experimental animal, results in a reduction in the blood pressure in most, but not all, patients. The effectiveness of the rice diet as advocated by Kempner (*27*) in lowering the blood pressure and causing a reversion in the characteristic manifestations of malignant hypertension, in some patients, is also now generally accepted. As already indicated, this response is a result of the low sodium content of the rice diet and can be duplicated by more varied diets containing equally small amounts of sodium (*18, 19*).

Not all patients respond with a decline in blood pressure when subjected to sodium restriction. In the original series of six patients reported by Grollman et al. (*19*), one failed to respond, three showed a moderate reduction, and two responded by a reduction in blood pressure to essentially normal levels. The latter two patients, incidentally, are the only surviving members of the group, 16 years later. Although attempts have been made to predict the response of a given patient to sodium restriction, there are no criteria by which this may be accomplished. In our experience the younger patient with moderate hypertension, in general, responds favorably, as opposed to the older patient with severe or malignant hypertension. However, exceptions to this rule are encountered and, as noted by Kempner (*27*), even patients with severe malignant hypertension may show a notable response. Approximately two-thirds of all patients respond with a reduction in blood pressure, although several months may elapse before this is attained.

Metabolism of sodium in hypertension

The demonstration that dietary restriction of sodium lowers the blood pressure led to the study of the metabolism of sodium in the hypertensive as compared to the normotensive individual. The results of such studies indicate definite deviations from normal in the electrolyte and water balance of the hypertensive in both the human as well as in the experimental animal. Eichelberger (*11*) first noted an increased sodium and chloride and a decreased potassium content of the muscle in the hypertensive dog. Laramore and Grollman (*29*) noted a general increase in sodium content of all tissues studied (blood, brain, heart, liver, gut, striated muscle, skin, and spleen) and a corresponding decrease in potassium content of these tissues. The change in chloride was variable, being increased in some tissues (heart, gut, striated muscle, and spleen) and decreased in others (brain, liver, and skin). In late stages of the disease, an increase in water content of the tissues was also demonstrable. This increased hydration of the tissues was only noted in animals with cardiomegaly and may therefore be attributed to edema or incipient congestive heart failure.

The question arises as to whether the changes observed in the water and electrolyte content of the tissues in hypertension reflect an alteration in intracellular composition or merely an increase in volume of the extracellular fluid. In view of the concomitant increase of chloride observed in tissues with a high muscle content (heart, gut, striated muscle, and spleen), one might explain the increased sodium and decreased potassium content of these tissues as reflecting some degree of extracellular edema. However, in the case of the other organs (liver, brain, skin) the observed decrease in chloride content would suggest an alteration in intracellular composition. The unchanged water content of the tissues during the earlier stages of hypertension, before cardiac dilatation had occurred, would also favor the conclusion that the changes observed reflect an actual alteration in composition of the intracellular phase. It is questionable if the changes in electrolyte content of the blood vessels (28) reflect any specific alteration concerned in the elevation of the blood pressure, rather than the changes observed in other tissues.

In addition to the change in electrolyte and water content of the tissues observed in hypertension, there is a demonstrable expansion of the extracellular space in the human as well as in the hypertensive dog (22). Although such changes are not noted when the less sensitive inulin space is measured (15), TENG, SHAPIRO and GROLLMAN (39), utilizing radiosulfate (42), demonstrated an appreciable expansion of the extracellular fluid in patients with essential hypertension. This was accompanied by an increase of the plasma volume in the hypertensive and a suggestive increase in the total body water. In dogs rendered hypertensive by a figure-of-eight ligature and contralateral nephrectomy (17), the antipyrine space was increased following the development of hypertension as compared to the pre-operative levels. Hypertensive dogs also had an increased deuterium oxide space as compared to normotensive animals (22, 39). It would appear, therefore, that the extracellular fluid volume is increased in hypertension with a probable increase in total body water as well as alterations in the electrolyte composition of the tissues (38).

Since the volume of the body fluid compartments and the electrolyte content of the tissues are regulated by the antidiuretic and adrenal cortical hormones, the rate of secretion of these in the hypertensive as compared to the normal has also been investigated. The rate of excretion of the antidiuretic hormone in the urine is increased in human as well as experimental hypertension (*12*). This may reflect a compensatory reaction, since this hormone is concerned in the maintenance of a normal tonicity of the extracellular fluid at the expense of an expansion in extracellular fluid volume.

Not only is the content and distribution of electrolyte and water different in the hypertensive from that of the normotensive, but the response of the two to a sodium load and to sodium restriction differs. Farnsworth and Barker (*13*) first demonstrated the abnormally rapid rate of excretion of chloride by the kidney in hypertension and subsequent observers have demonstrated that subjects with essential hypertension excrete an intravenously injected sodium load more rapidly than do normotensive individuals. Attempts have been made to correlate this observed difference with alterations in renal function, attributing it to a reduction in renal plasma flow and filtration factor. Cottier and his co-workers (*8*) have attributed the accelerated natriuretic response to the increased renal intravascular pressure, while Baldwin and his collaborators (*3*) consider it to be of extrarenal origin.

The abnormal pattern of excretion of sodium in the hypertensive reverts to normal when dietary sodium is restricted and is not present prior to the development of hypertension (*25*). Until the advent of an impairment of renal function, the response to a salt load is roughly proportional to the elevation of blood pressure.

Mechanism of the antihypertensive action of sodium restriction

There is ample evidence to indicate that hypertensive cardiovascular disease is a disorder induced by a humoral mechanism. Despite the efforts to implicate a pressor mechanism to account for the disease, there is no valid evidence to support this (*34*) except in the rare instances of so-called "unilateral" renal disease. The available evidence is more compatible with an alternative hypothesis which postulates that hypertension of the so-called essential type in man and its analogue, as induced in the experimental animal, is a consequence of a renal deficiency. According to this view the kidney, in addition to its excretory and other functions, is responsible also for the maintenance of the normotensive state, and in the abeyance of this function hypertensive disease ensues (*21, 23*).

It is difficult to envisage sodium depletion as counteracting the fundamental defect responsible for the appearance of hypertension. Were this the case, one would anticipate that such depletion would invariably result in a decline of blood pressure in every patient suffering from this disease, which, as already stated, is not the case.

Moreover, even in instances where the blood pressure declines, it is rarely reduced to normal except in patients with only mild elevations of blood pressure. In animals in which a severe degree of hypertension is induced, the decline in blood pressure is also often only moderate or may even fail to occur (24). Similar results are obtained following natriuresis induced by diuretic drugs (24).

It would appear logical, therefore, to conclude that the effects of sodium restriction on the blood pressure are only symptomatic in the sense that they influence this manifestation of the disease without affecting the fundamental disturbance responsible for the disorder. In this respect, therefore, sodium depletion resembles other presently available procedures used in the therapy of hypertension, such as the sedative and tranquilizing drugs and the autonomic blocking agents, which likewise only affect the blood pressure level without altering the basic pathologic process. Whether the reduction in blood pressure induced by sodium restriction is more conducive to the prolongation of life, as claimed by ALLEN and SHERRILL (1) and demonstrated in the rat (18), as compared to the effects of reducing the blood pressure by drug therapy, the beneficial effect of which, except in malignant hypertension, has been questioned (36), is problematical.

Experiments by the author (24) have indicated that sodium loss of a comparable degree, when induced either by dietary restriction or by the administration of diuretics, induces comparable declines in blood pressure in both human and experimental hypertension. However, since the administration of large doses of the diuretics induces a greater loss of sodium than can be achieved by dietary restriction, a more impressive and more rapid decline in blood pressure can be achieved by the use of the diuretics. The combination of dietary restriction and diuretic act together to accelerate the decline in blood pressure, particularly in the human in whom less drastic reduction in dietary sodium is possible as compared to the experimental animal. Because of the similar effects of sodium depletion, whether induced by dietary restriction or by the administration of natriuretic drugs, there is every reason to believe that both procedures act by the same mechanism (14).

As shown by WILSON and FREIS (45), chlorothiazide decreases the extracellular fluid volume of the hypertensive, which, as already indicated, is increased in hypertension. However, after prolonged therapy, this reduction of plasma and extracellular fluid volume and body weight are no longer demonstrable, although the blood pressure remains at its reduced level. Apparently, modifications occur in the organism which compensate for the initial change in the volume of the fluid compartments with the emergence of mechanisms which maintain the reduced blood pressure.

Conway and Lauwers (6) have also demonstrated a reduction in plasma volume of patients on chlorothiazide therapy, accompanied by a decrease in plasma volume, cardiac output and peripheral resistance. After a month or more of treatment, the plasma volume and cardiac output were restored to their pre-treatment levels, despite the maintenance of the fall in blood pressure.

It would appear that sodium depletion induces its hypotensive effect acutely by reducing the extracellular and plasma volume and that despite the homeostatic correction of these alterations, other changes occur, presumably in the tissues, which maintain the reduced blood pressure. The nature of the latter effect is unknown, but may consist in a correction of the increased sodium content of the tissues observed in hypertension. The negative sodium and water balance responsible for the decrease in plasma and extracellular fluid volume which follows sodium restriction is apparent within 3 or 4 days when drastic sodium restriction is supplemented by the administration of ammonium chloride (30), but may not become apparent for some weeks when natriuresis is not accelerated by an induced diuresis (32). However, there is no close correlation between the therapeutic response to sodium restriction, as reflected in the reduction of the blood pressure, and the change observed in plasma volume (7, 9, 32).

The total exchangeable sodium content of the body decreases with dietary sodium restriction (37). This loss is proportionately greater than the loss of water, suggesting the movement of water from the extracellular to the intracellular space (9, 38). To what extent these secondarily induced changes in hydration are responsible for the observed drop in blood pressure remains problematical.

Concomitantly with the decline in blood pressure induced by dietary sodium restriction, one observes a decrease in heart size as a consequence apparently of the decreased plasma volume, diminished venous return, and decreased cardiac output. The latter effects in turn are presumably responsible for the increased vasomotor tone observed and the greater responsiveness to the hypotensive action of ganglionic blocking drugs and sympathectomy.

Alterations in renal hemodynamics induced by sodium restriction include a decrease in renal blood flow and glomerular filtration rate (44), the decrease in the latter being out of proportion to that of the former. Retention of urea may also occur, particularly in patients manifesting a rapid diuresis.

It is apparent that sodium depletion induced either by dietary restriction or by the administration of natriuretic drugs induces hemodynamic changes which are responsible for the immediate decline in blood pressure observed when these measures are used in hypertension. It is unnecessary to assume the existence of a more intimate association between sodium metabolism and hypertensive disease. However, the chronic effect of such depletion may involve a more direct renal mechanism concerned in the reabsorption of sodium and the maintenance of blood pressure homeostasis.

Present status of sodium restriction in the management of hypertension

The availability of natriuretic drugs in the form of the potent, orally effective, relatively non-toxic benzothiadiazine and phthalimidine derivatives has relegated sodium restriction by dietary means to a lesser importance in the management of hypertension. The difficulties inherent in dietary restriction as compared to the relative ease with which comparable degrees of sodium depletion can be obtained by drug therapy has resulted in the displacement of the former by the latter as the preferred therapeutic measure. Nevertheless, sodium restriction has the advantage over the use of natriuretic drugs of being relatively free of side-effects, since it is less intensive in its sodium-depleting capacity and is not accompanied by such electrolyte disturbances as potassium depletion, such renal disturbances as uric acid retention, or the rare sensitization phenomena which give rise to hematological disturbances.

In view of these side-effects which accompany the use of natriuretic drugs, it would appear logical to use them only as a supplement to sodium restriction. The greater the degree of this restriction, the lower the dose of the drug necessary for eliciting the desired decline in blood pressure. On the other hand, the drastic restriction of sodium formerly required for eliciting a response and the use of onerous dietary restriction is no longer necessary. By utilizing sodium restriction, it is possible to obtain the desired response with a minimal dose of diuretic or other drugs and hence minimize the frequently serious side-effects inherent in their use. Following sympathectomy, patients often respond to sodium restriction, which like the diuretic drugs also exerts a synergistic action with other available procedures now used in the management of hypertension.

Although our presently available therapeutic measures for the management of hypertension are empirical and symptomatic, it is generally agreed with few exceptions (*36*) that lowering of the blood pressure is desirable if it can be effected without undue side-effects. Sodium depletion, by dietary restriction, by use of natriuretic drugs, or by a combination of these as well as other available measures, remains accordingly a desirable and at present our only available measure for use in the treatment of hypertension. Because of its relative freedom of side-effects and its demonstrated synergistic action when combined with other forms of therapy, sodium restriction, at least of a moderate degree, should be considered as a basic form of treatment in hypertension. For the mild and moderate degrees of hypertension, dietary restriction alone plus the usual measures of rest, phenobarbital, and reassurance will often yield as satisfactory and effective results, with less hazard and fewer undesirable side-effects, than will the use of more drastic measures.

Dietary sodium restriction is often referred to as impractical and impossible of application to the average patient population. This criticism is undeserved. Most naturally occurring foodstuffs are relatively sodium-free, their high sodium content being acquired by processing. By simply avoiding the latter, diets relatively low in sodium are readily procurable (*20*).

Undesirable reactions to the drastic restriction of sodium are rarely encountered. Such symptoms as anorexia, headache, lassitude, general malaise, nausea and muscle cramps secondary to hyponatremia, which develop in normal subjects whose intake of sodium is drastically restricted, are not observed in the uncomplicated hypertensive patient. This difference in reaction is presumably a consequence of the difference in the manner in which sodium is handled by the hypertensive as compared to the normal individual. Only in the presence of complicating factors, such as renal insufficiency with a propensity to wastage of sodium, is hyponatremia with its attendant symptoms encountered.

Summary

Salt restriction as a therapeutic measure in the management of hypertension, although advocated at the beginning of the century, has met with indifferent acceptance. There is ample evidence to indicate its effectiveness when adequately applied to a certain proportion of human patients. The exact mechanism whereby sodium depletion produces its antihypertensive effect is not clear. Such restriction induces demonstrable hemodynamic changes and may overcome the deviations in water and electrolyte metabolism and in the volume of the body fluid compartments which have been demonstrated to occur in hypertensive disease both in the human as well as in the experimental animal.

Although the availability of potent, orally effective, relatively non-toxic natriuretic drugs has made unnecessary the use of more drastic sodium restriction for reducing the blood pressure, a combination of moderate restriction with drug therapy is preferable to reliance on drug therapy alone.

Résumé

La restriction du sel alimentaire comme traitement de l'hypertension, encore que préconisée au début du siècle, n'a guère obtenu d'audience. Elle paraît néanmoins très efficace chez un certain nombre de patients quand elle est appliquée d'une façon adéquate.

Le mécanisme exact par lequel la déplétion sodique possède une action antihypertensive n'est pas nettement défini. La restriction sodique détermine des changements hémodynamiques indiscutables et permet peut-être de compenser les déviations du métabolisme de l'eau et des électrolytes, ainsi que du volume des compartiments liquidiens de l'organisme dont on a montré l'existence aussi bien chez l'homme hypertendu que chez l'animal de laboratoire.

Bien que l'apparition de médicaments natriurétiques puissants et relativement peu toxiques ait rendu inutile une restriction salée trop sévère, l'association d'une restriction modérée et d'une thérapeutique médicamenteuse reste préférable à l'utilisation exclusive de médicaments.

References

1. ALLEN, F. M., and J. W. SHERRILL: J. Metabol. Res. (U.S.A.) **2**, 429 (1922).
2. AMBARD, L., and E. BEAUJARD: Sem. méd. **25**, 133 (1905).
3. BALDWIN, D. S., A. W. BIGGS, W. GOLDRING, H. W. HULET, and H. CHASIS: Amer. J. Med. **24**, 893 (1958).
4. BIRCHALL, R., S. W. TUTHILL, W. S. JACOBS, W. J. TRAUTMAN JR., and T. FINDLEY: Circulation (U.S.A.) **7**, 258 (1953).
5. CHASIS, H.: J. Amer. Med. Ass. **142**, 711 (1950).
6. CONWAY, J., and P. LAUWERS: Circulation (U.S.A.) **21**, 21 (1960).
7. CORCORAN, A. C., R. D. TAYLOR, and I. H. PAGE: Circulation (U.S.A.) **3**, 1 (1951).
8. COTTIER, P. T., J. M. WELLER, and S. W. HOOBLER: Circulation (U.S.A.) **17**, 750 (1958).
9. DOLE, V. P.: J. Clin. Invest. (U.S.A.) **30**, 584 (1951).
10. DUSTAN, H. P.: J. Amer. Med. Ass. **172**, 2052 (1960).
11. EICHELBERGER, L.: J. Exper. Med. (U.S.A.) **77**, 205 (1943).
12. ELLIS, M. E., and A. GROLLMAN: Endocrinology (U.S.A.) **44**, 415 (1949).
13. FARNSWORTH, E. B., and M. H. BARKER: Proc. Soc. Exper. Biol. Med. (U.S.A.) **52**, 74 (1943).
14. FREIS, E. D.: Clin. Pharmacol. Therap. (U.S.A.) **1**, 337 (1960).
15. GRAEFF, J. DE: Acta med. Scand. **156**, 337 (1957).
16. GROLLMAN, A., T. R. HARRISON, and J. R. WILLIAMS JR.: J. Pharmacol. Exper. Therap. (U.S.A.) **69**, 76 (1940).
17. GROLLMAN, A.: Proc. Soc. Exper. Biol. Med. (U.S.A.) **57**, 102 (1944).
18. GROLLMAN, A., and T. R. HARRISON: Proc. Soc. Exper. Biol. Med. (U.S.A.) **60**, 52 (1945).
19. GROLLMAN, A., T. R. HARRISON, M. F. MASON, J. BAXTER, J. CRAMPTON, and F. REICHSMAN: J. Amer. Med. Ass. **129**, 533 (1945).
20. GROLLMAN, A.: J. Amer. Diet. Ass. **22**, 864 (1946).
21. GROLLMAN, A.: Recent Progress in Hormone Research **1**, 371 (1947).
22. GROLLMAN, A., and A. SHAPIRO: J. Clin. Invest. (U.S.A.) **32**, 312 (1953).

23. GROLLMAN, A.: Perspect. Biol. Med. **2**, 208 (1959).
24. GROLLMAN, A.: Unpublished observations.
25. HANENSON, I. B., H. H. TAUSSKY, N. POLASKY, W. RANSOHOFF, and B. F. MILLER: Circulation (U.S.A.) **20**, 498 (1959).
26. HOLLANDER, W., and W. E. JUDSON: J. Clin. Invest. (U.S.A.) **36**, 1460 (1957).
27. KEMPNER, W.: North Carolina Med. J. **5**, 125 (1944).
28. KOLETSKY, S., H. RESNICK, and D. BEHRIN: Proc. Soc. Exper. Biol. Med. (U.S.A.) **102**, 12 (1959).
29. LARAMORE, D. C., and A. GROLLMAN: Amer. J. Physiol. **161**, 278 (1950).
30. LYONS, R., S. D. JACOBSON, and N. L. AVERY JR.: Amer. Heart J. **27**, 353 (1944).
31. MOSENTHAL, H. O.: Med. Clin. North America **5**, 1139 (1922).
32. MURPHY, R. J. F.: J. Clin. Invest. (U.S.A.) **29**, 912 (1950).
33. PALMER, R. S.: J. Chron. Dis. (U.S.A.) **10**, 500 (1959).
34. PEART, W. S.: Erg. Physiol. (G.) **50**, 409 (1959).
35. PERERA, G. A.: Ann. Int. Med. (U.S.A.) **43**, 1195 (1955)
36. PERERA, G. A.: J. Amer. Med. Ass. **173**, 11 (1960).
37. ROSS, E. J.: Clin. Sc. (G.B.) **15**, 81 (1956).
38. SAPIRSTEIN, L. A.: Proc. Council High Blood Pressure Research **6**, 28 (1957).
39. TENG, H. C., A. P. SHAPIRO, and A. GROLLMAN: Metabolism (U.S.A.) **3**, 405 (1954).
40. THOMPSON, J. E., T. F. SILVA, D. KINSEY, and R. H. SMITHWICK: Circulation (U.S.A.) **10**, 912 (1954).
41. VOLHARD, F.: Handbuch der Inneren Medizin. Vol. VI, p. 1753. Berlin, 1931.
42. WALSER, M., D. W. SELDIN, and A. GROLLMAN: J. Clin. Invest. (U.S.A.) **32**, 299 (1953).
43. WATKIN, D. M., H. F. FROEB, F. T. HATCH, and A. B. GUTMAN: Amer. J. Med. **9**, 441 (1950).
44. WESTON, R. E.: J. Clin. Invest. (U.S.A.) **29**, 639 (1950).
45. WILSON, I. M., and E. D. FREIS: Circulation (U.S.A.) **20**, 1028 (1959).

Mechanism of hypotensive action of saluretics

By

E. D. FREIS[1]

The characteristic effects of chlorothiazide and other saluretic agents of similar potency on blood pressure are as follows: firstly, these drugs produce a moderate reduction of basal blood pressure in hypertensive patients (1, 2); secondly, they strikingly enhance the antihypertensive effects of other agents, particularly those of the ganglion blocking drugs; and, thirdly, in therapeutic dosages they do not reduce basal blood pressure in normotensive subjects (1, 2). An attempt will be made to formulate a concept of their mode of action which will encompass an explanation for each of the three clinical observations made above.

The various hypotheses that can be formulated to explain the mechanism of action of chlorothiazide include the following alternatives:

1. The antihypertensive effect is independent of the saluresis and represents a direct action of the drug on the cardiovascular apparatus or a specific metabolic antagonism such as neutralization or destruction of renin, as has been proposed by WILKINS and HOLLANDER (2).

2. The antihypertensive effect is dependent upon the sodium loss produced by the drug.

The second alternative, namely the sodium-loss theory, can be subdivided further in that the reduction of arterial pressure could be secondary to electrolyte changes, particularly sodium concentrations in vascular smooth muscle, leading to a decrease in total peripheral resistance; or the antihypertensive effect may be associated with a reduction in plasma and/or extravascular fluid volumes.

Evidence for dependence of antihypertensive effects on saluretic action

When chlorothiazide is administered to a non-edematous hypertensive on a constant salt intake there is a prompt increase in the

[1] Supported in part by U.S. Public Health Grant H-720 (National Heart Institute) and by research grants from Merck, Sharp & Dohme and Irwin Neisler & Company.

12*

urinary excretion of sodium and chloride. The saluresis is most pronounced during the first 48 hrs after drug therapy has been initiated and tapers off thereafter (*1, 4*). Potassium excretion is also increased but to a lesser degree and for a longer period. The major reduction of arterial pressure occurs during this first 48 hrs roughly paralleling the decline in body sodium (*1, 4*). In our experience (*1*) and also that of most others (*4, 5*) the blood pressure fall does not precede the saluresis, suggesting that the hypotension is not due to a direct depressant effect of the drug on the cardiovascular system. Nor does the reduction of arterial pressure begin after a significant interval following the saluresis, suggesting again that the salt loss and the blood pressure fall are related events at least in respect to time.

It is also well known that diets severely restricted in sodium lower blood pressure (*6*) and enhance the antihypertensive effects of ganglion blockade (*7*). In addition, parenteral mercurial diuretics reduce arterial pressure in hypertensive patients (*8*) and increase responsiveness to antihypertensive agents, particularly ganglion blocking drugs (*9*). Thus, it appears that various procedures which induce body sodium depletion have similar effects on blood pressure. It seems reasonable, therefore in the light of present knowledge, to postulate that the antihypertensive effects of the saluretic agents are dependent on their salt depleting action. For the purposes of the present discussion, this hypothesis will be accepted and further considerations will deal with the manner in which sodium loss produces antihypertensive effects.

Evidence that saluretic agents do not deplete cells of sodium

The sodium concentration of the plasma does not change significantly during treatment with the saluretic agents (*1, 10, 11*). Since plasma sodium is in equilibrium with extracellular fluid sodium it can be assumed that there is no change in the concentration of sodium in the extracellular fluids. The fact that the extracellular concentration of sodium is unchanged raises the possibility that the excess sodium lost from the body during saluresis may be derived from tissue cells, including those of vascular smooth muscle. However, it is equally possible that the sodium and chloride loss represents an extracellular dehydration, that is, a loss of *isotonic* extracellular fluid in sufficient volume to account for the negative salt balance. If the latter were the case one would expect to find a decrease in extracellular fluid volume of sufficient magnitude to account for the depleted body stores of sodium.

To estimate the extracellular fluid loss, we used the change in thiocyanate and radiosulfate spaces before and after chlorothiazide and correlated the change with the extent of weight reduction and cumulative negative sodium balance (*9, 10*).

The measurement of total extracellular fluid is notoriously variable. Its absolute value depends to a considerable extent on the time used for equilibration, molecular size and distribution of the indicator, and other factors. It is well known, for example, that thiocyanate enters certain cells, such as red blood cells. However, for the estimation of changes in extracellular fluid volume both thiocyanate and radiosulfate can provide useful estimates despite the fact that the space available to each indicator varies not only from the other but also from other indicators such as inulin. Thus, in non-edematous hypertensive patients the mean control extracellular fluid volume as estimated with thiocyanate was 21.8 l while the simultaneously determined radiosulfate space was 16.8 l (*10*). Nevertheless, both showed similar trends after chlorothiazide treatment, the reduction averaging -10.3% in the case of thiocyanate and -9.3% after radiosulfate (Table 1). Because of its greater simplicity we have relied on the thiocyanate space as a measure of the extent of change in the extracellular fluid space in most of these studies.

Table 1. *Comparative changes in extracellular volume after chlorothiazide as measured by 2 different indicators*

No. of cases	Mean control (liters)		Mean change after chlorothiazide (%)	
	SCN space	$S^{35}O_4$ space	SCN space	$S^{35}O_4$ space
9	21.8	16.8	-10.3 $\pm$ 5	-9.3 ± 7.3

In twenty non-edematous hypertensive patients treated for periods of 3 to 8 days (mean 6.4 days) with 500 mg of chlorothiazide three times daily there was a mean reduction of 2.1 ± 1.75 l of extracellular fluid volume as measured by the thiocyanate method. At the same time there was a loss of 1.8 ± 1.75 kg body weight. Although the standard deviations are large, reflecting the considerable variability in response of different patients, these changes were significant at the .001 level. It will be noted that the estimated change in available fluid space was sufficient to account for the decrease in body weight. In addition, it was observed that there was an approximate correlation between the degree of reduction in SCN space and in body weight in the different patients. These data suggest, therefore, that the weight loss which follows the administration of chlorothiazide is derived from the extracellular rather than the intracellular fluids. Parenteral mercurials also produce a decrease in the extracellular fluid space in non-edematous subjects (*12*).

It is important at this point to relate body sodium loss to the decrease in extracellular volume, since if chlorothiazide promotes an excretion of isotonic extracellular fluid one would expect that the negative balance of sodium would be approximately equivalent to the amount of sodium normally present in the volume of extracellular fluid lost. For example, if the extracellular fluid volume is reduced by 2 l following chlorothiazide treatment, then one would expect a negative sodium balance of 140×2 or 280 mEq. If significantly more sodium was lost than this, one would be justified in considering that some of the sodium was derived from the intracellular fluid. You will recall that the concentration of sodium in the extracellular fluid is unchanged after chlorothiazide, and, therefore, the excess sodium excreted could be derived either from a reduction in extracellular fluid volume or else could be extracted from tissue cells, or both.

Table 2. *Saluretic effect in hypertensives and normotensives*
After 3 days' chlorothiazide (500 mg 3 i.d.)

	No. of cases	Cumulative neg. balance (mEq.)		Decrease in bodyWt.(kg)	Hematocrit change	
		Na	K		No. of cases	per cent
Hypertensive .	6	257 ± 68	156 ± 71	3.0 ± 1.2	20	$+2.0$
Normotensive .	6	287 ± 103	108 ± 41	2.0 ± 0.7	14	$+3.7$

In six, hospitalized, hypertensive patients treated for 3 to 4 days with chlorothiazide who were on a constant daily intake of salt the cumulative negative balance of sodium averaged 257 mEq (*10*) (Table 2). In the same patients the mean decrease in thiocyanate space was 2.8 l and weight loss averaged 3.0 kg. Thus, the total loss of sodium from body stores could easily be accounted for on the basis of the extracellular fluid loss alone. This does not suggest a reduction in intracellular stores of sodium. ALEKSANDROW and his associates found a reduction of 3.8 mEq of sodium per kg of body weight and a mean loss of 2.9% of body weight in hypertensive subjects (*4*). Assuming that the weight loss represents body fluids, this would give an average sodium concentration of 133 mEq/l in the fluid lost from the body, a value closely approximating the sodium concentration in extracellular fluid. In six normotensive subjects, following three days of chlorothiazide treatment, we found an average cumulative sodium loss of 287 mEq and weight reduction of 2.0 kg (Table 2). This provides an estimated concentration of 143 mEq in the body fluids excreted during the saluresis. Such close correspondence to the normal concentrations of sodium in extracellular fluid must be considered fortuitous. However, these data do not indicate intracellular dehydration or significant loss of intracellular sodium content.

Of some importance also in this connection is the observation of HOLLANDER, CHOBANIAN and WILKINS (*14*) that during prolonged treatment with chlorothiazide the total exchangeable sodium does not decrease. During long-term therapy many other factors come into play, including possible depletion of body potassium. Under such circumstances sodium will move into cells to replace the lost potassium. Also, as will be seen later, extracellular fluid volume tends to be restored after prolonged treatment. Regardless of the factors involved, however, the observation of an unchanged total exchangeable sodium during prolonged therapy can be taken as evidence against the cellular depletion of sodium hypothesis, since there is no evidence, either in the initial or late responses to treatment, for such an event.

The most likely interpretation of the action of chlorothiazide in *non-edematous* subjects is that its effects are no different qualitatively than in edematous patients. In each there is a mobilizable pool of extracellular fluid which can be skimmed off by saluretic agents or by severely limiting the dietary sodium intake. Once this labile pool has been eliminated the saluretic agents are not able to deplete further the body's reserves of sodium and are effective only, and to a progressively diminishing degree with the passage of time, in maintaining the so-called "dry weight" of the treated subject.

In the absence of direct measurements of intracellular concentrations the present evidence cannot be regarded as absolute proof of unchanged cellular sodium content; but as a working concept we are led away from the hypothesis of reduced intracellular sodium toward a consideration of the volume changes in the mechanism of the antihypertensive effects of chlorothiazide.

Importance of changes in plasma volume

Since the extracellular space and the plasma volume are in equilibrium across capillary walls it is to be expected that a reduction in extracellular fluid volume will be accompanied by a fall in plasma volume (*1, 5, 15*). In the 20 hypertensive patients in whom simultaneous observations were made, the administration of chlorothiazide was followed by a reduction of 2.1 $\pm$ 1.75 l of available fluid and 358 $\pm$ 223 cc of plasma volume (*10*). Reduction in plasma volume has also been noted after mercurial diuretics in non-edematous subjects (*10, 16*).

If the reduction in plasma volume plays a role in the antihypertensive mechanism of chlorothiazide, then re-expansion of plasma volume should reverse the antihypertensive effects of the drug. Partial to complete reversal of the antihypertensive action of chlorothiazide was observed when the patients were infused with 500 cc of salt-containing or salt-free dextran (*9, 10*). This reversal was not limited to the patients who were taking ganglion blocking agents, but was also seen — although less regularly — in patients with moderate degrees of hypertension who were treated with chlorothiazide alone. Dollery has confirmed this effect of dextran infusion in patients receiving chlorothiazide and ganglion blocking drugs (*5*).

If plasma volume change rather than cellular depletion of sodium is important in determining the reduction of arterial pressure in hypertensive patients, then one would expect to find a reduction in right heart filling pressures and in cardiac output. Crosley and his associates were the first to report such changes following chlorothiazide (*17*). Unfortunately Crosley carried out the experimental studies only one hour after intravenous chlorothiazide when the saluretic effect was far from complete. His results, therefore, are difficult to interpret. Dustan and coworkers, using the dye method, observed a reduction of cardiac output averaging 23% in 9 hypertensive patients, 6 of whom also showed a decrease in mean arterial pressure (*18*). The total peripheral resistance was increased in 8 of the 9 subjects. Right heart pressures were not measured, but the transverse diameter was reduced by roentgenography. In the one case in which it was tried, dextran restored both the cardiac output and the pre-treatment level of blood pressure.

Using right heart catheterization and the Fick principle in 7 hypertensive patients we found an average reduction of 29% in cardiac output, all patients except one showing a decrease (*19*). Five of the seven exhibited a decrease in mean arterial pressure, while the total peripheral resistance increased in 5 of the 7 patients, the average change being + 33%. Right atrial pressure was measured in 3 cases and decreased 2, 5, and 8 mm Hg respectively following chlorothiazide. These results, which are in good agreement with those of Dustan et al., are at variance with the observations of Aleksandrow and his associates, where in 7 cases the cardiac output

decreased in two, increased in one, and was essentially unchanged
in four (*4*). The total peripheral resistance increased markedly in
one, decreased in five and was essentially unchanged in two. In
addition, VARNAUSKAS and WERKÖ (*4a*), while confirming the reduction in basal cardiac output, find a greater decrease in total peripheral
resistance during exercise after as compared to before chlorothiazide.
Perhaps it is premature to draw firm conclusions about the changes
in cardiac output and total peripheral resistance after chlorothiazide
except to state that the bulk of the available evidence does not
refute the hypothesis that the plasma volume change is important
in the antihypertensive effect.

Effect of chlorothiazide on blood pressure responsiveness in normotensive subjects

It will be recalled that normotensive subjects fail to show a
decrease in basal arterial pressure following acute salt depletion
(*1, 2*). Studies carried out in this laboratory on non-edematous,
normotensive subjects indicated that they exhibited a negative
sodium balance and decrease in body weight during 3 days of
chlorothiazide treatment which was quite similar to that seen in the
hypertensive patients (*13*) (Table 2). There was also a significant
elevation of the hematocrit, reflecting a decreased plasma volume.
Despite the similarity of the saluretic response in the two groups,
the hypertensive patients treated with chlorothiazide alone exhibited an average reduction of arterial pressure of 15%, while the
normotensive subjects showed no change in mean blood pressure
(Table 3). It is true that systolic pressure was slightly reduced, but
diastolic pressure was slightly increased and there was a moderate
elevation in heart rate, all of which probably represented normal
adjustments to a reduction in total circulating blood volume.

Table 3. *Changes in blood pressure on chlorothiazide*
alone (500 mg 3 i. d.) for 3 to 8 days

	No. of cases	Average change in blood pressure %	Change in mean blood pressure %
Hypertensive .	10	− 18 / − 9.5	− 15
Normotensive .	14	− 3 / + 3	0

Although the basal blood pressure was not changed in the normotensive subjects the pressor response to norepinephrine infusion
was altered significantly (*13, 20, 21*). Following chlorothiazide in 14
normotensive subjects the peak blood pressure response to duplicate

infusion rates of norepinephrine was reduced by an average of 13%
(*13*) (Fig. 1). This is strikingly similar to the 15% reduction in the
basal blood pressure of hypertensive patients (*1*) and suggests that
acute salt depletion affects similarly the elevated basal blood pressure of hypertensive patients and the transient elevation of blood

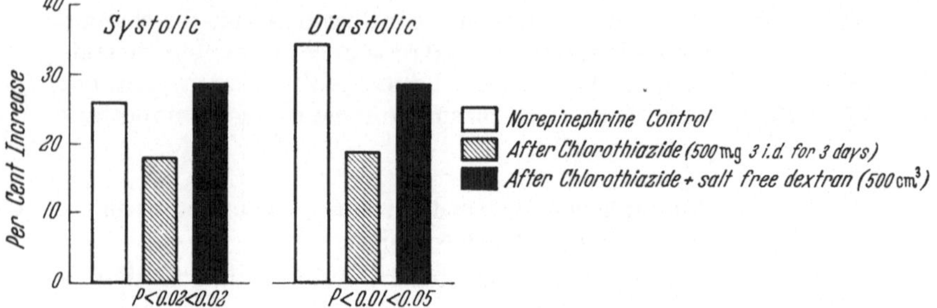

Fig. 1. Per cent changes in blood pressure during norepinephrine infusion before and after
chlorothiazide and after chlorothiazide plus dextran in 14 normotensive subjects

pressure induced by norepinephrine in normotensive subjects. In
this sense the antihypertensive effect of chlorothiazide used alone in
hypertension may be due to a decrease in the patient's responsiveness to the unknown pressor principles operative in that disease.
The moderating effect of chlorothiazide is not limited to norepinephrine alone but is also observed after a variety of pressor agents
(*22, 22a*). In addition, mercurials also share the ability to reduce
blood pressure responsiveness to pressor drugs (*20, 23*).

Aleksandrow and his associates found a diminished responsiveness to norepinephrine in hypertensive patients, but were unable
to correlate this with plasma volume reduction (*24*). Unfortunately
hematocrit changes were not published, so that it is not possible to
examine the consistency of their data. However, their observations
stand in sharp contrast to ours, where a significant increase in
hematocrit was observed in 13 of the 14 cases (*13*).

Each of these 14 normotensive subjects was given 500 ml of 6%
salt-free dextran immediately following the post-chlorothiazide
norepinephrine infusion. After completing the administration of
dextran, norepinephrine was again infused and its pressor effect
determined. The results indicated a significant return of blood
pressure responsiveness toward the control state (*13*). Thus the
difference between the hypertensives and the normotensives is not
as great as appears at first glance. Both show similar saluretic
effects and, in our experience at least, elevations of hematocrit

reflecting a decrease in plasma volume. If the blood pressure of the normotensive is artificially elevated saluretic agents will reduce the degree of elevation, and this effect can be neutralized to a considerable degree by replacing plasma volume just as in the case of the hypertensive patient.

Discussion

It is not too surprising that a reduction of plasma volume will alter the blood pressure responsiveness to norepinephrine infusion. There is ample evidence to indicate that catecholamines reduce the volume of the capacity vessels, thereby raising right heart filling pressures and, hence, cardiac output (25). The level of arterial pressure depends on a complex interrelationship between the pump and the peripheral resistance. Among the factors that are involved must be included constriction of arterioles, changes in contractility of the left ventricle, and the degree of filling of the ventricles. The latter is in large measure controlled by the venous return or right heart filling pressures. However, the venous return is dependent upon the relationship between the blood volume and the capacity of the post-arteriolar vascular bed.

If the blood volume is normal and post-arteriolar vascular capacity reduced, as after norepinephrine infusion or splanchnic nerve stimulation, the relationship between vascular capacity and blood volume will change so as to increase right heart pressures. If blood volume is normal and the vascular capacity increased, as after ganglion blocking drugs, right heart pressures will fall (25). In fact, the combined effects of increased vascular capacity with inability to reduce this capacity reflexly in the face of a smaller plasma volume probably explains the synergistic action of saluretic and ganglioplegic agents.

When the plasma volume is reduced this relationship is altered to favor a decline in right heart filling pressure. Reduction in tissue pressure through depletion of interstitial fluids following saluresis may also alter the transmural pressure sufficiently to produce a further increase in venous capacity. Both factors may produce a "flaccidity" of the capacity vessels which would make them less reponsive to constrictor stimuli and perhaps more responsive to dilator stimuli.

When his plasma volume is moderately reduced the normotensive individual appears to have no difficulty in making the homeostatic adjustments so that his mean basal arterial pressure remains unchanged. The changes in filling pressures and cardiac output that occur in the normotensive subject are not yet known, but from the slight fall in systolic and pulse pressures and the moderate increase in heart rate we may speculate that they are reduced, and that compensation occurs through the baroreceptor reflexes, which produce an increase in heart rate and total peripheral resistance.

In the normotensive subject whose blood pressure has been elevated temporarily by norepinephrine, the augmentor reflexes described above are inhibited. Under the influence of norepinephrine-induced hypertension, the baroreceptors will be stimulated to moderate the blood pressure. Without the homeostatic action of the augmentor reflexes, the depressor effect of a moderate reduction of plasma volume will be unmasked. For some unknown reason the basal blood pressure of the hypertensive subject reacts similarly in that his homeostatic mechanisms fail to recognize and respond to the plasma volume reduction. This is surprising in view of the fact that the moderator reflexes appear to react normally, at least to quick changes in blood pressure in hypertensive patients (25). Perhaps the gradual and persistent nature of the blood volume change, or the lack of red cell mass reduction, or the concomitant depletion of extracellular volume may account for the difference.

The profound effect of small changes in blood volume on arterial pressure, in the absence of adequate reflex homeostasis, may not be sufficiently appreciated. For example, we have observed that after hexamethonium in human subjects reductions of as little as 2 to 4% of the total blood volume can produce perceptible decrements of arterial pressure (26). There is no justification, therefore, in assuming that because the plasma volume change is relatively small there can be no effect on blood pressure.

In addition to the venous capacity it may also be pertinent to consider the arterial capacity. In fact, the presence of an elevated pressure necessarily implies that the ratio of the arterial blood volume to the arterial capacity is increased. More blood is packed per unit volume of arterial capacity than occurs normally. Perhaps reduction in plasma volume permits some relief of this abnormal disproportion.

These remarks are admittedly speculative. It would be unwise on the basis of present evidence to discard completely the hypothesis of sodium depletion in vascular walls. Such an explanation would be consistent with Tobian's observations of an increase in the salt and water content of arterial walls in human and experimental hypertension (27). Unfortunately, other investigators have not confirmed Tobian's findings. For example, Daniel and Dawkins found no disturbance in aortic wall concentrations of electrolytes in spontaneous, renal constriction, and long-standing DCA hypertension in rats (*28*). FREED et al. also failed to observe a significant elevation of sodium in the aortas of renal hypertensive rats, although they do report an increased potassium content (*29*). HADDY demonstrated a decrease in arteriolar resistance with increasing concentrations of sodium in the perfusing blood (*30*). FRIEDMAN believes that the tension developing in vascular smooth muscle varies directly with the ratio of sodium concentration inside the cells to that outside (*31*). LEONARD found that the tension in vascular smooth muscle is dependent on the potassium concentrations across the cell (*32*). It is obvious that the subject of the effects of electrolyte flux on vascular distensibility is extremely complicated and far from settled. There is no urgency, therefore, for clinical investigators to extrapolate TOBIAN's thesis to the conditions existing in the hypertensive patient under treatment with saluretic agents. For the moment, on the basis of the presently available evidence, the volume change hypothesis seems to explain best the actual observations made in hypertensive patients treated with saluretic agents.

Against the volume hypothesis is the observation that plasma volume, thiocyanate space and body weight tend to return to control values after months of continuous therapy (*10*). This could imply that volume changes predominate in the initial antihypertensive response, but that later some other mechanism takes over. However, it could also mean that prolonged therapy modifies the severity of the hypertension. Modification of even severe forms of hypertension occurs after intensive treatment with hexamethonium and hydralazine (*33*). Drug tolerance may also develop to further confuse the picture. It is very difficult to relate cause and effect under these circumstances.

Summary

The available evidence on the mechanism of the antihypertensive effects of saluretic agents has been partially reviewed and the conclusion reached that, of the various hypotheses considered, reduction in plasma volume appears to explain best the observed changes accompanying the initial antihypertensive response. Because the saluretic agents reduce blood pressure responsiveness to norpinephrine and other pressor amines it is suggested that they also decrease reactivity to the unknown pressor principles operative in hypertension. It is further speculated that the relationship between the vascular capacity and the contained blood volume may be important in this reaction, and that baroreceptor responses to the reduction in plasma volume may be defective in hypertensive patients.

Résumé

Les observations faites jusqu'ici concernant le mécanisme des effets antihypertenseurs d'agents salurétiques ont été passées en revue partiellement.

Nous parvenons à la conclusion que parmi les différentes hypothèses considérées, la réduction du volume plasmatique semble le mieux capable d'expliquer les modifications qui accompagnent la réponse anti-hypertensive initiale. Étant donné que les agents salurétiques réduisent la réponse tensionnelle à la nor-adrénaline et à d'autres amines vasopressives, nous suggérons qu'ils diminuent aussi la réactivité aux principes hypertenseurs inconnus qui interviennent dans l'hypertension.Nous supposons aussi que la relation entre la capacité vasculaire et le volume sanguin peut être importante dans cette réaction et que les réponses des baro-récepteurs à la réduction du volume plasmatique peuvent être inadéquates chez les hypertendus.

References

1. Freis, E. D., A. Wanko, I. M. Wilson, and A. E. Parrish: Ann. N. Y. Acad. Sc. **71**, 450 (1958).
2. Wilkins, R. W., W. Hollander, and A. V. Chobanian: Ann. N. Y. Acad. Sc. **71**, 465 (1958).
3. Freis, E. D., I. M. Wilson, and A. E. Parrish: Circulation (U.S.A.) **16**, 882 (1957).
4. Aleksandrow, D., W. Wysnacka, and J. Gajewski: N. England J. Med. **260**, 51 (1959).
4a. Varnauskas, E., and L. Werkö: Personal communication to the author.
5. Dollery, C. T., M. Harington, and G. Kaufman: Lancet (G.B.) **1959/I**, 1215.
6. Kempner, W.: Amer. J. Med. **4**, 545 (1948).
7. Stead, W. W., M. F. Reiser, S. Rapaport, and E. B. Ferris: J. Clin. Invest. (U.S.A.) **27**, 766 (1948).
8. Hollander, W., A. V. Chobanian, and R. W. Wilkins: Circulation (U.S.A.) **19**, 827 (1959).
9. Freis, E. D.: The effects of salt and extracellular fluid depletion on vascular responsiveness with particular reference to chlorothiazide. In: Hypertension Vol VII; Drug action, epidemiology and hemodynamics. Skelton, F. R., ed., Proc. Council High B.P. Res., Amer. Heart Ass. (publishers), Nov. 1958, p. 6.
10. Wilson, I. M., and E. D. Freis: Circulation (U.S.A.) **20**, 1028 (1959).
11. Esch, A. F., I. M. Wilson, and E. D. Freis: Med. Ann. District of Columbia **28**, 9 (1959).
12. Leard, S. E., and E. D. Freis: Amer. J. Med. **7**, 647 (1949).
13. Freis, E. D., A. Wanko, H. W. Schnaper, and E. D. Frohlich: J. Clin. Invest. (U.S.A.) In press (Aug. 1960).
14. Hollander, W., A. V. Chobanian, and R. W. Wilkins: Clin. Res. (U.S.A.) **6**, 21 (1958).
15. Tapia, F. A., H. P. Dustan, R. A. Schneckloth, A. C. Corcoran, and I. H. Page: Lancet (G.B.) **1957/II**, 831.
16. Lyons, R., S. D. Jacobson, and N. L. Avery jr.: Amer. Heart J. **27**, 353 (1944).
17. Crosley, A. P. jr., R. C. Cullen, D. White, J. F. Freeman, C. A. Castillo, and G. G. Rowe: J. Laborat. Clin. Med. (U.S.A.) **55**, 182 (1960).
18. Dustan, H. P., G. R. Cumming, A. C. Corcoran, and I. H. Page: Circulation (U.S.A.) **19**, 360 (1959).
19. Frohlich, E. D., H. W. Schnaper, I. M. Wilson, and E. D. Freis: N. England J. Med. In press.
20. Wanko, A., and E. D. Freis: Circulation (U.S.A.) **18**, 792 (1958).

21. MERRILL, J. P., A. GUINAND-BALDO, and C. GIORDANA: Clin. Res. (U.S.A.) **6**, 230 (1958).
22. BEAVERS, W. R., and W. P. BLACKMORE: Proc. Soc. Exper. Biol. Med. (U.S.A.) **98**, 133 (1958).
22a. BOCK, K. D., and F. GROSS: Naunyn-Schmiedebergs Arch. exper. Path. (G.) **238**, 339 (1960).
23. BLACKMORE, W. P., and W. R. BEAVERS: Proc. Soc. Exper. Biol. Med. (U.S.A.) **101**, 128 (1959).
24. ALEKSANDROW, D., W. WYSNACKA, and J. GAJEWSKI: N. England J. Med. **261**, 1052 (1959).
25. FREIS, E. D.: Physiol. Rev. (U.S.A.) **40**, 27 (1960).
26. FREIS, E. D., J. R. STANTON, F. A. FINNERTY jr., H. W. SCHNAPER, R. L. JOHNSON, C. E. ROTH, and R. W. WILKINS: J. Clin. Invest. (U.S.A.) **30**, 435 (1951).
27. TOBIAN, L., and J. T. BINION: Tissue cations and water in arterial hypertension. Circulation (U.S.A.) **5**, 754 (1952).
28. DANIEL, E. E., and O. DAWKINS: Amer. J. Physiol. **190**, 71 (1957).
29. FREED, S. C., S. ST. GEORGE, and R. H. ROSENMAN: Circulation Res. (U.S.A.) **7**, 219 (1959).
30. HADDY, F. J., D. EMANUEL, and J. SCOTT: Physiologist **1**, 131 (1958).
31. FRIEDMAN, S. M., J. D. JAMIESON, and C. L. FRIEDMAN: Circulation Res. (U.S.A.) **7**, 44 (1959).
32. LEONARD, E.: Amer. J. Physiol. **189**, 185 (1957).
33. PERRY, H. M., and H. A. SCHROEDER: Circulation (U.S.A.) **13**, 528 (1956).

Discussion

GROSS: I have one question to ask Dr. FREIS: Did you, in normotensive patients who were not treated with chlorothiazide, infuse the same amount of dextran as in your patients treated with chlorothiazide and did you observe the same increase of blood pressure as you found after infusion in patients with lowered blood pressure due to chlorothiazide?

FREIS: No, we haven't done that.

REUBI: I have also one remark to make to Dr. FREIS: I think your findings may well explain the acute change in blood pressure observed at the beginning of chlorothiazide treatment, i. e. after 3 to 6 days. You found a decrease in cardiac output, a slight decrease in blood pressure, and an increase in total peripheral resistance. But I am not sure that after 2 or 3 months of treatment you could get the same pattern, because we know that with almost every hypotensive substance the acute effects may be very different from the long-term effects. I would like to ask you whether you have been doing experiments on long-term treatment with chlorothiazide. This is my first question. Can you answer it?

FREIS: Yes, we have studied the same patients after 6 months and a year, and you are quite right that the volume changes are no longer present after 6 months or a year, although the blood pressure remains significantly reduced. One can explain this by saying that the blood pressure is reduced by one mechanism of action of chlorothiazide in the beginning and by an entirely different mechanism later on. This is difficult for me to believe. There is another explanation that I would like to propose and that is the one that PAGE and MCCUBBIN propose, namely that when you reduce the blood pressure for any length of time by any kind of therapy, you reset the baroreceptor mechanism or in some other way modify the hypertension. Therefore, you are not dealing with the same individual that you were dealing with initially, and this makes the attempt to relate cause and effect after such long-term control of blood pressure extremely difficult. For example, we have observed that the haemodynamic effects of ganglion blocking agents and Apresoline, after long-term therapy, may be quite different from what they are after short-term therapy. And yet I would not like to say that they are acting in a different way.

REUBI: I have a second remark. You did not mention in your paper HOLLANDER's studies, and I think his results are a bit different from yours. As far as I remember, HOLLANDER found that if he restored the plasma volume and the total exchangeable sodium to normal by adding fluorohydrocortisone to chlorothiazide, the blood pressure went up but not to the pre-treatment level. We might assume in this case that chlorothiazide has a vascular effect. What do you think about that?

FREIS: I must admit these studies are in opposition to ours. However, I think that the majority of the data available from various laboratories suggests that the volume change is the important factor in the initial antihypertensive effect.

HOOD: As you have calculated your cumulative negative sodium balances, did you ever re-infuse the sodium and water loss while you maintained the chlorothiazide treatment, and observe the effect of such a procedure?

FREIS: We are doing that at present, but we do not yet have enough patients to form any clear concept of what happens. So far, the results have been very sporadic and the infusions have not always restored the blood pressure to where it had been. In some of the cases the administration of salt solution failed to restore the blood pressure despite restoration of the fluid volume to where it had been in the pre-treatment period. A few days later we gave these patients dextran and the blood pressure was restored. So I am uncertain about the effects of extracellular fluid volume replacement on the basis of our present sparse data.

SCHROEDER: I would like to ask Dr. FREIS to emphasize a point which Dr. GROLLMAN mentioned, i. e. that about a third of hypertensive patients achieve a significant reduction of blood pressure on a low sodium diet. In 1937, when we first studied the effect of sodium chloride on the edema of congestive heart failure, we made many attempts to lower very high blood pressure with diets containing 0.5 g of NaCl. These studies were made on a metabolic ward and were controlled by daily 24 hr urinary chloride measurement, often for months. We were never able to convince ourselves that the diet was effective, except in occasional patients in whom it often had dramatic hypotensive effects. In general, when treatment was mandatory for prolongation of life, diet was ineffective, with rare exceptions. Since then, my experience with dietary salt restriction and the rice diet has failed to change these original opinions.

There is a group of people, mostly women with central obesity and low sweat sodium, who do respond dramatically to salt restriction and whose blood pressures rise with salt repletion. We have described them clinically and SOMERS is describing them pathologically, as they have adrenal cortical adenomata or hyperplasia. They probably represent a different disease than "essential" hypertension. If the chlorothiazides achieve their effects by natriuresis, one would expect their hypotensive effect to be no better and no worse than sodium restriction, with the expected dramatic results in those patients I described. I would also therefore like to ask Dr. FREIS: You showed that a mean diastolic fall of about 10% was produced by these agents. That is certainly not very much for a diastolic pressure of 130 or 140 mm Hg and would result in normotension only if the diastolic was 100 mm Hg. How many patients have strict normotension with the use of chlorothiazide alone? Or the drug plus moderate salt restriction? In other words, is this agent actually as relatively ineffective in severe hypertension as is salt restriction?

GROLLMAN: In Dr. FREIS' chart comparing the effects of chlorothiazide in hypertensive and normotensive individuals, the loss of weight in the former was 3 kg as compared to only 2 kg in the latter. This loss in the normotensives corresponded to the loss of extracellular fluid; the extra loss of a liter of fluid by the hypertensives was attributed by Dr. FREIS to errors in measurement. I would suggest that the loss unaccounted for in the hypertensives may represent the excretion of water derived from the intracellular space. If this is the case, the response of the two groups to the drug as well as to the replacement of the reduced blood volume are not comparable.

It seems to me that the available experimental data indicate that sodium depletion induced by either dietary restriction or by natriuretic drugs exerts its immediate hypotensive effects by a different mechanism than that operative later. The immediate effect as shown by Dr. FREIS is a consequence of hemodynamic changes of an acute nature. Adjustments in the distribution of electrolyte and water between the extracellular and intracellular spaces then occur which perpetuate the lowering of the blood pressure with a lowering of peripheral resistance from its initially elevated value.

SARRE: We can confirm the experiments of Dr. FREIS. Dr. MERTZ at my clinic made a determination of the extracellular fluid with the method of the inulin space. In 20 or more hypertensive patients on a normal diet we found an extracellular volume of 15.2% of body weight, but on a low salt diet only 11,9% of body weight. This is a difference of 2.0—2.5 kg! Afterwards we made some experiments with chlorothiazide, and found the same as with the low-salt diet.

SCHMID: I would like to make some remarks on Dr.FREIS' statements. I am not sure whether only the loss of intravascular fluid is responsible for the blood pressure decline. In a couple of non-edematous patients I treated with hydrochlorothiazide, I observed that they lost during the first 2—3 days about 2 kg of weight. However, the blood pressure drop was in no way related to this. It seemed to me, however, that it was related to the dosage of hydrochlorothiazide. In some patients you may get rather an important a drop of blood pressure with only 25 mg of hydrochlorothiazide, but in other patients only with 100 mg. Nevertheless, there was always the same loss of weight. Now I wonder how this haemodynamic feature and the weight loss could be correlated to the hypothetical plasma volume diminution, because I think that in all patients there should be the same plasma volume loss but not the same hypotensive effect.

FREIS: Dr. SCHROEDER asked what percentage obtained a reduction of blood pressure to normal levels; very few showed a reduction to normal levels. We did not study the most severe types of hypertension, because we were trying to stay away from people with severe renal damage or heart failure. Reduction of blood pressure with chlorothiazide alone was not very marked. Indeed, its main clinical effect, as we stated in our earliest reports, is that it enhances the activity of other antihypertensive agents. I do not believe, Dr. GROLLMAN, that there is an increased water loss in the hypertensives. The cases reported here were only 6 hypertensives and 6 normotensives. In larger groups, in which we determined weight loss, the weight loss was the same in 20 hypertensives and 14 normotensives. This loss was about 2 kg body weight on the average. I think the discrepancy was probably due to the small series and the approximate nature of balance studies. As to the question of the relationship of the blood pressure fall to the degree of body weight loss, we too failed to observe a close relationship between weight loss and the degree of blood pressure reduction. This did not surprise us too much, because there are many other factors involved in vascular responsiveness. The relationship between plasma volume and vascular capacity is only one of the factors involved, and the response will vary from one individual to another depending on the relative importance of these other factors in each patient. All we are trying to say is that in the initial reduction of arterial pressure, plasma volume and vascular capacity relationships play an important part. We do not say this is the only factor involved in blood pressure control. However, we did not find any evidence that chlorothiazide has any specific effect that was independent of the salt losing action.

HOOBLER: I would like to ask whether chlorothiazide has been shown by any investigator to lower blood pressure in the renal hypertensive animal. So far as Dr. FREIS' report is concerned, results obtained by Dr. LAUWERS and Dr. CONWAY are at variance. They studied ambulatory patients at several months rather than a few days or weeks after chlorothiazide treatment was started. Cardiac output, at this later time interval, was not reduced. A report by Dr. LAUWERS soon to be published in the J. of Lab. Clin. Med. also indicates that, in this later phase of chlorothiazide treatment, plasma volume and total exchangeable sodium are not reduced. Total body water, measured by antipyrine space, was, however, consistently lower after treatment, and I suppose total body potassium had fallen although he did not measure this parameter. He did a few short-term experiments and found the same changes as Dr. FREIS has reported. Therefore we believe there must be a change in mechanism during prolonged therapy. I doubt whether this represents a resetting of the baroceptor or some other body readjustment to a reduced cardiac output, as suggested by Dr. FREIS, since even after a year or so of treatment, the blood pressure rises and the body weight increases as soon as chlorothiazide is stopped. I would not expect such a rapid reversal if the body had adapted itself to the lower pressure.

COTTIER: I want to ask Dr. FREIS how long he could find a saluretic effect in hypertensives treated by chlorothiazide, because after four weeks' therapy we already found antinatriuresis — perhaps the expression of a compensatory mechanism. On the other hand, after 4 weeks' therapy potassium clearance was still elevated. We also did studies on the extracellular volume change (inulin space) under therapy. We found[1] after four weeks' treatment with chlorothiazide in 10 hypertensive patients an average decrease of the inulin space (extracellular fluid volume) of 0.5 l/70 kg body weight, a decrease of the body weight, however, of 1 kg on the average. Could the greater fall of body weight than of the extracellular fluid volume be due to a loss of intracellular fluid volume?

We also calculated the renal resistances, and there was a mean fall after four weeks of treatment of 8.7%.

SCHETTLER: We did the same experiments as Dr. COTTIER just outlined with the inulin space and the blood pressure, and we got the same results in the reduction of the extracellular fluid.

HOOBLER: What kind of treatment?

SCHETTLER: Chlorothiazide.

HOOBLER: How long?

SCHETTLER: 3 to 14 days.

BOCK: In agreement with the results of Dr. FREIS we found[2] that in the trained non-anaesthetised dog after 8-days' oral treatment with hydrochlorothiazide the pressor response to adrenaline, nor-adrenaline, and angiotensin is significantly reduced. The fact that the effects of pressor agents with different peripheral sites of action are diminished in the same way seems to indicate a non-specific change in vascular reactivity. HOLLANDER[3], however, has shown in a patient with essential hypertension that the reduced pressor response to nor-adrenaline, observed after 8 days' treatment with chlorothiazide, returned to the control values after 8 weeks' treatment, indicating too that there exists a difference between the early and the late effect of saluretics on vascular reactivity.

WILSON: I have been wondering whether this response to saluretics may throw some light on the mechanism of essential hypertension. We may have been overlooking some disturbance of blood volume distribution which, combined with a cardiac factor, may be involved in the change from acute to

---

[1] COTTIER, P.: Therap. Umschau (Switz.) **16**, 30 (1959), Helvet. med. Acta, Suppl. 39 ad Vol. 27 (1960).

[2] BOCK, K. D., and F. GROSS: Naunyn-Schmiedebergs Arch. exp. Path. Pharmak. (G.) **238**, 339 (1960).

[3] HOLLANDER, W., A. V. CHOBANIAN and R. W. WILKINS: In "Diuresis and Diuretics, an International Symposium". Berlin-Göttingen-Heidelberg, Springer 1959.

chronic hypertension. For some years now, Dr. LEDINGHAM in our laboratory has been examining the function of the isolated heart in the hypertensive rat. There seems to be a difference in the relationship of cardiac output to auricular filling in the hypertensive animal. Recently Dr. FLOYER in our laboratory made a very interesting chance observation on the relationship between blood pressure differences and sodium excretion in the parabiotic rat preparation. The rats had normal blood pressures and normal sodium excretion before they were united in parabiosis. After being united, although their blood pressures might be within the normal range, there were slight differences between the two, and the rat with the slightly higher pressure was excreting the greater part of the total sodium excretion of the pair. The blood pressure in one rat was raised to 165 mm Hg, while in the other member of the pair, it was 105 mm Hg. In this pair the hypertensive rat excreted over 90% of the total.

Dr. FLOYER did red-cell volume measurements in the two rats and found a higher volume in the rat with the greater sodium excretion. When the renal artery of one rat was clipped, the degree of hypertension produced was different on the two sides and so was the degree of crossed hypertension in the other member of the pair. It is possible that this experimental model may enable us to clarify the relationship between changes in blood pressure and blood volume.

TAQUINI: I fully agree with the interpretation given by Dr. FREIS on the results obtained in his short-term experiments. The lowering of the blood volume and subsequent fall in cardiac output are indeed the best explanation for the reduction of the blood pressure in his cases. I do not believe that changes in blood volume followed by changes in cardiac output can be involved in the long-term depressor action of the drug. The chronic increase in blood volume can hardly be accepted as a cause of hypertension. This does not appear in diseases such as cardiac failure or polycythemia, in which the blood volume is frequently very high.

The alteration of the relationship between vascular-bed capacity and blood volume is a frequent cause of changes in cardiac output, but the alteration or disequilibrium, even physiological, pathological or experimentally induced, is rapidly compensated in different ways and cannot by itself be the cause of a chronic modification of the cardiac output and the blood pressure. Moreover, there must be another mechanism involved in the long-term reduction of the blood pressure seen in patients treated with saluretics, since, as Dr. FREIS pointed out, the blood volume return, later to normal values.

FERRERO: I would like to make one point. We have done investigations in the cardiac laboratory of Prof. DUCHOSAL on the hemodynamic effects of chlorothiazide during heart catheterisation in a group of ten patients with congestive heart failure; after intravenous administration of $^1/_2$ g or 1 g of chlorothiazide, we did not observe consistent modifications in hemodynamics during the control period of 30 to 80 min.

PLUMMER: Dr. FREIS suggested in his talk that the vasculature may become more responsive to depressor agents after chlorothiazide. We can give some information in that direction. The depressor response to histamine is intensified in the dog following chlorothiazide or hydrochlorothiazide. Also Apresoline, in doses which normally did not lower the blood pressure in the dog, became depressant after hydrochlorothiazide. It required about 3 hr after the intravenous administration of hydrochlorothiazide for these effects to develop.

SARRE: Did you see any cases without response of the blood pressure but with reduction of extracellular fluid or hemodynamic factors?

FREIS: There have been a great deal of comments to the fact that the hemodynamic changes are different after long-term therapy. In the paper Dr. WILSON and I published last year, we agreed that the changes after long-term therapy are not the same as after short-term therapy. I do not know why that is; but there is no need to conclude that chlorothiazide is acting differently. Did we see hypertensive patients who got no reduction of blood pressure with a reduction in body weight? Yes, occasionally, but not usually. Lack of hypotensive response tended to occur in the more severe cases. Did we measure total body water? No, we did not. But we did not see any particular need to measure it, at least in the acute studies, because we could account for the weight loss by the extent of the extracellular fluid volume change. What was the spread in pre-treatment blood-pressure levels between hypertensives and normotensives? It was quite wide. The hypertensive patients were of the type that might be classified as moderately severe with established hypertension. The saluretic effect lasted for 48 hrs after chlorothiazide was started in a dose of 500 mg three times per day. After that, the daily excretion of salt parallels the intake. However, the loss of body stores of sodium which occurs during the first 48 hrs is maintained. There seems to be a certain labile pool of extracellular fluid which is excreted during the first 48 hrs, after which the drug maintains this so-called "dry weight", but seems unable further to deplete body stores of salt.

REUBI: I am afraid we shall have to stop this discussion. To sum up, I would say that Dr. FREIS' explanation seems at first to be the most attractive, but cannot be accepted for long-term studies, so that we still do not know how to explain the hypotensive action of chlorothiazides on a long-term basis. Do you agree?

FREIS: I agree.

The natural history of benign hypertension

By

P. BECHGAARD

By now, it is nearly 50 years since the first natural history of hypertension was written by JANEWAY (*10*). His work was both comprehensive and thorough, and it has been highly inspiring to review it and to see to what extent his opinions still hold good in the light of subsequent developments.

JANEWAY's series was characterised by the fact that many of his hypertensive patients were in a late phase of the disease, and that many of them had renal disease. Consequently, he found that the prognosis was very poor. Four years after the occurrence of the initial symptoms one half of his patients had died. In his efforts to make early diagnosis possible, he attached great significance to the disclosure of early symptoms.

The fact that JANEWAY's paper was justly considered for a long time to be the best description of untreated hypertension caused the views taken of the prognosis of essential hypertension to be very pessimistic for many years afterwards and resulted in too much attention being focused on the symptoms. Hence, most investigators were far too willing to ascribe discomforts of varying severity to the consequences of elevated blood pressure.

To-day, when attempting to describe the picture of untreated essential hypertension, we are still faced with some of the same difficulties as JANEWAY. He knew that he was not working with just one disease, an aetiological entity; we know this also. The picture we paint of the disease to-day will not remain valid in the future. The concept of essential hypertension will be constantly narrowed down. This has been done most recently by the demonstration (*20*) that involvement of the renal artery is far more common than was previously thought.

This discovery will reduce the value of the series to which we at the present time attach the greatest importance — series in which urography, and not aortography, has marked the approximate peak of what has been attained by technical investigations; and yet we must presumably also in future be content with the best series that are available to-day. It will become practically impossible to get an opportunity to follow up a large, representative series of untreated hypertensives for 20 years or more, which is necessary in order to assess the prognosis.

Blood pressure

In the diagnosis of hypertensive disease the definition of normal blood pressure has always been a great problem which is still partially unsolved.

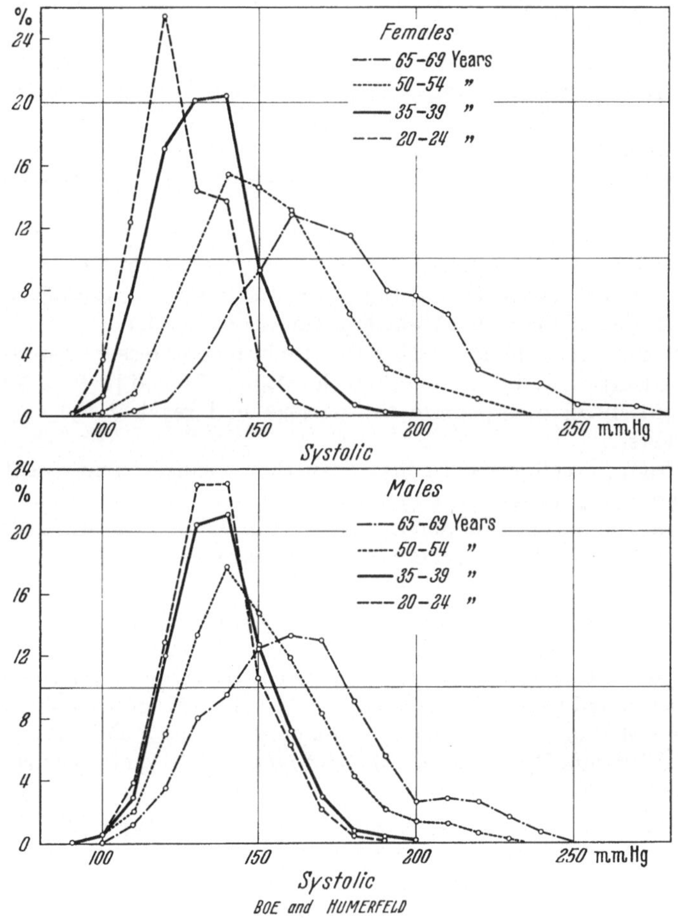

Fig. 1. Frequency distribution of systolic blood pressure

Although I do not intend to enter into a discussion on the nature of high blood pressure, I wish to call your attention to the great Norwegian investigation by Bøe and Humerfelt (8), whose figures are based on the study of the blood pressure in about 68,000 persons representing almost the entire population of the city of Bergen.

Here is one of their figures which gives a good impression of the distribution of blood pressures at different ages (Fig. 1).

The peaks of the different age curves show a tendency towards higher blood pressures and the bases of the curves are broadened with advancing age.

These findings are in support of Pickering's view (18) that, strictly speaking, it is impossible to use a single value in order to delimit normal blood pressure. What we really want is the generally unobtainable observation that a person's blood pressure leaves a fairly stable level and, within a short time, rises to a new and much higher one.

As far as I know, Perera (15) is the only investigator who has been able to use this method in a follow-up study of 200 cases of benign hypertension and at the same time has given us a new and better idea of the ages at which hypertension starts.

In most cases he found that the rise in blood pressure appeared in the thirties, and that abnormal elevations of blood pressure were evident in all cases before the persons had reached the age of 48 years.

From these findings we may draw the conclusion that essential hypertension, in most cases, develops between the ages of 35 and 45 years, and that a sudden rise in blood pressure in the age groups before 30 and after 50 years must always arouse suspicion of being not essential but secondary hypertension.

But even if we accept a fixed value which has been necessary in all follow-up studies, the incidence of hypertension is still open to discussion. Generally, 25% of the population over forty years of age are estimated to be hypertensives, a view which is supported by the figures of Master, Marks, and Dack (11) showing a blood pressure of 150/100 mm Hg or more in 30% of men and 40% of women over forty.

This view does not agree with the experience gained by those who have made comprehensive follow-up studies. As Perera (15) puts it, after having made repeated analyses in different age groups, he never observed an incidence of essential hypertension greater than 6% in any series.

This is in accordance with my own experience. I found my own 1,000 hypertensive patients among 21,000 records in a medical out-patient clinic, which represents 5%, and in order to get a control series for sympathectomised patients HAMMARSTRÖM and I (*3*) had to go through 120,000 records, and we found a frequency of serious hypertension of only $^1/_2\%$ suitable for this purpose.

The comprehensive Norwegian investigation probably illustrates the situation best of all.

Although these pressures were measured as thoroughly as possible, they can only be taken as casual pressures, giving too high an incidence as compared with patients kept under observation for some time before the diagnosis of hypertension is made.

Table 1. *The frequency of high blood pressure in a population* (HUMERFELT and Bøe).

Systolic blood pressure 160 mm Hg and more

	—40 years %	—50 years %	—60 years %
Men . . .	10	20	40
Women. .	5	35	50

Diastolic blood pressure 100 mm Hg and more

	—40 years %	—50 years %	—60 years %
Men . . .	4	7	12
Women. .	3	10	18

Unfortunately, we cannot pick out from the investigation a group having both a systolic blood pressure of 160 mm Hg and a diastolic of 100 mm Hg or more, the figures used in most follow-up studies. But the figures must be considerably smaller than those in the diastolic group, where the highest incidence in the sixty-year-old group is 12% for men and 18% for women.

With the exception of PERERA's 200 cases (*15*) our knowledge of the natural history of hypertension is based on a number of follow-up studies, in which the hypertensive patients were followed not from the start of the rise in blood pressure but from a chance point in time generally rather late in the clinical course. Looking at these studies, you will find that there is a great difference in the evalua-tion of the prognosis. It is important to make the reason for this difference clear at once.

One group consists of patients in the late stage of the disease; the majority are being looked after in hospitals or hypertensive clinics because of symptoms and complications. In the other group, an attempt has been made to combat the hypertension in an earlier stage, and the patients are generally out-patients, not specially seeking medical advice for hypertensive disease.

Table 2. *Follow-up studies of hypertension*

		Number of patients	Years of observation	Dead %
JANEWAY	1913	458	10	75
TOP (hosp.)	1919	157	2— 5	83
BENNI (hosp.)	1926	148	4	77
BLACKFORD	1930	222	5—11	50
ROSLING	1934	450	8	30
BECHGAARD	1946	1,038	4—11	28
PALMER	1948	430	8	39
FRANT	1950	418	8— 9	32
MATHISEN	1959	290	10	33
BECHGAARD	1956	1,038	16—22	65
PALMER	1959	453	19—24	83

To take another example, if you want to outline the natural history of polio you cannot just describe the paralytic cases.

Whether hypertension, as a rule, is a progressive disease, or whether it is apt to stabilise quickly at the level at which it is going to stay in future, as suggested by PICKERING (*18*), is another open question.

I had hoped to be able to illustrate this by applying PICKERING's scores to my series, but it appeared that my series was not quite ideal for this purpose.

In follow-up studies, I gained the impression that, on the whole, the blood pressure level did not rise in the group of patients who were alive at the second examination. I found that the diastolic blood pressure was the same in 61%, higher in 12%, and lower in 27%. In order to see what had happened between the second and the third examination in 1956, I went through the records of a group of 80 patients and found that the diastolic pressure had increased only in 7, i.e. in about 9%. But, obviously, this applies only to the group which has the best prognosis. In those who died — the severe cases — the blood pressures recorded before death were not reliable enough to allow a similar investigation.

Classification of benign hypertension

In our study of the surgical and medical treatment of malignant hypertension it has been of the greatest value that in group 4 of KEITH and WAGENER's classification we have had a well-defined group of patients with a well-known prognosis.

In investigating the prognosis and results of treatment for benign hypertension we are not fortunate enough to be in possession of a clear and universally accepted classification.

Although it has been used to a great extent, the classification of
KEITH and WAGENER has not been of much value here. In benign
hypertension it is not possible to base a classification on the eyegrounds only. The documentation supporting this view will be given
later.

The sex, age, and the condition of the heart and kidneys are not
taken into account in KEITH and WAGENER's classification, but in
benign hypertension these factors are of such great significance that
they must be considered. Group 3 of KEITH and WAGENER is relatively well defined, but there is no doubt that this group contains
some cases both of definite malignant hypertension without papilloedema and of retinal thrombosis and latent diabetes, especially
when only unilateral lesions are found without extremely high
blood pressures.

In collaboration with an ophthalmologist (23) I have investigated
the ophthalmological appearance of the eyegrounds in elderly persons with arteriosclerosis and normal blood pressure. We found that
10% of the patients in the 40—50 age group showed slight changes
in the retinal arteries. Over the age of fifty, these changes increased
in severity and frequency, and many cases of constricted arteries
and irregularities of calibre were observed.

Table 3. *Eyeground findings in 124 elderly persons with normal blood pressures*

Age group	40—49	50—59	60—69	70—79	80+
No. of patients	26	25	24	25	24
Arteries constricted	0	1	9	13	18
Irregularities of calibre	3	9	18	25	24
Abnormal reflex	0	4	15	22	23
Venous depressions	4	6	12	10	12

No haemorrhages, exudates, or papilloedema.

These two types of changes correspond to the alterations occurring in patients with hypertension in KEITH and WAGENER's
groups 1 and 2.

Haemorrhages and retinopathy were not seen.

Classifications of benign hypertension more suitable for the purpose are given by PALMER (13), SMITHWICK (21), HAMMARSTRÖM
and BECHGAARD (3), and others, but none of these have been
generally accepted, and perhaps they are not quite ideal. Would it
not be worth while to agree on one single classification and to try to
combine the different series of untreated patients to make a big
control series while it is still possible ?

Symptoms

In 1913, Janeway was anxious to analyse the symptoms of hypertension. In his opinion, early symptoms were dyspnoea on exertion, urinary disturbances, fatigue, oedema, headache, dizziness and vertigo, failure of eyesight, haemorrhages, especially nose-bleed, intermittent claudication, depression, anaemia, anorexia, and loss of flesh.

We cannot approve of these as early symptoms; yet I have the impression that too many of them are still accepted and their disappearance taken as proof that treatment is having good results, although it has never been sufficiently shown that they are direct consequences of the elevated blood pressure itself.

Table 4. *Symptoms in hypertension of more than 10 years' duration*

Headache	23%
Dizziness	30%
Depression	7%
Nervousness	35%
Encephalopathy	3%
Precordial pain	26%
Angina pectoris	7%
Palpitation	32%
Functional dyspnoea . .	42%
Resting dyspnoea . . .	4%
Nose-bleed	3%

Total 840 patients.

At least in my country, such symptoms as headache, nervousness, and vertigo have prompted treatment which was not otherwise indicated.

In hypertensive patients you will find a lot of minor symptoms. In my series the frequency of these symptoms was as shown in Table 4.

In 1946, I was ready to accept the greater part of these symptoms as being due to high blood pressure, but to-day I think that most of them, with the exception of dyspnoea on exertion and encephalopathy, do not differ very much from those seen in series of non-hypertensive persons of the same age.

Of Janeway's patients with severe hypertension, 15% complained of headache. Most of these cases were found in the group of malignant hypertension. This means that he did not register many instances of typical morning headache among his patients with benign hypertension.

Headache is a very common complaint in many grown-up persons. When a hypertensive patient complains of headache, other causes must be carefully ruled out, especially the neurotic headache, which according to Stewart (22) is the most common cause, and also vasomotor and cervical headaches. When all this is taken into consideration, the real hypertensive headache becomes a rare symptom, even in cases with a very high blood pressure.

Theoretically, too, it is not so easy to explain why high blood pressure of medium degree should cause headache. Experimental evidence is lacking.

I should like to mention two of the patients who aroused my interest in the problem. A middle-aged man had been under treatment for malignant hypertension for seven years. He had not previously complained of headache. One day he consulted me on account of a very severe headache. Finding that his diastolic blood pressure was 150 mm Hg, I feared a relapse of his malignant hypertension. An examination disclosed a sore region in his neck. After anaesthesia in this region his headache disappeared, and it has not returned during the last three years.

Shortly afterwards I had the same experience with another patient who at that time had a diastolic blood pressure of 140 mm Hg.

I shall not deny that very high blood pressure may cause headache, especially of JANEWAY's morning type, but I think that in benign hypertension this symptom is rarely caused by the high blood pressure itself, and no series showing the real frequency are available.

As soon as the blood pressure rises, it puts a strain on the heart, and therefore we find that dyspnoea on exertion is the first symptom. In my series, it was present in 40% at the beginning of the observation period. There is a fairly good correlation between the height of the blood pressure and the size of the heart. In the case of permanent hypertension this correlation is very remarkable.

However, PERERA (15) found that even after a long period of observation, 32% of his patients did not have an enlarged heart. In my series, the figure is still higher, namely 50%.

These figures are high as compared with those of other series relating to more severe hypertension, but they show the important fact that in many cases of hypertension the heart is not affected, even where the disease has been present for a long time. On the other hand, all investigators agree that the chance of a real improvement of the heart in untreated hypertension is minimal if a large heart or electrocardiographic signs of degeneration are present.

The elevated blood pressure can only be an indirect cause of the other symptoms and complications.

Vertigo (dizziness) is another symptom which is often found. We have no positive evidence that it is directly caused by the blood pressure. On the contrary, BORRI and MAROBBIO (7), who tested 40 hypertensives suffering from vertigo, found no symptomatology of vestibular disorders which might be regarded as typical of the hypertensive patient. Nor is there any correlation between the blood pressure level on the one hand and the extent and location of the vestibular disorder on the other. Vertigo must be regarded primarily as an arteriosclerotic symptom accelerated by hypertension.

Transient encephalopathy has given rise to much discussion. Without going into details concerning the pathogenesis, it may reasonably be presumed that both organic changes in the vascular system and spasms, either separately or in combination, are of significance here.

In clinical practice, these cases are a problem on account of the uncertainty surrounding their diagnosis, treatment, and prognosis. In hospitalised patients under 50 years PIERSON and HOOBLER (*19*) found that 5% had experienced transient unconsciousness, convulsions, unilateral paralysis, paraesthesia, and temporal aphasia. They reported a duration of up to seven days.

In my out-patient series of older patients there were 3.5% with similar cerebral insults, as a rule of a slighter degree and a duration of up to 24 hrs.

These two rather different series may aptly illustrate the problem.

The cases of long duration presage a bad prognosis. PIERSON and HOOBLER found that 30% died from apoplexy within five years, and that 45% had died before ten years.

Only 20% of my patients died from cerebral insults.

PIERSON and HOOBLER have compared their series with KAHN and ISBERG's (*19*) patients treated by sympathectomy. Among the patients who had a fall in blood pressure of at least 20 mm Hg they had a death rate of only 5% from apoplexy. A difference of that order should be of statistical significance, indicating that it must be correct to aim at a lowering of the blood pressure, at least in the group where it is very high.

The frequency with which essential hypertension develops into the malignant variety has always been a subject that has attracted much attention. While previous investigators were inclined to assume that the transition from benign to malignant hypertension was a relatively frequent occurrence, my series of 1946 suggested that this occurred in less than 1% of the cases. At the last follow-up examination I was therefore anxious to see if new cases of malig-

Table 5. *Length of clinical history in malignant hypertension* (BJÖRK, SANNERSTEDT, ANGERVALL, and HOOD, 1960).

	Men	Women
1 year	50	12
1—3 years	38	31
4 years and more	38	43

nant hypertension had developed. In spite of personal examination of patients, hospital records, and death certificates, it could not be demonstrated that any additional cases of malignant hypertension had developed.

By proceeding in the opposite direction in an analysis of the duration of the disease in a series of patients with malignant hypertension, Hood et al. (*6*) showed that the duration of symptoms was less than 12 months in 62 patients, from 1 to 3 years in 69, and more than 4 years in 81 (Table 5).

I think we may conclude that only one-half of the patients with malignant hypertension have had a long period of benign hypertension.

Prognosis

As in other chronic diseases, it has proved difficult to make a simple estimate of the prognosis of essential hypertension.

Recently Palmer (*14*) has given a good account of his 450 hypertensive patients, divided into his 4 groups, and followed for up to 23 years.

Fig. 2 provides at a glance a good idea of the fate of the different groups.

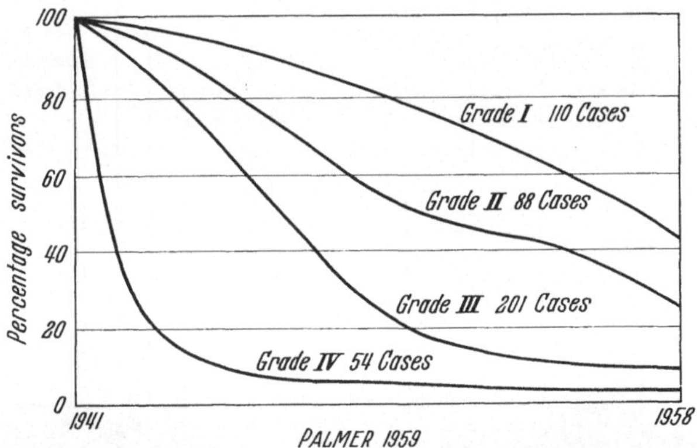

Fig. 2. Percentage of survivors by grade since closing the series to additional patients in 1941, most of the patients having been first studied between 1935 and 1940. The majority of Grade IV patients, without prolonged rice diet or sympathectomy available at that time and without the hypotensive drugs now available, died in less than 2 years. In this group the median duration of known hypertension was 1.5 years, and the time of actual observation in this study prior to death was slightly over 4 months

Only the first part of the observation can be regarded as a period without specific treatment, and perhaps the slight bulge of curve II is a result of the institution of drug therapy.

In diseases of such long duration and where the patients observed are of different ages, survival curves are only of limited value. Therefore, a calculation of the mortality as used in vital statistics gives a better evaluation. The figures are given in per cent, one hundred being the normal death rate in Denmark.

I should like to present briefly my series which has now been followed for up to 22 years. It is remarkable that one-third are still alive after such a long time. The patients may still be regarded as untreated, since sympathectomy has been performed in only two patients and only another two have been treated with ganglion blockers. More than one-third of the surviving women are more than 70 years old, 21 over 80 years. Many of these persons are in relatively good health and are not seriously troubled by their high blood pressure.

From these calculations it is quite clear that the outlook is much better for women than for men, and the difference is so great that it is necessary to make the calculations separately. It is most remarkable that women with a blood pressure of up to 200 mm Hg show almost a normal mortality rate.

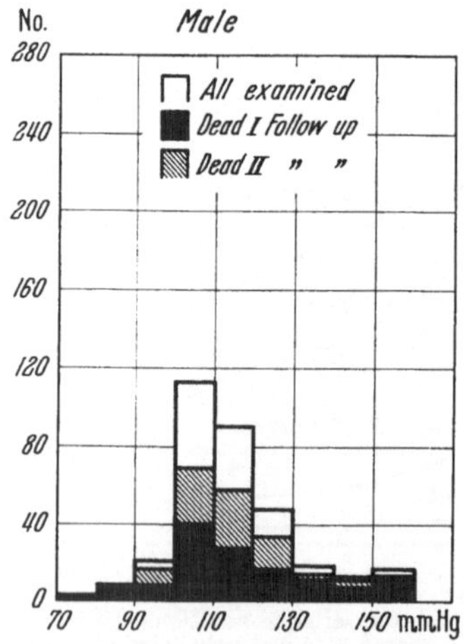

Fig. 3. Diastolic blood pressure at first examination

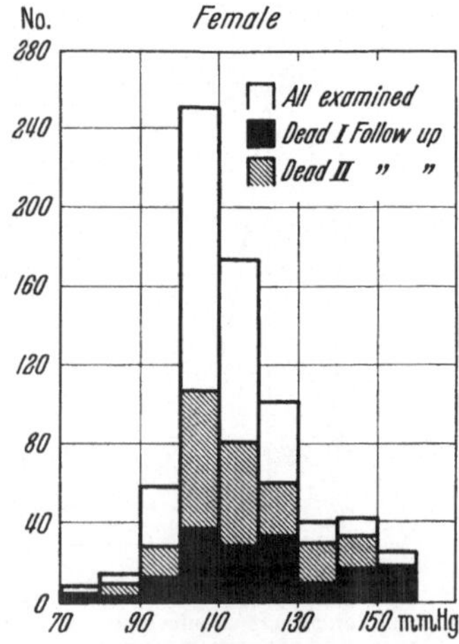

Fig. 4. Diastolic blood pressure at first examination

There is one group of women for whom the outlook is less favourable. Together with Dr. Andreassen and Dr. Hertel (5), I have followed a group of 265 patients who during the years 1925 to 1933 had toxaemia of pregnancy. They were followed up in 1943,

Table 6. *Patients*

	Men	Women	Total
Original series	325	713	1038
Dead after 4—11 years . . .	133	160	293
Dead after 16—22 years . . .	229	367	596
Living after 16—22 years . . .	60	297	357
Unidentified			31
Normal blood pressure at first follow-up			54

Table 7. *Mortality in essential hypertension*
828 cases: 248 men, 580 women

Age	Men %	Women %	Time of observation	Men %	Women %
—49	500	200	— 2	411	189
50—59	319	153	3— 5	292	133
60—	159	106	6—10	243	153
			11—	176	116
Total	238	133	Total	238	133

Table 8. *Mortality in relation to age and diastolic blood pressure*

Age	Men		Women	
	mm Hg ≤ 119 %	mm Hg ≥ 120 %	mm Hg ≤ 119 %	mm Hg ≤ 120 %
—49	500	750	170	286
50—59	320	317	120	250
60—	144	200	92	139
Total	221	295	111	189

and at that time 93 had a blood pressure of 160/100 mm Hg or more.
They were examined again in 1958, which gives an observation
period of at least 25 years. When you compare this group with a
group of patients with essential hypertension, you will find that it
has about twice the mortality rate of the female group and nearly
the same mortality rate as the male group with essential hypertension.

It is easy to show that, as expected, myocardial degeneration and
albuminuria are the most important prognostic factors.

Table 9. *Mortality in high blood pressure following toxaemia*

Age	Toxaemia		Essential Hypertension	
	mm Hg ≷ 119 %	mm Hg ⋚ 120 %	mm Hg ≷ 119 %	mm Hg ⋚ 120 %
—39	400	500	214	667
40—49	156	714	148	295
50—	267	400	136	262
Total	224	562	142	280

Table 10. *Mortality in relation to myocardial degeneration*

Age	Men		Women	
	Present %	Absent %	Present %	Absent %
—49	(1,600)	462	350	181
50—59	1,800	245	475	136
60—	288	135	171	96
Total	544	203	239	121

Table 11. *Mortality in essential hypertension in relation to albuminuria*

Age	Men		Women	
	Present %	Absent %	Present %	Absent %
—49		375		158
50—59	700	270	133	152
60—	200	145	167	95
Total	467	206	200	121

In 1946, I was surprised to find that no extra increase in the mortality rate was observed when hypertension was combined with obesity. This curious finding which has been confirmed by others (*9, 12*) cannot be explained as being merely due to a fat arm. We may therefore consider whether fat people, like middle-aged women, are blessed with a special benign hypertension. The life assurance companies have been rather slow in drawing the proper conclusions from this fact, I think.

Looking back to the days of Janeway, we must admit that the concept of essential hypertension has changed considerably. High blood pressure is found more frequently and in more younger people than expected, but the disease also has a longer and more symptom-free course. In the young group we find the highest relative mortality, but, as shown by Perera (*15*), the outlook is not too bad, since a duration of 20 to 30 years is not unusual, and 10 years was the minimum. In older age groups the mortality rate is closer to that of the non-hypertensive portion of the population. 12% of my 1,000 patients were alive at an age of 70 years or more, and there is good reason to believe that their blood pressure had been elevated from their forties. On the other hand, we also know that especially among men there are cases characterised by a high and fixed diastolic blood pressure which run a serious and rapid course. When these patients develop organic changes in the brain, heart, or kidneys, all investigators agree that after 5 years 50% are dead, which is just the same as JANEWAY found 50 years ago.

Early differentiation between these groups is still one of the most important problems facing the clinician, as it is his principal duty, if possible at an early phase of the disease, to protect his hypertensive patients against the development of serious vascular disease, without having to subject too many of them to troublesome treatment. To a certain extent the study of the natural history of hypertension has given us much valuable new information. This applies, in particular, to the observation that a high proportion of middle-aged women have a relatively favourable prognosis.

I doubt, however, whether we shall be able, by direct observation of the patients at an early phase of hypertension, to pick out those who are specially threatened by vascular disease. Further pathological, physiological, and biochemical studies are needed before this becomes possible.

Summary

The following facts make it difficult to give a true account of the natural history of benign hypertension: 1. New causes of hypertension constantly appear; 2. It is difficult to obtain long-term observations of untreated series; 3. Opinions differ as to the range of normal blood pressure; 4. The onset of essential hypertension is free of symptoms.

Essential hypertension generally develops between the ages of 35 and 45 years. The incidence of hypertensives is estimated at about 15% in the grown-up population.

At first the patients are generally free of symptoms for many years. Later, a lot of minor symptoms are found, but few can be looked upon as direct consequences of the elevated blood pressure, and more criticism concerning the origin of symptoms is desirable.

Half of the cases of malignant hypertension develop from benign, essential hypertension. The other half develops *de novo*.

The relation between malignant and benign hypertension is less than 1 to 200.

The lack of an ideal and generally accepted classification must be regretted.

The course of benign hypertension is from 10 to 50 years. Important prognostic factors are sex, degree of blood-pressure elevation, and organic changes, especially of the heart, kidney, and brain.

The good prognosis in women is a remarkable feature; here a near-normal mortality for systolic blood pressures up to 200 mm Hg is observed.

On the other hand, high blood pressure following toxaemia of pregnancy has just as bad a prognosis as hypertension in men.

Résumé

Vu les faits ci-après, il est difficile de donner une idée exacte de l'évolution naturelle de l'hypertension bénigne:

1. on découvre constamment de nouvelles causes d'hypertension,
2. il est difficile d'obtenir des observations portant sur une longue période pour des séries de malades non traités,
3. les opinions divergent quant aux limites dans lesquelles la tension artérielle peut être considérée comme normale,
4. le début de l'hypertension essentielle ne se signale par aucun symptôme.

L'hypertension essentielle se développe en général entre 35 et 45 ans. Le pourcentage des hypertendus est estimé à environ 15% dans la population adulte.

Pendant les premières années, il n'y a en général pas de symptômes. Plus tard, on trouve un bon nombre de symptômes mineurs, mais rares sont ceux qui peuvent être considérés comme une conséquence directe de l'élévation tensionnelle; il serait souhaitable qu'on fît preuve de plus de sens critique en indiquant l'origine de ces troubles.

La moitié des cas d'hypertension maligne se développe à partir de l'hypertension essentielle bénigne; l'autre moitié est maligne dès le début.

Le rapport entre hypertension maligne et hypertension bénigne est inférieur à 1:200.

On doit sérieusement regretter le manque de toute classification généralement acceptée.

La durée de l'hypertension bénigne est de 10—50 ans. Les facteurs importants pour le pronostic sont le sexe, le degré de l'hypertension et les altérations organiques, en particulier du coeur, des reins et du cerveau.

Une particularité remarquable est le pronostic favorable chez la femme, où la mortalité reste presque normale pour des tensions systoliques s'élevant jusqu'à 200 mm Hg.

Au contraire, lorsque l'hypertension résulte d'une toxémie gravidique, le pronostic est tout aussi sombre chez la femme que chez l'hypertendu du sexe mâle.

References

1. BECHGAARD, P.: Acta med. Scand., Suppl. 172 (1946).
2. BECHGAARD, P.: Brit. Med. J. 1089 (1949).
3. BECHGAARD, P., and S. HAMMARSTRÖM: Acta chir. Scand., Suppl. 155 (1950).
4. BECHGAARD, P., H. KOPP, and J. NIELSEN: Acta med. Scand. **154**, Suppl. **312**, 175 (1956).
5. BECHGAARD, P., C. ANDREASSEN, and E. HERTEL: The ultimate prognosis of hypertension following toxaemia. Non-toxaemic hypertension in pregnancy. Ed.: NORMAN MORRIS and MCCLURE BROWNE. London: Churchill 1958, p. 192.
6. BJÖRK, S., R. SANNERSTEDT, G. ANGERVALL, and B. HOOD: Acta med. Scand. **166**, 175 (1960).
7. BORRI, G., and C. MAROBBIO: Minerva med. (It.) **50**, 1977 (1959).

8. Bøe, J., S. Humerfelt, and F. Wedervang: Acta med. Scand. **157**, Suppl. **321**, 1 (1957).
9. Frant, R., and J. Groen: A.M.A. Arch. Int. Med. **85**, 727 (1950).
10. Janeway, T. C.: A.M.A. Arch. Int. Med. **12**, 755 (1913).
11. Master, A. M., H. H. Marks, and S. Dack: J. Amer. Med. Ass. **121**, 1251 (1943).
12. Mathisen, H. S., D. Jensen, E. Løken, and H. Løken: Amer. Heart J. **57**, 371 (1959).
13. Palmer, R. S., D. Loofbourow, and C. R. Doering: N. England J. Med., **239**, 990 (1948).
14. Palmer, R. S.: J. Chron. Dis. (U.S.A.) **10**, 500 (1959).
15. Perera, G. A.: The natural history of hypertensive vascular disease. Hypertension. A symposium. Ed.: E. T. Bell. University of Minnesota Press 1950, p. 363.
16. Perera, G. A.: Ann. Int. Med. (U.S.A.) **49**, No. 6 (1958).
17. Perera, G. A.: Primary hypertension in the elderly. Ann. Int. Med. (U.S.A.) **51**, No. 3 (1959).
18. Pickering, G.: High blood pressure. London: Churchill 1955.
19. Pierson, E. C., and S. W. Hoobler: Med. Bull. Univ. Michigan **23**, No. 12 (1957).
20. Poutasse, E. F.: J. Urol. (U.S.A.) **82**, 403 (1959).
21. Smithwick, R. H.: Surgical measures in hypertension. American Lecture Series No. 61, 1951. Springfield (Illinois).
22. Stewart, J. Mc. D. G.: Lancet (G.B.) **1953/I**, 1261.
23. Vogelius, H., and P. Bechgaard: Brit. J. Ophth. **34**, 404 (1950).

The natural course of malignant hypertension

By

P. Milliez, P. Tcherdakoff, P. Samarcq and L. P. Rey

Clinical findings

Fixed elevated systolic and diastolic blood pressure with high, stable levels

Eye-grounds revealing papilloedema, spastic arteriolitis, and haemorrhagic and exudative retinitis

Appreciable changes in renal function

Rapid progression towards a fatal outcome, death usually occurring in azotaemic coma.

Histological findings

Diffuse lesions chiefly affecting the kidneys and taking the form of fibrinoid necrosis of the arterioles and endarterial proliferation of the fine-calibre arteries.

These are the characteristic criteria of malignant hypertension as listed by Volhard and Fahr in their papers published between 1914 and 1919. The list continues to be valid in its entirety and few new factors have been added since, but the diagnostic value of each element in the syndrome has been the subject of impassioned discussion.

A marked rise in diastolic blood pressure is generally accepted as a reliable sign of malignant hypertension. Nevertheless, Kincaid-Smith points out that just as high blood pressure levels may be encountered in cases of benign hypertension. Moreover, stability of the diastolic blood pressure is not a constant factor even in this author's own patients.

Papilloedema is regarded as an essential sign of malignant hypertension by the Mayo Clinic investigators, who draw their inspiration from Keith and Wagener; and Murphy in 1958 also selected his cases of hypertension on the basis of papilloedema. Perera, on the other hand, does not consider papilloedema to be an indispensable diagnostic criterion.

Renal insufficiency, for PERERA and for GOLDBLATT (1957), is an important and constant sign of malignancy, but its diagnostic value is held to be of only secondary importance by McMAHON and PRATT, SCHOTTSTAEDT and SOKOLOW, as well as McMICHAEL and MURPHY, because renal failure is not always present in malignant hypertension.

In 1958 a study group, formed with the aim of establishing a classification of the various types of arterial hypertension (BRUST, PERERA, and WILKINS), defined malignant hypertension as follows:

Diastolic blood pressure usually elevated and not very labile
Papilloedema and retinopathy common but not constant
Rapidly progressive renal changes.

These authors do not believe that the presence of lesions due to necrotising arteriolitis is an indispensable diagnostic factor.

In short, the combined presence of the three major clinical symptoms can be regarded today as sufficient evidence of malignant hypertension, but in cases where one of them is lacking, only a rapidly progressive course terminating in death can provide sufficient grounds for diagnosing the condition, since there are no structural lesions which are absolutely specific for malignant hypertension. Ultimately, therefore, the only valid criterion is the course taken by the illness.

The patients in our particular study were selected in accordance with the following principles: where the blood pressure was very elevated and generally stable, the combined presence of papilloedema and renal changes prompted a diagnosis of malignant hypertension. If one of these elements was missing, malignant hypertension could only be confirmed by rapidly progressive deterioration in the angiopathy or by the discovery at subsequent examinations of the element that was lacking initially.

Of the 641 hypertensive patients admitted to Professor PASTEUR VALLERY-RADOT's department between 1942 and 1959, 79 (12.3%) were found to satisfy these criteria. This proportion may appear large when compared with the figures quoted in other papers, viz. 5% (PERERA), 2.5% (MURPHY and GRILL), and 1% (KINCAID-SMITH et al.). We do not suggest in any way that the incidence of the disease can be deduced from our figure, since we hospitalise only those patients who are seriously ill.

The average *age* of our patients with malignant hypertension is 41.1 years for males (minimum 18 and maximum 55 years), and 37.5 years for females (minimum 9 and maximum 60 years). The overall average for both sexes is 39 years and tallies with the average age in other studies. BECHGAARD emphasises that with age hypertension tends less and less to become malignant. Malignant hypertension is indeed a disease of young adults.

Like other authors we, too, have found the *highest incidence among men*. In fact, we encountered 35 cases of malignant hypertension among 232 male hypertensives (i. e. 15%), whereas the figure for the female sex was 44 out of 409 (i. e. 10.7%). Admittedly, hypertension is more frequent among females (70% of 60,000 hypertensives examined by Perman were women), but it is generally more severe in men.

The existence of *previous benign hypertension* has often been reported. We encountered it in 48 of our 79 cases, i. e. in 60.7%. Where malignant hypertension is preceded in this way by a benign phase, the duration of the latter varies, averaging 7.7 years for our patients, but ranging from 1 to 30 years. A deterioration may therefore set in at any time during the course of the disease, but becomes much rarer as the patient grows older.

It is often difficult to obtain information about the previous blood pressure levels, either because the patient, in the absence of symptoms, never sought medical advice, or because the doctor did not tell the patient how high his blood pressure was. Thus, we were unable to find out the pre-morbid blood pressure level in 25 patients (31.6%); it is therefore impossible to say exactly whether the hypertension was malignant from the outset or whether, on the contrary, it developed after a long period of benign hypertension.

Only in 6 cases (7.7%) can we state that the blood pressure was normal shortly before the appearance of functional signs indicative of a malignant course; what is more, in 5 of these 6 cases, there were special aetiological circumstances (2 cases of periarteritis nodosa, 2 of phaeochromocytoma, and 1 of thrombosis of a renal artery). The occurrence of malignant hypertension "de novo", as it has been called by certain authorities, seems therefore to be a rare event which is observed only under certain aetiological circumstances.

The manner of onset of the malignant phase of hypertension seems to have attracted hardly any attention. Nevertheless, in the course of our study, we were struck on many occasions by the exceptional suddenness with which the malignant syndrome appeared. In 34 patients (43%) it was possible to establish with very great accuracy the date of the first alarm signals. Some patients even managed to note the exact hour when it started: for example, one patient, a 54-year-old coalman, experienced while at work on 5th December 1946 a sudden bout of severe giddiness accompanied by nausea, vomiting, and headache, although he had hitherto been in perfect health and had never consulted a doctor. A few days afterwards, examination revealed obvious signs of malignant hypertension. Another patient, who had suffered since the age of 48 from benign hypertension discovered at a systematic examination and causing no functional disorder, developed at age 55 at 3.30 p.m. on 15th February 1958 a violent headache accompanied by blurred vision and paraesthesia; when admitted to our department a fortnight later, he showed all the signs of malignant hypertension. The abrupt onset does not appear to be connected with a particular aetiology, nor do such cases seem to be more common in patients already suffering from benign hypertension.

In other cases, admittedly, the onset is gradual; in one of our female patients moderate hypertension was discovered in the course of a systematic examination at the age of 50 years. Moderately severe headaches, a few bouts of giddiness, and occasional slight blurring of vision gradually developed. Little by little these signs became worse, and when we examined the patient 3 years later there was no doubt that the hypertension was malignant. This gradual appearance of malignant signs seems to be less frequent and less characteristic, and to be more often encountered in older patients.

In a not insignificant number of patients (15, i. e. about 19%) the malignant phase of hypertension seems to be precipitated by an epiphenomenon: 7 patients had contracted an infectious disease a fortnight before the appearance of the first signs of malignancy; 3 of them had had influenza, 1 acute localised pneumonia, another diphtherial tonsillitis, another an infectious syndrome thought to be typhoid fever, and the last viral hepatitis; in 3 women who had long been known to have hypertension and had completed previous pregnancies without incident, the course of renewed pregnancy was marked by the appearance of malignant signs which persisted after the delivery. Another of our hypertensive patients completed a pregnancy without any serious trouble. Signs of malignant hypertension appeared one week after a normal delivery and persisted subsequently. Another female patient showed signs of aggravation following the inhalation of toxic products, the nature of which could not be defined. Finally, 2 patients reported a period of physical overwork and another of mental overstrain in the months preceding the appearance of malignant signs. We are wary of asserting that there is a cause and effect relationship between these various episodes and the occurrence of a malignant syndrome in patients who already have hypertension but tolerate it well. Nevertheless, these cases can be compared with those of malignant hypertension developing after an abrupt change in climate or altitude (DE GENNES) or following events of grave national importance (LAUBRY). REISER, ROSENBAUM, and FERRIS, who studied the psychological factors in 12 cases of malignant hypertension, found in all the patients a correlation between the abrupt transition from the benign to the malignant stage and an unusual emotional tension. These authors noted that changes in blood pressure were often more pronounced under the influence of emotional factors than under that of physiological (cold pressor test) or pharmacological stimuli.

It thus seems possible that a non-specific episode — infection pregnancy, physical, mental, or emotional strain, change of climate — may be a precipitant factor in the occurrence of the malignant syndrome and may trigger off a remorseless deterioration in a patient who has hitherto tolerated his hypertension well.

There are a very great number of *functional and systemic disorders* which, singly or jointly, may herald the malignant stage of hypertension. Five of these disorders deserve particular attention.

Headache is by far the most common and most constant sign. Encountered in 66 cases, i. e. 83.5%, it varies in type, being usually occipital, dragging, continuous, and subject to sudden intensification; sometimes it is frontal, but the other characteristics remain the same. In a certain number of cases the headache is purely paroxysmal, pulsatile, and resembles migraine. The abrupt occurrence of headache or the sudden aggravation of a previously mild headache are in the great majority of cases the first signs to attract the patient's attention.

Visual disorders, usually accompanying the headaches and consisting of blurred vision or decrease in visual acuity, are likewise very common (44 cases, i. e. 55.6%), and, in a great number of instances, it is on their account that the patient first seeks medical advice.

Profound asthenia may be the first sign (24 cases, i. e. 30%).

Loss of weight, as much as 10—20 kg in a short space of time (18 cases, i. e. 22.7%), is an unusual symptom in the course of benign hypertension. When assessing this loss of weight, allowance must be made for the effect of the diet prescribed for the hypertension; but considerable loss of weight may also be encountered in the absence of any dietary restrictions.

Finally, we consider it worthwhile to dwell a little on the question of *nocturia*. This disorder is common, for we have observed it in 30 cases, i. e. 38%. It is rare for this sign to alarm the patient and cause him to consult a doctor. But systematic questioning reveals that this nocturia may develop at an extremely early date; it precedes the other manifestations by several weeks or months and, whether due to renal dysfunction, autonomic nervous disorder or insomnia, it is one of the reliable precursors of malignant hypertension.

Here are some other prodromal signs:

Vomiting (15 cases), giddiness (10 cases), tinnitus aurium (8 cases), anorexia (7 cases), low back-ache (7 cases), haematuria (7 cases), nosebleed (7 cases), cryaesthesia (6 cases), haemoptysis (5 cases), nocturnal insomnia and diurnal drowsiness (5 cases), sexual impotence (4 cases), acute pulmonary oedema (3 cases), nocturnal muscular cramp (3 cases), digestive tract haemorrhage (1 case).

A study of the *past history* of these patients does not provide any particular evidence which might have a bearing on the malignant hypertension. In the past histories of our 79 patients we found scarlet fever or repeated sore-throats on 18 occasions (22.7%), acute pyelonephritis on 9 (11.3%), and various urinary tract disorders of long standing in 13 (16.4%). In one case, anamnesis revealed albuminuria in childhood, and in another the malignant hypertension was superimposed on a nephrotic syndrome which was in the course of developing.

22 (50%) of our female patients had had pregnancies. In 18 of them, all the pregnancies had been normal. Only 2 had had toxaemia during one pregnancy after previously completing normal pregnancies, while 2 others had developed toxaemia with every pregnancy. The low incidence of toxaemia may be surprising. In fact, it clearly indicates that before the syndrome of malignant hypertension appeared, the women were either in good health or, if suffering from benign hypertension, were nevertheless perfectly capable of tolerating and completing a pregnancy.

We made a systematic search for evidence of hereditary hypertension or nephropathy. In 5 cases, however, this investigation could not be carried out (patient could not be questioned, no relatives available). Among the 74 remaining cases, evidence of a direct hereditary trait was found in 25, i. e. 33.7%. This proportion hardly differs from that observed in benign hypertension.

Neither a study of the past history (pathological and obstetrical) nor an inquiry into the family history revealed any distinctive factors which might have made it possible to explain or foresee the development of malignant hypertension.

The entire clinical, biological, and radiological investigations were governed in all the cases by two main aims:

To evaluate the effect of the hypertension on the internal organs.

To discover the exact aetiology of the condition.

The blood pressure seemed almost constantly to be at a very high level. We give below the highest and lowest figures recorded for each patient during his stay in hospital:

Highest figures
Systolic: average: 232 mm Hg — minimum and maximum: 190—345
Diastolic: average: 150 mm Hg — minimum and maximum: 100—220

Lowest figures
Systolic: average: 197 mm Hg — minimum and maximum: 160—250
Diastolic: average: 126 mm Hg — minimum and maximum: 100—170

Bearing in mind that these figures do not take account of the different therapeutic measures employed — whether dietary or medicamentous — it would appear that the diastolic level, in accordance with the classic view, is fairly stable.

Functional disorders indicative of a cardiovascular effect are not very often in the forefront of the clinical picture, except for *attacks of acute pulmonary oedema*, which we encountered on 10 occasions. Mere questioning of the patient yielded evidence of dyspnoea on exertion (14 cases), dyspnoea in the supine position (2 cases), atypical precordial pain (4 cases), or intermittent claudication (1 case), but these disorders were seldom sufficiently marked to constitute by themselves the reason why the patient sought medical advice. Like Kincaid-Smith et al., we have been struck by the rarity of heart attacks in our patients: in no cases have we been able to discern any evidence of angina on exertion, and only one of our patients had an infarction demonstrable in the E.C.G. Clinical examination of the heart regularly revealed tachycardia and, in 18 cases (22.7%) a pre-systolic gallop rhythm. Kincaid-Smith et al. seem to us perfectly justified in regarding this gallop rhythm as a sign of ill omen for the prognosis.

The almost absolute constancy of the cardiac changes, however, is clearly revealed by examination of the teleroentgenogram and the electrocardiogram. We shall leave out of account 8 patients examined during war-time, when it was not possible to perform these investigations. Of the 71 others only 4 had normal E. C. G. patterns. In 67 cases there was left-ventricular hypertrophy which varied in degree but was often considerable. Signs of myocardial ischaemia were noted in 12 cases and incomplete block of the right branch in 3. We find this absence of marked coronary atheroma most interesting and believe it may have a bearing on the absence of malignant hypertension in the elderly; it is as if the vascular sclerosis prevented arteriolar failure — a typical sign of malignancy.

Eye-ground changes were found to be regularly present at the first examination. They can be classified as follows:

Papilloedema	none	4
	slight	28
	moderate	27
	pronounced	20
Arteriolar spasm	slight	28
	moderate	25
	pronounced	26
Retinopathy (haemorrhages and cotton-wool	none	6
exudates):	slight	32
	moderate	22
	pronounced	19
Star figure in the fovea centralis		19
Retinal arterial pressure	100 and above	29
	less than 100	24
Atrophy of the optic nerve		1

Thus, spastic arteriolitis is usual, while papilloedema is absent in only 4 cases and retinopathy in only 6. We do not believe there is any strict parallel to be drawn between the different types of retinal lesions; in particular, there is hardly any correlation between the severity of the oedema and that of the retinopathy. It is worth noting that in the cases in which oedema was absent, retinopathy was always present, and vice-versa: all our patients had eye-grounds of at least Grade III, almost all of them being Grade IV. Retinal arterial pressure was 100 mm H_2O or more in half the cases; the minimum and maximum figures were 50 and 140 mm H_2O.

Questioning and examination revealed that the course of the disease had been marked by *neurological episodes* in 37 (46.8%) of our patients; 7, as we shall see later, died of cerebromeningeal haemorrhage. 4 of the remaining 30 had had several such episodes. Thus, 37.9% of the cases (a proportion which is similar to that found in other studies of malignant hypertension) showed at some time during the course of the illness various neurological disorders: hemiplegia (9 cases), transient amaurosis (7 cases), generalised convulsive seizures (5 cases), aphasia (3 cases), central facial paralysis (3 cases), or peripheral facial paralysis (2 cases), temporary loss of consciousness (1 case), rotatory vertigo (1 case), meningeal haemorrhage (1 case), and scotoma (1 case). The 7 cases in which a fatal incident brought the course of the illness to a sudden end have not been included in this survey; the majority of these episodes regress as a rule. Permanent lesions were found only in 3 cases of hemiplegia and in the case with a scotoma. Transient amaurosis is a relatively common alarm signal which often prompts the patient to consult a doctor.

The anatomical study of Rosenberg, who examined the brains of 17 patients who had died of malignant hypertension, demonstrated the almost constant finding of functional or organic changes; the brain would thus seem to be the organ most commonly affected after the kidney.

Changes in renal function were assessed on the basis of a certain number of examinations: urea clearance, phenolsulphonphthalein excretion test, enumeration of the red and white blood cells excreted per minute, and intravenous urography.

Proteinuria seems to be extremely frequent, as many authors have observed. We encountered it on 48 occasions, i. e. in 60.5% of the cases; this figure, however, relates only to the first examination. In cases where we were able to follow the course of the angiopathy, we found that if albuminuria was absent at the first examination it invariably appeared subsequently. In 3 of our patients, 2 of whom are not included in this series, proteinuria assumed massive proportions and led to a nephrotic syndrome.

We have divided our cases into 3 groups, according to the severity of the renal involvement:

Slight changes (blood urea between 0.3 and 0.5 g/l, van Slyke between 50 and 70%, P.S.P. between 45 and 60% in 70 min): 35 cases, i. e. 44.3%.

Moderate changes (blood urea between 0.5 and 0.7 g/l, van Slyke between 30 and 50%, P.S.P. between 30 and 45% in 70 min): 18 cases, i. e. 22.7%.

Severe changes (blood urea in excess of 0.7 g/l, van Slyke below 30%, P.S.P. below 30% in 70 min): 22 cases, i. e. 27.8%.

Tests of renal function yielded absolutely normal results in only 4 cases. Here again this applies only to the first examination, and in each case we observed subsequently a progressive deterioration in renal function.

Hence, renal involvement seems to be almost regularly apparent even at the very first examination of a patient suffering from malignant hypertension, but the severity of this renal involvement varies. In rare cases it is lacking initially, but it is bound to appear sooner or later.

It was not possible to carry out a full *aetiological investigation* in 11 patients for various reasons, e. g. because the patient was in too poor a general state of health to tolerate the examinations or because he left the hospital of his own accord before they could be completed. Of the 68 patients who were properly examined 39 (57.3%) had essential hypertension. Of the 29 others 10 had atrophy or complete failure of one kidney, 3 thrombosis or constriction of the renal artery, 9 bilateral renal lesions, 2 lesions of the lower urinary tract, 2 periarteritis nodosa, 2 phaeochromocytoma, and 1 polycystic disease. The extremely variegated results of this aetiological investigation, in which most of the known causes of hypertension are represented, clearly show that malignant hypertension constitutes only one particular mode of development, and that it is a syndrome and not a disease in its own right.

It was impossible to follow the *course* of the illness after the first stay in hospital in 33 cases (including 3 patients who underwent an ordinary bilateral Smithwick operation and 1 who had a bilateral Smithwick with total adrenalectomy on one side and subtotal on the other). The reason why such a large proportion of the patients were lost sight of is that quite a number of them were referred to us from the provinces and did not return to consult us after their first stay in hospital. Moreover, relatives, having been warned that the illness will probably run a severe course, prefer to take the patient away so that he can spend his last days in the bosom of his family; our requests to relatives for subsequent information frequently remain unanswered.

We were able therefore to follow the long-term course of the disease in only 46 patients.

In 33, treatment, whatever form it took, brought no regression in the malignant syndrome.

27 of the patients died. The average duration of the illness can be assessed in two ways:

Average duration since discovery of Grade IV eye-grounds: Survival time 11.1 months; the minimum and maximum duration was 3 days and 5 years respectively. The detection of papilloedema is an objective criterion, but it will be realised that varying lengths of time may have elapsed before the first ophthalmoscopic examination was performed.

Average duration since the appearance of the first functional signs suggestive of malignant hypertension: 22.3 months, the minimum and maximum being 3 weeks and 5 years respectively. Here, the initial criterion is evidently more subjective and less reliable, but it may perhaps better reflect the real duration of the illness.

Consequently, if we accept the second assessment, the natural course of malignant hypertension is such that death occurs in about 2 years. The maximum survival time observed was 5 years.

In the 27 patients in whom the course could be followed until the end, the immediate causes of death can be divided up as follows:

Uraemic coma alone	11
Uraemic coma + heart failure	7
Cerebro-meningeal haemorrhage	7
Death during operation	1
Intercurrent accident (acute peritonitis)	1

It thus seems clear that renal insufficiency, whether accompanied or not by heart failure, was the major cause of death in these patients. Disregarding the last two deaths, which may be considered as accidental, uraemic coma preceded the fatal outcome in 18 out of 25 cases, i.e. in 72%. Only in 7 patients (28%) was the course of the illness suddenly interrupted by fatal cerebromeningeal haemorrhage. These data tally approximately with those of other studies (McMahon and Pratt, Schottstaedt and Sokolow, Kincaid-Smith, McMichael and Murphy). Furthermore, we would point out, that in our series of patients death was never due to myocardial infarction — an odd finding which has already been reported by other authors (Kincaid-Smith).

19 out of 46 patients are still alive at the present moment. In 6 of them the disease is becoming progressively worse (3 of these 6 have undergone an ordinary bilateral Smithwick and 2 a bilateral Smithwick with total adrenalectomy on one side and subtotal on the other). The survival time of these 6 patients, calculated from the apparent onset of the malignant syndrome until today (June 1960) has been 2 years in 3 cases, 3 years in 2, and 5 years in 1. But these survivors are in a precarious state; all of them have renal failure of varying degree.

In only one of our cases did we observe a spontaneous regression in the malignant syndrome. This patient was a 43- year-old man in whom malignant hypertension began to develop, it seems, one year before his first examination in our department. At this examination, which took place in 1957, he was found to have Grade IV eye-grounds not connected with any recent neurological episode; blood urea was 0.37, but a Van Slyke of 50% and a P. S. P. of 45% in 70 min. indicated renal involvement. Retrograde ureteropyelography had revealed bilateral hydronephrosis and had been followed by temporary anuria. The prognosis was extremely bleak. However, a spontaneous improvement set in, the patient's general condition is now excellent, and there are no signs of functional disorders. His blood pressure is 220/120, eye-grounds Grade II, retinal arterial pressure 55 mm, blood urea 0.52, and both the clinical and electrocardiographic signs of cardiac involvement are regressing. A similar spontaneous regression of malignant signs was observed by KEITH and WAGENER in 15 of their patients. Our single case may seem very little in comparison with these authors' series, but we must point out that:

1) KEITH and WAGENER encountered this spontaneous regression on only 15 occasions in the course of their vast experience extending over a period of 20 years.

2) We have systematically excluded from our study patients who developed papilloedema immediately following a cerebrovascular accident. The authors mentioned above, on the other hand, seem to have included a certain number of such cases in their study.

In any case, a spontaneous regression is certainly a *very rare* occurrence which cannot be relied upon. The natural course of malignant hypertension remains, in the absence of treatment, rapid, progressive, and remorseless. There should be no modification of the dogma which advocates energetic and, especially, early treatment before any sign of severe renal insufficiency has appeared.

The signs of malignant hypertension disappeared in 12 patients who underwent surgical treatment of an aetiological or symptomatic nature.

In 6 of these patients (aged 9, 11, 18, 26, 46, and 47 years — 3 nephrectomies, 1 phaeochromocytoma, and 2 bilateral Smithwicks with total adrenalectomy on one side and subtotal on the other) the blood pressure returned completely and permanently to normal levels.

In the 6 others (2 ordinary bilateral Smithwicks and 4 bilateral Smithwicks with total adrenalectomy on one side and subtotal on the other) all signs of malignancy disappeared and the moderately severe hypertension re-assumed a benign form.

The results of renal tests were satisfactory in all these patients at the time of operation. As soon as any appreciable degree of renal insufficiency appears, all treatment, surgical or otherwise, is illusory. This means that malignant hypertension may be sometimes curable, but only if it is treated, and therefore diagnosed, at an early stage.

An anatomico-pathological study of the kidney was carried out in 17 of our patients. The material for the study was obtained on 7 occasions from biopsies performed during operation or from surgical specimens, and on 10 occasions from autopsy specimens.

In only one case were renal vascular lesions virtually absent: this patient was a boy of 18 years in whom hypertension had suddenly developed 6 months previously. The aetiology of the condition had been ascertained: thrombosis of the left renal artery due to the presence in the renal pedicle of a mass which histological examination revealed to be a phaeochromocytoma. This patient has completely recovered from his hypertension.

All the other cases had vascular lesions, though their extent and severity varied:

Sclerosis of the small-calibre arteries with reduction or obstruction of the lumen: . . . . .8 cases
Arteriolar hyalinisation and sclerosis: . . . . .6 cases
Arteriolar necrosis: . . . . .6 cases

In all these patients the lesions affected selectively or with particular intensity the smallest arteries (distal part of the interlobular arteries) and the afferent arterioles. It must be emphasised that these vascular lesions differed only in intensity and extent from those observed in all cases of hypertension. No special type of lesion was encountered in the patients with malignant hypertension.

Glomerulosclerotic lesions were present in 9 cases out of 17; tubular atrophy was noted in 8 cases. These changes in the renal parenchyma were manifestly due to the vascular lesions.

On the whole, the lesions were obviously less severe in the biopsy material than in the autopsy specimens; they were, of course, less marked in the patients who succumbed to cerebromeningeal haemorrhage than in those who died in uraemic coma. This suggests that the histological picture described by Fahr only appears if the clinical course of the illness has been sufficiently long and if it has not been interrupted before reaching its normal end — i. e. renal insufficiency — by an intercurrent accident, particularly a neurological episode.

A renal biopsy performed at an early stage does not reveal any histological signs which will entitle the investigator either to diagnose or to exclude malignant hypertension. A biopsy performed at a later stage makes it possible to confirm the malignancy of the hypertension and to gauge the seriousness of the case on the basis of the severity and extent of the lesions.

From the *aetiological point of view,* anatomical studies afforded corroborative evidence that malignant hypertension may be due to a variety of causes: chronic pyelonephritis in 9 cases, glomerulonephritis in 1, thrombosis of the renal artery in 1, adrenal adenoma in 2, phaeochromocytoma in 2, periarteritis nodosa in 2. These examples confirm that there is no specific aetiology for malignant hypertension and indicate that *the cause of the disease may nevertheless be ascertained by means of histological examination or at autopsy.*

Conclusions and summary

1. Having completed this study, we can only re-affirm what we said as far back as 1954: "All cases of hypertension, whatever the cause, whatever the age of the patient, and whatever the form the hypertension has assumed hitherto, may suddenly become malignant. Malignancy is nothing more than a sign of the progression of the disease, as indicated by the varying aetiologies which have been suggested for those cases of hypertension decribed as 'malignant' ". BRUST, PERERA, and WILKINS have also expressed the same idea, preferring the definition "accelerated form of hypertension" to the term "malignant hypertension".

2. There seems to be no point in discussing the regularity and relative diagnostic value of ocular lesions or renal changes. Both will inevitably appear at some stage in the course of the illness, unless the latter is interrupted by an intercurrent episode. The same applies to structural changes, which only become evident if the illness has run its full course.

3. Malignant hypertension occurs chiefly in young patients who have no atherosclerosis but are usually already suffering from benign hypertension. More rarely it develops suddenly in a hitherto normotensive subject.

4. The first signs of malignancy are frequently preceded by non-specific episodes.

The onset of malignant hypertension is often extremely sudden.

Headache and visual disorders are the most common alarm signals; nocturia is an even earlier sign in a good many cases.

5. The course of malignant hypertension continues remorselessly until the patient dies in uraemic coma with or without heart failure. More rarely the course of the disease is suddenly interrupted by a neurological episode, but never, in our experience, by a heart attack. Spontaneous regression of malignant hypertension is exceptional.

Removal of the cause of the hypertension or certain symptomatic forms of surgical treatment sometimes prevent the condition from progressing towards death and bring about a return to the benign form.

6. In the future, thorough examination will no doubt always make it possible to discover the aetiology of so-called essential hypertension, whether malignant or otherwise; this is indicated by the fact that the cause of the hypertension is being ascertained more and more frequently in patients subjected to a full examination, particularly in young subjects and in cases which are malignant from the very outset.

Résumé

1. Au terme de cette étude, nous ne pouvons que réaffirmer ce que nous disions déjà en 1954: «Toute hypertension artérielle, quelle que soit sa cause, quel que soit l'âge du sujet, quel que soit le type évolutif revêtu jusqu'alors, peut devenir brusquement maligne. La malignité n'est qu'un signe de l'évolutivité, comme l'indiquent les étiologies variées relevées à l'origine des hypertensions dites malignes.» C'est ce qu'expriment également BRUST, PERERA et WILKINS lorsqu'ils préfèrent, au terme d'hypertension maligne, celui de «forme accélérée d'hypertension artérielle.»

2. Il paraît vain de discuter sur la constance et la valeur diagnostique relative des lésions papillaires ou des altérations rénales. Les unes et les autres feront inévitablement leur apparition à un moment quelconque de l'évolution, à moins que celle-ci ne soit interrompue par un accident intercurrent. Il en va de même des lésions anatomiques qui ne sont évidentes que si la maladie a parcouru tout son périple.

3. L'hypertension maligne survient de préférence chez les sujets jeunes, indemnes d'athérosclérose et le plus souvent porteurs d'une hypertension artérielle bénigne préalable. Plus rarement elle s'installe d'emblée chez un sujet jusque-là normotendu.

4. Les premiers signes de malignité sont souvent précédés d'agressions non spécifiques. Le début de l'hypertension artérielle maligne est souvent extrêmement brutal. La céphalée et les troubles oculaires sont les signes d'alarme les plus fréquents; la nycturie est un signe encore plus précoce dans bon nombre de cas.

5. L'évolution de l'hypertension artérielle maligne se poursuit inéluctablement vers la mort dans la grande azotémie avec ou sans défaillance cardiaque associée. Plus rarement un accident neurologique vient brutalement interrompre le cours de la maladie et jamais, dans notre expérience, un accident coronarien. La régression spontanée de la malignité est un phénomène exceptionnel. La suppression de la cause de l'hypertension artérielle ou certains traitements chirurgicaux symptomatiques entravent parfois l'évolution vers la mort et entraînent le retour à la bénignité.

6. Un examen complet permettra sans doute à l'avenir de découvrir toujours l'étiologie des hypertensions artérielles dites essentielles, malignes ou autres, comme le prouve la découverte de plus en plus fréquente de la cause de l'hypertension artérielle chez les malades soumis à des investigations complètes, en particulier chez les sujets jeunes et au cours des hypertensions malignes d'emblée.

Work done at the Hypertension Research Centre, Hôpital Beaujon-Clichy (Professor Paul Milliez), with the assistance of the National Institute of Hygiene (Professor Bugnard) and the Research Fund of the Social Security Board.

Literature

Aitken, R. S., and C. W. Wilson: Quart. J. Med. (G.B.) 4, 14, 179—190 (1935).

Bechgaard, P., H. Kopp, and J. Nielsen: Acta med. Scand. Suppl. 312, 154, 175—184 (1956). — Bernheim, M., R. François, F. Larbre, and A. Perrin: Pédiatrie (Fr.) 11, 2, 281—287 (1956). — Brust, A. A., G. A. Perera, and R. W. Wilkins: J. Amer. Med. Ass. 166, 640 (1958). — Byrom, F. B.: Lancet (G.B.) 1954/II, 201—211.

Castex, M. R.: Prensa méd. argent. 42, 49, 3683—3692 (1955).

Degoy, A., and L. Schuller: J. méd. Bordeaux 135, 9, 971—973 (1958). — Derow, H. A., and M. D. Altschule: N. England J. Med. 213, 20, 951—960 (1935). — Derow, H. A., and M. D. Altschule: Ann. Int. Med. (U.S.A.) 14, 10, 1768—1780 (1941).

Elwyn, H.: Bull. N.Y. Acad. Med. 28, 3, 145—158 (1952).

Gennes, L. de, D. Mahoudeau, and P. Desvignes: Bull. Soc. méd. hôp. Paris 59, 35, 457—459 (1943). — Goldblatt, H.: J. Exper. Med. (U.S.A.) 67, 5, 809—826 (1938). — Goldblatt, H.: Circulation (U.S.A.) 16, 5, 697—699 (1957). — Grob, D.: J. Chron. Dis. (U.S.A.) 1, 5, 546—562 (1955). — Gros, Cl., J. Mirouze, B. Vlakovitch, and A. Pages: Sem. hôp. Paris 35, 23, 1015—1022 (1959).

HANLEY, H. G.: Brit. J. Urol. **29**, 4, 359—361 (1957). — HOLTEN, C., and V. POSBORG-PETERSEN: Lancet (G.B.) **1956/II**, 918—922.

KEITH, N. M., H. P. WAGENER, and J. W. KERNOHAN: A.M.A. Arch. Int. Med. **41**, 2, 141—188 (1928). — KEITH, N. M., H. P. WAGENER, and N. W. BARKER: Amer. J. Med. Sc. **197**, 3, 332—343 (1939). — KEITH, N. M., and H. P. WAGENER: A.M.A. Arch. Int. Med. **87**, 1, 25—47 (1951). — KINCAID-SMITH, P., J. McMICHAEL, and E. A. MURPHY: Quart. J. Med. (G.B.) **27**, 105, 117—153 (1958). — KLEMPERER, P., and S. OTTANI: Arch. Path. (U.S.A.) **11**, 1, 60—117 (1931).

LEISHMAN, A. W. D.: Brit. Med. J. **1959/I**, 1361—1368. — LEVITT, W. M., and S. ORAM: Brit. Med. J. **1956/II**, 910-912. — LOCKET, S., P. G. SWANN, and W. S. M. GRIEVE: Brit. Med. J. **1951/I**, 778—784. — LUNSETH, J. H., L. A. BAKER, and A. SHIFRIN: A.M.A. Arch. Int. Med. **88**, 6, 783—792 (1951).

MACMAHON, H. E., and J. H. PRATT: Amer. J. Med. Sc. **189**, 2, 221—235 (1935). — McMICHAEL, J., and E. A. MURPHY: J. Chron. Dis. **1**, 5, 527—535 (1955). — MANDLOWITZ, M., A. D. PARETS, T. GOLD, and S. R. DRACHMAN: J. Chron. Dis. (U.S.A.) **7**, 6, 484—492 (1958). — MANLOVE, F. R.: A.M.A. Arch. Int. Med. **78**, 4, 419—440 (1946). — MARTIN-NOEL, P., Y. MAZARE, and M. REVOL: J. méd. Lyon **39**, 922, 511—519 (1958). — MILLIEZ, P.: Les hypertensions artérielles permanentes curables. Acquisit. Méd. Récentes 65—71. Ed.: Méd. Flammarion. Paris 1954. — MURI, J. W.: Acta med. Scand. **158**, 3—4, 173—180 (1957). — MURPHY, E. A.: Bull. Johns Hopkins Hosp. (U.S.A.) **102**, 158—159 (1958). — MURPHY, F. D., and J. GRILL: A.M.A. Arch. Int. Med. **46**, 1, 75—105 (1930).

NEWMAN, M. J. D., and J. I. S. ROBERTSON: Brit. Med. J. **1959/I**, 1368—1373.

PAGE, I. H.: Ann. Int. Med. (U.S.A.) **12**, 7, 978—1004 (1939). — PAGE, I. H.: J. Chron. Dis. (U.S.A.) **1**, 5, 536—545 (1955). — PALMER, R. S., D. LOOFBOUROW, and C. R. DOERING: N. England J. Med. **239**, 26, 990—994 (1948). — PEET, M. M., and E. M. ISBERG: Ann. Int. Med. (U.S.A.) **28**, 4, 755—767 (1948). — PERERA, G. A.: Amer. J. Med. **4**, 3, 416—422 (1948). — PERERA, G. A.: J. Chron. Dis. (U.S.A.) **1**, 5, 472—476 (1955). — PERMAN, E.: Acta med. Scand. Suppl. **312**, 154, 214 — 215 (1956). — PERRY, H. M. jr., and H. A. SCHROEDER: A.M.A. Arch. Int. Med. **102**, 3, 418—425 (1958). — PICKERING, G. W.: Clin. Sc. (G.B.) **1**, 4, 397—413 (1934). — PICKERING, G. W.: Circulation (U.S.A.) **6**, 4, 599—612 (1952). — PORGE, J. F.: Arch. mal. coeur (Fr.) **41**, 9, 449—451 (1948).

REISER, M. F., M. ROSENBAUM, and E. B. FERRIS: Psychosomat. Med. (U.S.A.) **13**, 3, 147—159 (1951). — ROSENBERG. E. F.: A.M.A. Arch. Int. Med. **65**, 3, 545—586 (1940).

SCHOTTSTAEDT, M. F., and P. SOKOLOW: Amer. Heart J. **45**, 3, 331—362 (1953). — SCHROEDER, H. A.: J. Chron. Dis. (U.S.A.) **1**, 5, 497—515 (1955). — SHAPIRO, P. F.: A.M.A. Arch. Int. Med. **48**, 2, 199—233 (1931). — SHELBURNE, S. A., D. BLAIN, and J. P. O'HARE: J. Clin. Invest. (U.S.A.) **11**, 3, 489—496 (1932). — SIGLER, L. H.: Amer. J. Cardiol. **1**, 2, 176—180 (1958). — SMIRK, F. H., and E. G. McQUEEN: J. Chron. Dis. (U.S.A.) **1**, 5, 516—526 (1955). — SMITHWICK, R. H.: J. Chron. Dis. (U.S.A.) **1**, 5, 477—496 (1955).)— SMITHWICK, R. H., R. D. BUSH, and D. KINSEY: J. Amer. Med. Ass. **160**, 12, 1023—1026 (1956).

TAYLOR, R. D., A. C. CORCORAN, and I. H. PAGE: A.M.A. Arch. Int. Med. **93**, 6, 818—824 (1954).

WAGENER, H. P.: J.Amer. Med.Ass. **101**,18, 1380—1384 (1933).—WERT-
HEIM, A. R., and Q. B. DENNING: J. Chron. Dis. (U.S.A.) **1**, 5, 574—588
(1955). — WESSELOW, O. L. V. S. DE, and W. J. GRIFFITHS: Brit. J. Exper.
Path. **15**, 1, 45—52 (1934). — WILKINS, R. W.: J. Chron. Dis. (U.S.A.)
1, 5, 563—573 (1955). — WILSON, C., and G. W. PICKERING: Clin. Sc.
(G.B.) **13**, 3, 343—351 (1938). — WILSON, C., and F. B. BYROM: Lancet
(G.B.) **1939/I**, 136—139. — WOLFERTH, C. C., W. T. FITTS, W. A. JEFFERS,
and A. M. SELLARS: Bull. N.Y. Acad. Med. **33**, 3, 151—170 (1957). —
WOODS, W. W., and M. M. PEET: J. Amer. Med. Ass. **117**, 18, 1508—1515
(1941).

Discussion

REUBI: I would like to make a suggestion. Like Dr. BECHGAARD, I think that we should try to agree on a classification and a definition of malignant hypertension. It is no problem to define malignant hypertension from an anatomical point of view: I think we all agree that there is arteriolar necrosis in different organs, for instance in the kidney. But to separate malignant from benign hypertension from a clinical point of view is difficult. Essential hypertension usually shows a rather benign course, but a small group of cases may go into malignant hypertension. On the other hand, known causes of elevated blood pressure, like glomerulonephritis or periarteritis nodosa, may also lead to malignant hypertension. The question which arises is whether it is possible to diagnose malignant hypertension on the basis of clinical criteria only. Shall we use the word "malignant" only when arteriolar necrosis is established or already prior to its development? How can we diagnose clinically arteriolar necrosis? Dr. MILLIEZ said he would diagnose malignant hypertension when the diastolic blood pressure is higher than 120, when the eyegrounds show changes of grade IV and if there are signs of renal insufficiency. But he also said that in his series he had sometimes to make the diagnosis on the basis of grade III retinal changes, and he stated that renal insufficiency was not always present at the beginning. So I think that it is a little confusing. I should like to say how we diagnose malignant hypertension in my department. We do not think that our criteria have any absolute value, but they usually are: diastolic blood pressure higher than 130, retinal changes grade III or IV, and marked alteration of the general condition. I think this last criterion is very important. Most patients lose weight. Even if they were obese, they lose weight, the general condition is altered, the central nervous system often shows signs of involvement. Of course, there is also albuminuria. When albuminuria is very marked, that is an important sign, but you can find cases of essential hypertension which certainly do not have malignant lesions and yet show fairly marked albuminuria, up to 3 g/l. We believe, therefore, that moderate albuminuria is not a reliable sign of a malignant course. I should like to hear what the competent authors in this assembly think about that.

MILLIEZ: The term "accelerated hypertension" strikes me as being a more accurate description for the syndrome described by VOLHARD than the term "malignant hypertension". The criterion of malignancy lies in the fact that the disease progresses. True, arteriolar necrosis is a specific sign of malignancy, but only a secondary one. Biopsies carried out in the initial stages of malignancy reveal no arteriolar necrosis. Arteriolar necrosis is, however, always discovered at death in cases where the patient dies of renal insufficiency.

I personally do not believe in the idea of trying to split up essential hypertension into an ever-increasing number of categories. I think we should do our utmost to find out the cause, especially where the hypertension is malignant.

There are certain causes of hypertension which are always sought for nowadays: an adrenal tumour, unilateral renal atrophy, thrombosis of the renal artery, glomerulonephritis, polycystic disease of the kidneys.

But there are other causes that are overlooked. Let me quote a few examples: in patients with only one kidney, in whom cystoscopy confirms the absence of a ureter on the side which shows up blank in the urograph, one should always bear in mind the possibility of a purely endocrine kidney with no ureter — a possibility which should be explored retropneumoperitoneally; in a patient who has sustained an abdominal trauma, had a severe fall, or suffered from phlebitis of the legs, one must always suspect the possibility that his hypertension may be of venous origin. In such cases, phlebography via the femoral or humeral route is indispensable as a means by which to confirm or disprove this diagnosis.

Ascending nephritis may lead to severe or even malignant hypertension without ever at any time having presented the classic picture of a major febrile infection of the urinary tract. One must therefore know how to look for the functional signs and symptoms of this condition (besides the usual manifestations associated with cystitis, difficulty at the start of micturition, pain occurring at the moment of micturition as a sign of a reflux of urine towards one or both of the renal pelvises, absence of the need to urinate). These symptoms, of course, merely indicate dyskinesia of the urinary tract; where a reflux of infected urine from the bladder occurs, this dyskinesia leads to ascending renal infection as postulated by the classic authors.

Proof of this unilateral or bilateral mechanism in ascending hypertensive nephritis can easily be furnished, either by radiocinematography carried out during micturition using a brilliancy amplifier, or by simple retrograde cystography (40 ml of contrast agent instilled into the bladder, plus 300 or 400 ml of saline, radiographs being made of the whole urinary tract before, during, and after micturition).

REUBI: I think we all agree with you that in this disease a downhill course is a good criterion of malignancy. However, I must say, if you treat such patients early, you may alter the course and stop the progression. This may make the diagnosis difficult.

PICKERING: Sir, I think that this is an extremely important and interesting problem. I think one needs two types of classification of hypertension. The one is by kind. I need not give you a list of all these, but may I just mention a few: there are the renal causes, of which Dr. MILLIEZ gave us some in his talk; and there is phaeochromocytoma. I am not going to give all the causes, because they are generally agreed on. We know there is a residuum which we call essential. Now the course of any of these diseases may be, as VOLHARD first pointed out, one of two kinds: it may be quite stable, which we call benign hypertension. That is what Dr. BECHGAARD told us about so excellently in his first talk. Or it may be rapidly downhill, and for that reason VOLHARD called it malignant. And these two courses may ensue in any of these kinds of hypertension; Dr. MILLIEZ showed us the malignant course occurring in a variety of kinds of renal hypertension and in phaeochromocytoma; it also occurs in Cushing's syndrome, and we know that it occurs further in essential hypertension. Now what is the nature of the malignant course ? The essential feature of the malignant course is the fibrinoid necrosis of the arterioles. It is that that kills the patient. But clinically the first evidence is often the changes in the eyegrounds, and the first change may be either a large ill-defined exudate, or it may be papilloedema. The full-blown picture, of course, has both. Now, unfortunately, as GOLDRING and CHASIS pointed out, some patients who have arteriolar necrosis in their kidneys after death have never shown retinopathy during life, and in those the first sign of the onset of the malignant phase is haematuria or proteinuria. Now, it seems extremely likely that the malignant phase is an expression of a very severe hypertension, particularly one of rapid and recent onset, and we all know that we can now reverse the malignant phase. Dr. MILLIEZ showed us how this could be done by removing the cause, if we can find the cause, and if we cannot, by bringing down the blood pressure by sympathectomy or by hypotensive drugs. Now, my point is this — that the success of our treatment of malignant hypertension depends on how early we get the patient. If we wait until the eyegrounds are absolutely characteristic, until there is no doubt that renal function is failing, then we wait too long. As Dr. PAGE and others have so clearly shown, renal failure gets the patient. Therefore I think that from a practical point of view one should suspect the outset of the malignant phase in any patient whose hypertension is severe, and the higher the blood pressure the more one ought to be on the lookout. There are two things that one ought to look out for: one is the sudden development of an exudate in the eye, another is the sudden development of haematuria or proteinuria; and if either of those happens, then it is time to treat the patient. I think I just ought to say that you cannot diagnose the malignant phase on just the eyegrounds. I have been extremely interested in eyegrounds, and you see a condition exactly resembling the retina of the malignant phase of hypertension in patients who have severe gastro-intestinal haemorrhage and who have perfectly normal blood pressures, and you may also see it in the presence of a perfectly normal blood pressure in disseminated lupus erythematosus.

SCHROEDER: I think that we must differentiate between the pathological and clinical diagnoses of malignant hypertension. Many pathologists make such a diagnosis only when necrotizing arteriolitis is present. Necrotizing arteriolitis develops only in the presence of azotemia, with rare exceptions. Therefore, by the time necrotic lesions are found, the disease is in terminal stages.

Clinical and especially therapeutic considerations, on the other hand, require earlier diagnosis of the malignant stage in order that treatment can be effective. Before the advent of specific therapy, prognostic considerations required early diagnosis. I can only give you our own criteria. For all cases, exudative and/or hemorrhagic lesions in the ocular fundi, a fixed, high diastolic pressure (over 120 mm Hg average) at bed rest and during sleep induced by sodium amytal, and some diminution of renal function is necessary for the diagnosis of Stage IV, or malignant hypertension. We divide Stage IV into three sub-groups: Stage IVa: Early malignant hypertension. Ocular fundi Grade III without frank papilloedema but disc margins may be blurred. Phenol red excretion less than 25% and at least 15% in 15 min after intravenous dye. Proteinuria usually present. Occasionally this stage may regress spontaneously. Stage IVb: Severe malignant hypertension. Diastolic pressure 140 mm Hg or over. Papilloedema and exudative and/or hemorrhagic lesions in fundi (grade IV). Renal function reduced without or with border-line azotemia. State IVc: Malignant hypertension with renal insufficiency. Usually a terminal stage akin to the pathological criteria of the disease.

I agree with Dr. PICKERING that we must use our clinical judgment in making the diagnosis and we cannot rely on any one sign. I do not think we can diagnose this stage without signs of renal damage and without acute fundal changes, but for therapeutic purposes we must be aware of the earliest signs of malignant deterioration of the disease and treat vigorously before irreversible renal damage has occurred.

GOVAERTS: I wish to call attention to the fact that it is possible in the dog to create the whole syndrome of malignant hypertension. This was done by GOLDBLATT, and I had the opportunity to observe it repeatedly while studying experimental renal hypertension. When, in the dog, you clamp too tightly the renal arteries on both sides, some animals may occasionally develop a high blood pressure, a severe renal insufficiency, and survive say 10 to 20 days with increasing uraemia. They develop during that time the whole syndrome of malignant hypertension with haemorrhages in their intestines or in the peritoneum, and necrotic lesions are found in the arteries. Therefore, at least in the dog, the syndrome of malignant hypertension may have a purely renal origin, and accordingly it is very interesting to see that in the clinical observations of Dr. MILLIEZ the development of malignant hypertension, in man, is linked with a pathological condition of the kidney, such as a reduction in renal blood flow or a reflux of urine into the ureters. As I showed you yesterday, a severe reduction of the kidney function can increase the response to substances like renin and angiotensin by a mechanism which ought to be more closely investigated.

PLATT: I am sure we all agree that it is most rare to see the malignant phase start after the age of 55. I can remember two cases, a woman of 57 who was a doctor's wife, who suddenly developed malignant hypertension and died and we had no post-mortem. The other case was a woman of 67 who developed malignant hypertension with the typical fundi, and she had a non-functioning kidney. But it is most rare to develop malignant hypertension at that age. We cannot diagnose malignant hypertension simply on the height of the blood pressure, because I am sure we all know, particularly in woman at 55 to 60, how often we see alarmingly high blood pressures sustained over years without the development of any of the signs of malignant hypertension. If we wait for the papilloedema and so on, we wait too long, says Dr. PICKERING; of course, quite right, you should certainly treat them before that, if you can, but as Dr. MILLIEZ pointed out, the majority, or a large number, present because they have already developed the eye lesions, so that is a counsel which it is impossible to keep. Now, as to the criteria of diagnosis, I agree that pathologically there are cases in which the arteriolar lesions are present and yet no papilloedema, but from the point of view of assessing other people's results in the literature, it is much easier if we say: we do not count the cases to be malignant hypertension unless they have the typical retinopathy, papilloedema and everything. Otherwise, you get lists of cases in which, when you look carefully at them, two thirds have no papilloedema, and you wonder whether the other man's criteria are the same as your own. So, I do not say this is right pathologically, but for the convenience of the medical literature it is a very good thing. Finally, Dr. BECHGAARD's interesting notes on toxaemia of pregnancy: I think they had mostly gone through it before he ever saw them, and I suppose he does not know really whether they were cases which developed hypertension for the first time during pregnancy or whether perhaps they were early hypertensives who were discovered because of pregnancy. In a series which GIBSON and I reported — really studied by GIBSON, but the results were analysed by myself — it was very common for women who had gone through a toxaemic pregnancy to end up with a blood pressure somewhat higher than it had been before. It was extremely rare for them to develop a severe form of hypertension in that series.

WILSON: On this question of diagnosis I agree entirely with Dr. PLATT. I think we must regard papilloedema as the pathognomonic sign of malignant hypertension. It is not justifiable to include patients with grade III retinopathy, since we do not know the natural prognosis in these patients;

some may develop malignant hypertension, but the majority do not. If therefore such cases are included in a treatment series of "malignant hypertension", the therapeutic response cannot be compared with that in other series. It is therefore impossible to diagnose cases in the early stage before papilloedema has developed. The presence of necrotising arteriolitis in the kidney in my view is not sufficient for the diagnosis of malignant hypertension. Occasionally such lesions are found in patients who do not subsequently develop papilloedema. Other speakers have suggested that nitrogen retention is necessary for the production of arteriolar necrosis. I do not know of any evidence for this. In acute nephritis and early malignant hypertension these lesions are found before renal impairment develops and this is certainly true of experimental hypertension. BYROM's observation of focal vasoconstriction in the cerebral arteries during attacks of encephalopathy in rats with experimental hypertension, is to my mind convincing evidence that malignant hypertension is qualitatively different from benign hypertension, in that it produces severe regional vascular spasm, which I believe to be the cause of fibrinoid necrosis in various organs. A point which needs explanation is the very different incidence of the malignant phase in essential hypertension and renal hypertension. KIMMELSTIEL and I found that about 3% of all cases with left ventricular hypertrophy at autopsy showed the histological features of malignant hypertension. This was obviously a selected hospital series and I think essential hypertension becomes malignant in probably less than 0.1% of cases. On the other hand, in our series of chronic glomerular nephritis, 50% of patients developed malignant hypertension. In this latter group there is no evidence that nitrogen retention is the cause of the malignant phase, nor is the blood pressure higher than in essential hypertension, Furthermore, papilloedema seems to be reversible by hypotensive therapy more easily in renal than in essential hypertension.

BECHGAARD: So much has been said about the diagnosis of malignant hypertension. I think we can agree that in KEITH and WAGENER's group IV we have had a well-defined group which has been valuable in the evaluation of surgical and medical treatment of malignant hypertension, but at the same time we must admit that this group is too limited and does not contain all cases of malignant hypertension.

Concerning the group of toxaemia, I want to say that the patients whom I have followed were all well examined at the beginning of the study because the material is taken from a Danish thesis by Dr. HERTEL. All the patients who had hypertension before or at the beginning of their pregnancy or who were suspected to have renal disease were taken aside.

The group of toxaemia is as pure as possible. From that group (256 patients) we picked out those who 10—15 years afterwards had hypertension and followed them for at least another 10 years.

As to the figure of 1% of conversion from benign to malignant hypertension, I agree that it is too high. The reason why I came to this figure was that in my 1,000 patients there were 13 cases of malignant hypertension, but they were all diagnosed at the beginning of the investigation and no other cases were found during the observation time.

The malignant group had reported to the out-patient clinic on account of their disease, but at that time (1946) it was generally estimated that about 10% of the benign cases were converted to malignant cases. Therefore I did not dare to go further down than 1%, but now I agree that the figure is not more than a few $^o/_{oo}$.

BROD: We have been very interested in the differential diagnosis of malignant hypertension. In our series of cases, most of them confirmed by either peroperative biopsy in the course of an exploratory lumbotomy or sympathectomy or by autopsy, we made a queer finding which, so far, I have not succeeded in explaining and which might be very much in accord with what has been said by Dr. WILSON. While in cases of chronic pyelonephritis with grave hypertension we see the onset of malignant change mainly in those cases which are far progressed, the malignant change in essential hypertension occurs irrespective of the level of functional disturbance of the kidneys. There I disagree with Dr. MILLIEZ that we would have to postulate renal insufficiency to diagnose malignant hypertension. As for the differential diagnosis between chronic pyelonephritis and essential hypertension with malignant change, there are several important criteria. One is the comparison of a restriction of glomerular filtration rate and concentrating power. While in chronic pyelonephritis the concentrating power is always much more restricted than would correspond to the degree of restriction of glomerular filtration, it is just the reverse in cases of essential hypertension with a malignant course, where the degree of restriction of glomerular filtration is in advance of the degree of the restriction of concentrating power. That is one criterion. The second one is in the Addis count, where in over 75% of cases we find usually a discrepancy between the excretion of leucocytes and erythrocytes, but we should never rely on this criterion alone. This I would like to stress: much misunderstanding has been caused by others who have relied solely on this criterion. One must take this criterion together with the disbalance between glomerular and tubular balance and other criteria. The third one is that in cases which are far progressed, where glomerular filtration is restricted to values of 30 ml per min or below, in cases of essential hypertension which do not show — in autopsy or histology — any changes of pyelonephritic origin, the concentrating power is still above 1,012, while we have not seen a single case of chronic pyelonephritis which would bring the urine concentration to 1,012 in thus far advanced cases. And one final remark about nocturia, to which Dr. MILLIEZ has referred. Dr. FENCL and I have been studying the day and night rhythm of renal function in hypertensive subjects, and we found that even essential hypertensives without the slightest indication of malignancy — about 30 or 40% of them — had nocturia, even if they did not complain of it.

HAMBURGER: We have made some observations on the evolution of blood pressure in patients with chronic nephritis treated by transplantation of a normal kidney. These observations could give a partial answer to some of the questions presented by Dr. WILSON and by Dr. PICKERING. One year ago, we transplanted the kidney of a non-identical twin to his brother. This one was suffering from severe renal insufficiency after a long history of chronic pyelonephritis. Blood urea was 400 mg %, blood pressure was 165/110 and the eyegrounds grade III. A lethal prognosis was estimated to be a matter of weeks. The patient received a total body irradiation of 460 r. Then one of the normal kidneys of his brother was transplanted. Three months later, the blood pressure was normal, the urea was normal, and the eye lesions had vanished. After six months the eyes were still normal, but the blood pressure began to go up again. Then we decided to nephrectomize the patient's own two kidneys. Once more the blood pressure went back to normal. That was six months ago. Now blood urea and function tests are normal. But during the last weeks the blood pressure has been going up again, between 160/100 and 170/110. The eyegrounds are still normal. I thought that perhaps this rather exceptional case could be of some interest to people interested in the natural course of hypertension and the relation between kidney and blood pressure.

SARRE: In my opinion, the diagnosis "malignant hypertension" does not depend on whether or not "malignant nephrosclerosis" as described by FAHR and VOLHARD is present, i. e. nephrosclerosis with necrotic arteriolitis and periarteriolitis. As renal biopsy studies carried out on sympathectomised hypertensives by SMITHWICK, ZENKER, myself, and others have shown, all degrees of renal vascular damage — ranging from mild to very severe — are liable to be encountered in malignant hypertension. I shall be referring to this again to-morrow in my paper. It is my view that the diagnostic criteria for malignant hypertension are the severity and rapidity of progress of the clinical course. Among the clues to look for here are the eyeground findings (Grade III or IV), resting diastolic blood pressures above 120 or 130 mm Hg, headache, dizziness, and rapid worsening of the disease. In the early stages of malignant hypertension, renal insufficiency may still be absent. In 89 cases from the hospital in Frankfurt with a clinical diagnosis of "malignant hypertension" which resulted in death, the pathologist's post-mortem findings were as follows:

Renal findings at autopsy:

No pathological findings whatsoever . .	3.3%
Renal arteriosclerosis	1.1%
Renal arteriolosclerosis	42.7%
Malignant nephrosclerosis (FAHR) . . .	41.6%
Pyelonephritis	0 %
Adrenal adenoma	3.4%
Hypernephroma	1.1%
Chronic nephritis	6.7%
Syphilitic endarteritis	1.1%
Atheroma of a renal artery	0 %

Thus, true "malignant nephrosclerosis" as defined by FAHR was found in only 41.6% of the cases with malignant hypertension, while in 3.3% the renal vessels showed no pathological signs whatever.

HILDEN: Can I just come back to your question about malignant hypertension and its criteria? I think it is very important to have as sound and well-defined a group as possible in order to compare the different treatments, and therefore I think it is dangerous to include too many criteria. I agree with Dr. WILSON and Dr. PLATT that we should first of all look at the eyegrounds and take those with papilledema. Now as to those within the third degree of retinopathy you suggested, I am sure that there are some which are nearly as grave as those with papilledema, i. e. younger patients with fresh exudates which we usually call premalignant. Those with retinal haemorrhages or hard spots I think have a far less grave prognosis. I think we have only to take those with papilledema. I do not think that fits in with diastolic blood pressure, because this depends on the patient's age. If he is a very young patient, it may be 110 or 115 and that may be a malignant case. As to renal function, I do not think this need necessarily be severely depressed. I am sure that if you take a large group you will find slightly depressed renal function, but I do not think we need have depressed renal function to diagnose a malignant phase.

To Dr. PICKERING: I think it is very important from the therapeutic point of view to look for those symptoms pointing to an acceleration, and albuminuria is important. When it disappears after treatment, we feel that

this is very nice, but if it then reappears, we begin to wonder if we have
been doing the right thing or not. Haematuria is a very important sign, too.
I have stressed several times that the appearance of the malignant phase
very often starts with haematuria.

REUBI: Thank you. May I make a final remark? I may have been mis-
understood. I never said we should consider every patient with grade III retinal changes to belong to the malignant group. But I think it is worth while
emphasising that we always have a bunch of symptoms, and we have to
consider all of them in making the diagnosis. I agree with Dr. PICKERING
that blood pressure is most important, but as Dr. PLATT pointed out, and
I think that is an excellent point, many women who have a diastolic blood
pressure over 150 never develop so-called malignant hypertension. Therefore
on the basis of the blood pressure alone you cannot diagnose malignant
hypertension. You have to wait for changes in the eyegrounds, in the kidney,
in the heart or in the general condition. As these signs may come earlier or
later, but not all at the same time, in one given case it seems advisable to
base one's assessment on a combination of the symptoms which are present.
As to Dr. SCHROEDER's remark, I would not agree that azotemia is a very
early sign. However, I have never seen normal kidney function in a patient
with malignant hypertension. There is always a marked reduction of the
glomerular filtration rate and of the PAH-clearance. On the whole, I think
we can say that there are no absolute criteria for a clinical diagnosis of
malignant hypertension.

SCHROEDER: I did not mean to imply that azotemia was a prerequisite
of the clinical diagnosis. It is not. On the other hand, because of its association with necrotizing arteriolitis, it usually is a requisite of the diagnosis
as made by pathologists. The clinical diagnosis is made differently than is the
pathological, but is just as valid.

REUBI: I would like to take the opportunity of asking Dr. PAGE what he
has to say about malignant hypertension.

PAGE: Well, I can tell you how I diagnose it. I think that number
one, you cannot make a spot diagnosis of any chronic disease, and you
cannot make it on the basis of one examination. To me malignant
hypertension is a syndrome that steadily advances. It is the rate of
advance which is one important facet. We actually accept papilledema,
hemorrhage, and exudate as essential criteria for making the diagnosis.
We do not think that renal function as measured by clearances need
necessarily be depressed, but we also believe that if it really is malignant
hypertension, the clearances will soon become depressed. I have seen a good
many patients at the beginning of this disease when both inulin and diodrast
clearances were normal only to become abnormal in the course of a few months.
I must confess that when we have looked for widespread necrotising arteriolitis, we have repeatedly been disappointed. We do not think that this
lesion must necessarily be found widespread to make the diagnosis. I am
intrigued by the fact that nobody seems to have any very reasonable explanation as to how it comes about. I would certainly believe that an abnormally high diastolic pressure over a sufficient length of time might lead
to malignant hypertension, and I am equally certain that many people have
extremely high diastolic pressures of 180 or 190 over a long period of time
and do not develop it. I am always much impressed from a therapeutic point
of view that we have our greatest successes in the treatment of malignant
hypertension. I remember the thing that impressed me most about sympathectomy, even when we did it in the form of the anterior nerve-route sections'

was that it was the first time I ever saw malignant hypertension reversed. That was in 1931—32; we did not believe it was possible at that time. But malignant hypertension can on occasion reverse without great fall in blood pressures, and for this reason I cannot accept the height of the blood pressures as the only cause. There are some rather interesting experimental prototypes which might be called malignant hypertension or might not. You know WILSON and BYROM's very important work. Years ago WINTERNITZ injected kidney extract into animals and got what looked like a malignant type lesion, which, as far as I know, has never been followed up. It ought to be. The other one that happens to come to my mind is some work that GEORGES MASSON did in our laboratory. He gave DOCA and salt to rats, and then gave them injections of renin or angiotensin. These animals tripled their weights within a few hours. Fibrinoid was precipitated in the blood vessels. The animals looked as though they had toxemia of pregnancy with hypertension. Hemorrhages in the brain and throughout the body also occurred. What the syndrome was due to, we have no idea. I suppose, however, one can always question whether this is or is not malignant hypertension.

To me malignant hypertension as I saw it thirty years ago was a frightening and discouraging disease. My patients always died. Today I know of no aspect of hypertension that is more satisfying to treat. At the moment we at the Cleveland Clinic are very interested in the appearance of the renal blood vessel as demonstrated by aortograms. Over 1,500 have now been done without a single fatality. If malignant hypertension appears suddenly in a patient with essential hypertension, there is a good possibility that an arteriosclerotic plaque may be obstructing the renal circulation. We now have both surgical and medical means of reversing this dangerous disease. It is interesting that the first clear evidence of reversal came from the very early and, I must confess, very traumatizing sympathectomies. To me, then, malignant hypertension is a state which in most cases is easily recognizable at the bedside and has a characteristic course. The problem is, what is its mechanism ? I think it significant that the lesions of malignant hypertension can appear in a normal twin's kidney transplanted into the twin's partner when that individual suffers from this disease.

Pharmacology of new hypotensive drugs

By

A. J. PLUMMER

One of the more notable accomplishments resulting from the continuing intensive search for effective therapeutic agents of all kinds has been the discovery of several compounds of benefit in lowering the blood pressure in human essential hypertension. This success, attained in the span of slightly more than a decade, is the more remarkable when it is realized that the underlying physiological aberration responsible for essential hypertension is not as yet entirely clarified. Nonetheless, much insight has been acquired as to the nature of the disorder, and this in turn has facilitated recent advances in the drug therapy of hypertension. The opinions of various investigators differ concerning the relative importance of the roles played by renal, adrenal, or nervous influences in the initiation of essential hypertension; yet there is unanimity that increased peripheral arteriolar resistance of uncertain etiology is the immediate mechanical factor leading to the elevation of the diastolic blood pressure. Since the sympathetic vasoconstrictor nerves were known to regulate the peripheral resistance of the arterioles, especially in the splanchnic region and in the skin, it was logical that agents which suppressed the sympathetic nervous system should receive early attention as potential antihypertensives.

Although there is no evidence that the increased peripheral resistance of essential hypertension is due to exaggerated sympathetic nervous activity, it has been established by SMITHWICK (*1*) that the therapeutic bilateral excision of portions of the thoraco-lumbar sympathetic ganglionic chains serves to lower the blood pressure in essential hypertension by restoring the peripheral resistance toward the normal range. It was undoubtedly this observation which suggested the possibility of securing this therapeutic advantage pharmacologically through a so-called "chemical sympathectomy".

The emphasis of this presentation will be on the pharmacology of the newer antihypertensive agents. Since all are of such recent origin, however, an adequate treatment will require a discussion

of the pharmacologic basis for the actions of several earlier types
of hypotensive agents.

Adrenergic blockade. The first substances to receive serious
consideration as antihypertensive agents were the adrenergic
blocking and ganglionic blocking agents. Adrenergic blockade was
well known since the work of BARGER, CARR and DALE in 1906 (2)
with ergotoxin. However, this substance, a vasoconstrictor in its
own right, was too toxic for therapeutic application. Yohimbine,
another naturally occurring adrenergic blocker, was a convulsant
with a narrow therapeutic index. Of the several synthetic compounds exhibiting adrenergic blocking action, phentolamine,
prepared in 1939 by HARTMAN and ISLER (3), may be mentioned
as a prototype.

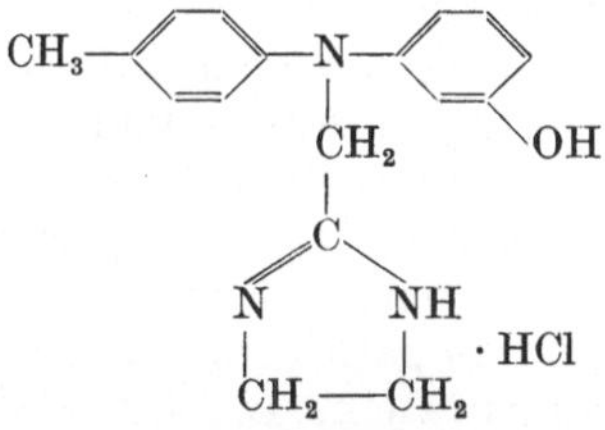

$$CH_3 - \underset{}{\bigcirc} - N - \underset{}{\bigcirc} - OH$$

Phentolamine

Pharmacologically phentolamine diminished the augmentory
effects of epinephrine and norepinephrine upon the blood pressure
(4). In fact, the pressor effect of injected epinephrine was inverted
in the so-called "epinephrine reversal". Somewhat larger doses
of phentolamine were required to antagonize the pressor effect
following direct sympathetic nervous stimulation. The inhibitory
effects of epinephrine on the smooth muscle of the intestine and
bronchi and the stimulatory effect upon cardiac rate and amplitude
were not impeded by phentolamine. Although it had been thought
that this group of agents might have a beneficial action in human
hypertension, this hope has not been realized. The blood pressure
could be lowered but the concurrently developing reflex tachycardia tended to be excessive because the sympathetic cardioaccelerator pathways escaped the inhibitory influence of the adrenergic blocker.

An important clinical use has been found for phentolamine, which
serves as a means for the diagnosis and temporary palliative treatment of a pheochromocytoma, an adrenal medullary tumor
secreting norepinephrine and epinephrine into the circulation in
excessive amounts. In this diagnostic test a properly selected

intravenous dose of phentolamine promptly lowers the hypertension due to excess circulating catecholamines but is without effect in essential hypertension.

Ganglionic blockade. Ganglionic blockade as a pharmacological mechanism was described in 1889 by Langley and Dickinson (*5*) in their classical experiments with nicotine. The diffuse stimulating effects of this alkaloid on the central nervous system, on the chemoreceptors of the carotid sinus and on the skeletal system interfered with its use as a specific blocking agent. It was not until 1946 that Acheson, Moe and Pereira (*6*) pointed out the specific autonomic ganglionic blocking action of tetraethylammonium chloride. It was later shown by Paton and Perry in 1953 (*7*) that there was a distinct difference between the mechanisms of action of nicotine and of tetraethylammonium chloride (TEA), the former blocking by irreversibly depolarizing the ganglionic cells and the latter acting competitively to raise the threshold of the ganglionic cells to stimulation by acetylcoline. Since TEA was not well absorbed from the gastrointestinal tract, its antihypertensive potential was restricted. The excellent hypotensive response due to the blockade of the sympathetic nervous pathways by TEA was achieved only upon parenteral administration. In the effort to obviate this disadvantage, Barlow and Ing in 1948 (*8*) and Paton and Zaimis in 1949 (*9*) independently worked on a class of substances known as the methonium compounds, which were also quaternary. Hexamethonium, the most interesting bisquaternary compound resulting from the effort, was composed of two trimethylammonium centers separated by six methylene groups. The formulae of hexamethonium and of several other bisquaternary ganglionic blocking substances are shown in the text.

$$CH_3N^+(CH_3)_2{-}(CH_2)_6{-}N^+(CH_3)_2{-}CH_3 \cdot 2Cl^-$$

Hexamethonium

$$N^+CH_2CH_2N^+(CH_3)_3 \cdot 2Cl^-$$

Chlorisondamine

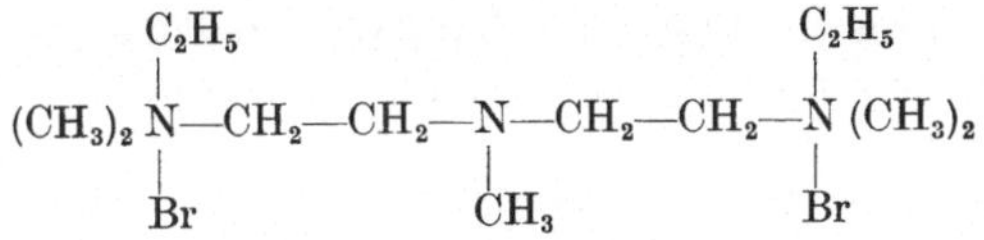

$$\text{(CH}_3)_2 \overset{\overset{\displaystyle C_2H_5}{|}}{\underset{\underset{\displaystyle Br}{|}}{N}}\text{—CH}_2\text{—CH}_2\text{—}\overset{\overset{\displaystyle}{|}}{\underset{\underset{\displaystyle CH_3}{|}}{N}}\text{—CH}_2\text{—CH}_2\text{—}\overset{\overset{\displaystyle C_2H_5}{|}}{\underset{\underset{\displaystyle Br}{|}}{N}}\text{(CH}_3)_2$$

Pendiomide

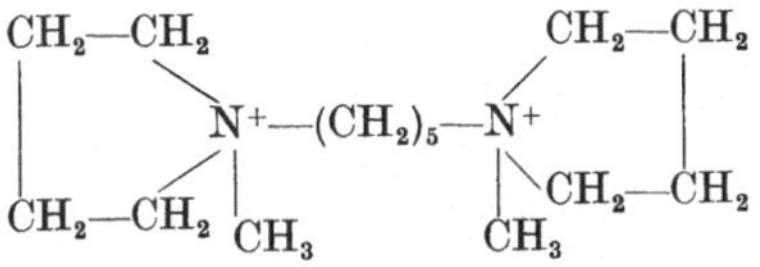

Pentolinium

It will be noted that among the quaternary derivatives the optimal distance between the nitrogen atoms for maximal ganglionic blockade is dependent upon the type of substituent groups on the nitrogen atoms. Although the absorption of hexamethonium from the gastrointestinal tract represented an improvement over that of TEA, it still amounted to but ten per cent of the ingested dose with unpredictable daily fluctuations. LEVINE (*10*) has suggested the possibility that the oral absorption of quaternary compounds generally is limited by binding with intestinal mucin to yield a complex transported with difficulty across the intestinal cell wall. If such is the limiting factor, the more potent quaternary derivatives should possess the greatest oral efficacy. This, in fact, seems to be the case, because chlorisondamine, the most potent of the quaternary blockers, has also provided the most effective and most long-acting ganglionic blockade upon oral administration (*11*). Mecamylamine, which is a secondary amine (*12*), and pempidine (*13*), which is a tertiary amine, are more readily absorbed from the gastrointestinal tract. Although they were less potent than chlorisondamine, their more complete absorption has provided a degree of ganglionic blockade comparable to that of chlorisondamine when given orally.

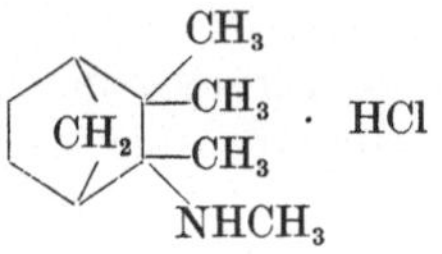

Mecamylamine 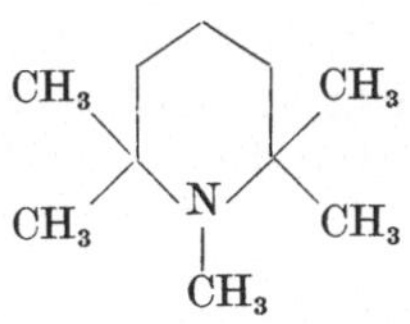   *Pempidine*

The ganglionic blockers provided a successful transition between the laboratory and the hypertension clinic, since it was demonstrated for the first time that hypotensive activity produced by a drug in the normotensive animal in the laboratory could be translated into useful controlled antihypertensive action in the human. Since ganglionic blockers affected all of the organs innervated by both the sympathetic and parasympathetic systems, their widespread actions have limited their therapeutic applicability. The effects of parasympathetic blockade which are the most annoying include visual blurring, dry mouth, constipation, dysuria and impotence. The ganglionic blocking agents succeeded clinically where the adrenergic blockers failed chiefly because they blocked the sympathetic cardioaccelerator pathways at the sympathetic ganglia. This action, however, has proven to be a double-edged sword, since the blockade of pressor reflexes mediated by the sympathetic nervous system is responsible for the excessive postural hypotension caused at times by the ganglionic blocking agents. Nevertheless, the reduction in peripheral resistance, the decreased cardiac output related to the increased capacity of the vascular space, and the resultant lowered diastolic blood pressure stamped ganglionic blockade as the initial demonstrable success in the search for a chemical sympathectomy.

Veratrum. Various alkaloids of veratrum cause a sustained hypotensive effect when administered to laboratory animals. This action is associated with a peripheral vasodilation and bradycardia. The postural pressor reflexes are not depressed. The action of these alkaloids is due in part to an activation of the Bezold reflex with sensory receptors located in the left ventricle and lungs and with afferent pathways following the vagus nerves to the brain. Some direct central action has been suggested, since not all of the actions of the drug are eliminated by atropine or vagotomy.

Unfortunately the hypotensive dose of the veratrum derivatives was found to lie precariously close to the emetic dose when they were applied in human hypertension, a finding which has seriously limited the development of a potentially useful group of compounds.

The continued quest for more effective and better tolerated antihypertensive agents led to the appearance within a short interval of two interesting new types of antihypertensive compounds. The first of these included hydralazine, (1-hydrazinophthalazine) and Nepresol (1,4-dihydrazinophthalazine), synthetic preparations first described by Gross, Druey and Meier in 1950 (*14*), and the other was reserpine, a crystalline alkaloid of plant origin isolated from *Rauwolfia serpentina* by Mueller, Schlittler and Bein in 1952 (*15*). The formulae of hydralazine and Nepresol are shown:

Hydralazine *Nepresol*

Hydrazinophthalazines. The type of blood pressure fall in experimental animals following the administration of hydralazine and of the related 1,4-dihydrazinophthalazine, known as Nepresol, differed considerably from that seen after ganglionic blocking agents. The drop in blood pressure following hydralazine was slower in onset, more gradual, and more sustained than that following ganglionic blockade (*16*). Regularly there was an increase in heart rate associated with the hypotension, suggesting that the sympathetic cardioaccelerator fibers were intact. The vasoconstrictor pathways also appeared to be functional, since postural hypotension which was common with ganglionic blockers was unusual with hydralazine.

The observation by REUBI in 1950 (*17*) that hydralazine increased renal blood flow both in the dog and the human did much to spur interest in the substance because of the potential significance of renal ischemia in the development of human hypertension. In this connection, RENZI (*18*) has shown in the rat that hydralazine prevents the damaging effect of renin, a substance produced by the ischemic kidney, on the whole vascular system, and especially on that of the kidneys.

The site of action of hydralazine appears to be primarily peripheral since it interferes with the hypertensive effect of several peripherally-acting pressor substances including serotonin, epinephrine, norepinephrine and pitressin. BEIN (*19*) has also shown that hydrazinophthalazine antagonizes the constrictor effect of ergotamine and ephedrine after transection of the spinal cord, providing further evidence that hydralazine acts at a peripheral site close to the blood vessels where these two substances were known to act. The pressor effect following bilateral carotid occlusion was also decreased or eliminated by hydralazine. Similarly, the rise in blood pressure caused by faradization of the central end of the divided vagus or sciatic nerves or of the peripheral end of the divided splanchnic nerve was diminished. The latter effect is consistent only with a peripheral action of hydralazine.

In further support of a peripheral site of action, it may be mentioned that hydralazine, in a concentration of 1 μg/ml of perfusate, was capable of increasing the coronary blood flow in the isolated cat heart (*19*) or in the dog heart-lung preparation (*20*). In the latter preparation, hydralazine also potentiated and prolonged the coronary dilating action of epinephrine. This latter effect is of interest, since Wilkinson et al. (*21*) have suggested that a portion of the clinical antihypertensive action of hydralazine may be related to its property of increasing the reactivity of the vasculature to the sympathetic vasodilator component of epinephrine.

It has been proposed by Schroeder (*22*) that the hypotensive action of hydralazine may be related in part to its capacity to chelate with trace metals in the body. It is of interest in this regard that Jaques, Tripod and Meier (*23*) have shown that hydralazine is capable of preventing the coronary constrictor action of copper salts on the isolated perfused rabbit heart.

In view of the many possibilities, it is not possible to assign a definitive mode of action to hydralazine. The available evidence, however, does point to a resultant dampening of sympathetic vasoconstrictor activity, and, by the same token, to a degree of chemical sympathectomy.

Reserpine. Reserpine differed from all the previously known antihypertensive agents since it provided quieting and sedation in addition to a subtle hypotensive action. The mechanism of action of reserpine was also unique among those of all the previously known antihypertensive agents. The central and circulatory effects of reserpine first noted by Bein (*24*) were of gradual onset and of long duration, lasting not uncommonly several days after oral administration to laboratory animals. In acute experiments in rabbits, dogs and cats, the reflex pressor responses following carotid occlusion and central vagal stimulation were decreased by reserpine, while bradycardia characteristically accompanied the fall in blood pressure. The nictitating membrane was also regularly relaxed. These actions as a group pointed toward a general dampening of the sympathetic nervous system at a locus which was believed at first to be exclusively within the central nervous system. This concept was supported by the work of Bein (*25*), who showed that a much larger dose of reserpine was required to block the carotid occlusion reflex after brain stem transection than before this procedure. A supramedullary locus of action for reserpine was also indicated when it was observed that the pressor response to elevated intracranial pressure was not suppressed in view of the fact that the mediation of this pressor function was ascribed to the medullary region (*26*). When PLETSCHER, BRODIE and SHORE (*27*) made the interesting observation in 1955 that reserpine caused the liberation of serotonin from binding sites in various organs including the central nervous system, it was proposed that this action was causally related to the hypotensive and sedative actions and that the gradual onset of effect of the substance was related to the time required for displacement of the amine from its binding sites. However, the later observation by HOLZBAUER and VOGT (*28*) that reserpine also freed norepinephrine from binding sites not only within the hypothalamus but also at peripheral sympathetic nerves raised the question of the role played by depletion of this sympathetic nervous neurohumor for the hypotensive action of reserpine. Continuing studies by BRODIE (*29*), by CARLSSON (*30*), by MUSCHOLL and VOGT (*31*) and by BURN and RAND (*32*) have indicated a striking correlation between depletion of the catecholamines from peripheral sympathetic nerves and ganglia and the hypotensive activity of reserpine. Therefore, this mechanism appears to be involved in the decrease in peripheral resistance responsible for the hypotensive effects of reserpine. From a practical standpoint, however, the quieting aspect of the action of reserpine may well be of importance for its effect on blood pressure, since sedation may be desirable where anxiety is contributory to the elevation of the blood pressure; for it is well recognized that man by his thoughts alone may raise his blood pressure.

It had been noted earlier that reserpine caused a potentiation of the pressor effect of norepinephrine in the dog and also caused a tachycardia in the Starling heart-lung preparation (*33*). These effects, which were at first inexplicable, are probably related to the increased sensitivity of the blood vessels and heart (*34*), which are in a sense "denervated" through the loss of norepinephrine from the nerves by which they are innervated. Neither hypertension nor tachycardia are associated with the clinical use of reserpine, probably because the removal of norepinephrine is less precipitate and less complete with the small doses sufficient for human antihypertensive activity.

IGGO and VOGT (*35*) have recently reported that the spontaneous action potentials of the cervical sympathetic nerves of the cat are not reduced by reserpine. Bradycardia, which was not noted in the animals in these experiments, appears to be a less common finding in the cat than in the dog. In view of this species difference, it does not appear possible at present to exclude the central

248 A. J. Plummer:

nervous system as one of the sites of action for the "chemical sympathectomy" produced by reserpine.

Syrosingopine. The appearance of syrosingopine, a reserpine analogue, in 1959, constituted a further important advance in antihypertensive therapy. Since reserpine was first studied, investigators had been concerned with the problem of trying to separate its sedative and hypotensive effects by appropriate structural modification.

Reserpine

Syrosingopine

It was only after the preparation of more than a hundred ester analogues of reserpine by Lucas (*36*) that one was found which provided adequate hypotensive action with minimal sedative properties in several laboratory animal species. In the dog, for example, syrosingopine and reserpine had equal hypotensive activity, while the sedative effect of syrosingopine was but one-tenth that of reserpine. It was thus possible to maintain the mean blood pressure of the unanesthetized dog at 30 to 40 mm Hg below its resting level without attendant drowsiness with a daily oral dose of 40 μg/kg of syrosingopine (*37*).

The availability of syrosingopine has also provided essential clues to the relative importance of the release of serotonin and catecholamines for the lowering of the arterial blood pressure. ORLANS, FINGER and BRODIE (*38*) have found that syrosingopine, administered to the dog or rabbit, caused marked reduction of peripheral cardiac catecholamines and moderate reduction of brain catecholamines, but no detectable lowering of brain serotonin levels in hypotensive doses in the dog. The hypotensive action of syrosingopine, and, as mentioned previously, of reserpine as well, appears on the basis of such evidence to depend on their effects upon catecholamines rather than on serotonin. Studies by GARATTINI (*39*) have similarly indicated a linkage between the cardiovascular effects of syrosingopine and catecholamine release rather than serotonin depletion. Biochemical evidence has therefore served to substantiate and explain the earlier pharmacological assessment of syrosingopine as a compound with predominantly hypotensive and minimally sedative activity. Syrosingopine appears to be capable, therefore, of producing a more specific peripheral "chemical sympathectomy" than reserpine by virtue of its reduced central action.

Guanethidine. Within the past year a novel synthetic compound with a unique antiadrenergic mechanism has been described by MAXWELL, MULL and PLUMMER (*40*). This substance, which was synthesized by MULL, is known as guanethidine:

$$N-CH_2CH_2NH-C{\overset{NH}{\underset{NH_2}{}}}$$

Guanethidine

On the basis of the pharmacological actions of guanethidine, as described by MAXWELL (*41*) and PAGE (*58*), it may be most properly described as a specific peripheral sympathetic nervous suppressant which impedes sympathetic efferent transmission. The characteristic sympathetic nervous inhibition caused by guanethidine is gradual in onset but is prolonged and is preceded in the dog and cat by a brief period resembling sympathetic stimulation which may be due to a period of active catecholamine release. Following the oral or parenteral administration of guanethidine to a dog, a marked relaxation of the nictitating membrane developed after a latent period of about six hours and persisted usually for several days; concomitantly there was a gradual drop in blood pressure and also a bradycardia which, too, lasted for several days. Significantly, the fall in blood pressure which was produced by guanethidine was considerably greater in the neurogenic or renal hypertensive dog than in the normal animal. This attribute is, of course, a potential asset for antihypertensive applicability. The rise in blood pressure accompanying annoying stimulation of unanesthetized neurogenic

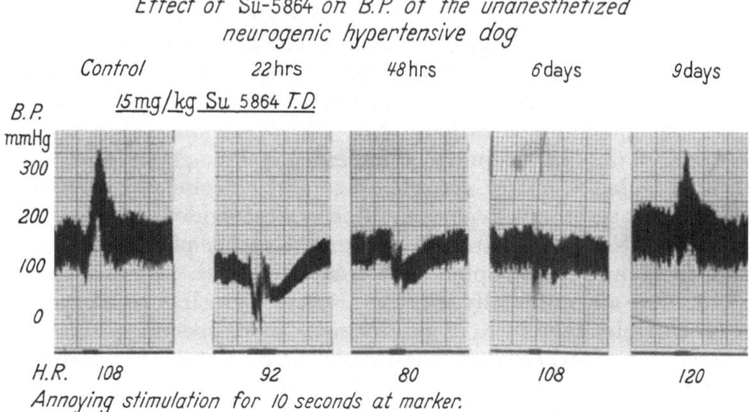

Fig. 1. The long-lasting hypotensive and bradycardic effect of guanethidine is shown in the neurogenic hypertensive dog. The pressor effect of annoying stimulation is abolished for more than six days

hypertensive dogs was also abolished by pretreatment with guanethidine (Fig. 1). Renal hypertension in the rat is also antagonized by guanethidine (42).

The pressor response to carotid occlusion was reduced by guanethidine for a period of four to seven days; in contrast, the pressor effect of norepinephrine was greatly augmented. During the prolonged hypotensive state induced by guanethidine, the nictitating membranes were relaxed and were but weakly stimulated by faradization of their postganglionic sympathetic nervous supply, while, as in the case of the blood vessels, the membranes were hypersensitive to intravenously administered norepinephrine (Fig. 2). At this stage, also, faradization of the splanchnic nerve produced very weak pressor spikes, while the pressor responses to intravenously injected norepinephrine were augmented above control levels (Fig.3).This parallelism of events in two sympathetically innervated structures pointed to an inhibition of the transmission of impulses from the terminals of postganglionic sympathetic nerves, possibly by interfering with the availability of norepinephrine at these terminals. In support of this view it has been shown by Maxwell (unpublished) that the reflexly induced rise in blood pressure due to asphyxia was reduced by guanethidine

in the cat under pentobarbital anesthesia, while at the same time
the characteristic electrical potentials induced in the splanchnic
nerve by the asphyxia were undiminished. In still further support

EFFECT* OF 10mg./Kg SU-5864 I.V. ON:

A.

NICTITATING MEMBRANE

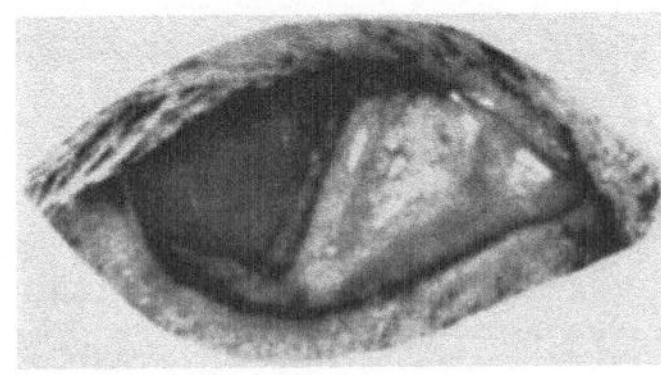

B.

POST GANGLIONIC POTENTIALS
EVOKED BY PREGANGLIONIC
STIMULATION

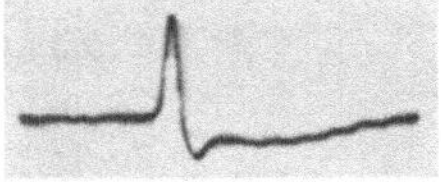

C.

CONTRACTIONS OF THE NICTITATING MEMBRANES
ELICITED BY PREGANGLIONIC FARADIZATION AND
INJECTED NOR-EPINEPHRINE

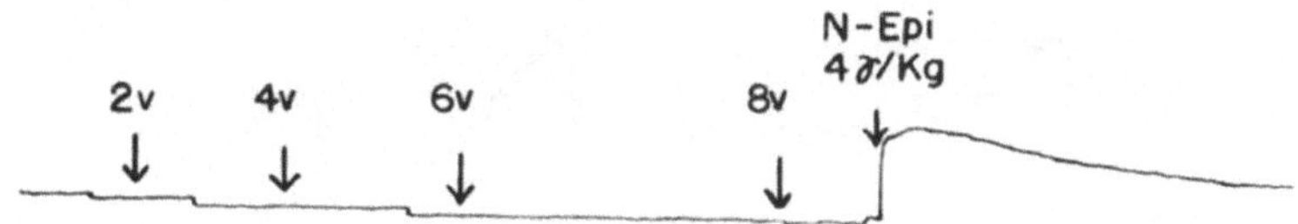

* IN THE CAT AT 24 HOURS FOLLOWING DRUG ADMINISTRATION

Fig. 2. (1) relaxed nictitating membrane, (2) unimpaired transmission by postganglionic
sympathetic nerve, (3) refractoriness of nictitating membrane to nervous stimulation,
(4) responsiveness of nictitating membrane to injected norepinephrine, indicate site of action
of guanethidine at the periphery of the sympathetic nervous system

of this thesis, it has been established that guanethidine caused
neither ganglionic nor peripheral adrenergic blockade at the time
of maximum sympathetic nervous inhibition. In fact, when

administered after a peripheral adrenergic blocking agent such as
phentolamine, the reduced pressor response to parenteral norepinephrine reverted to normal, while epinephrine reversal was

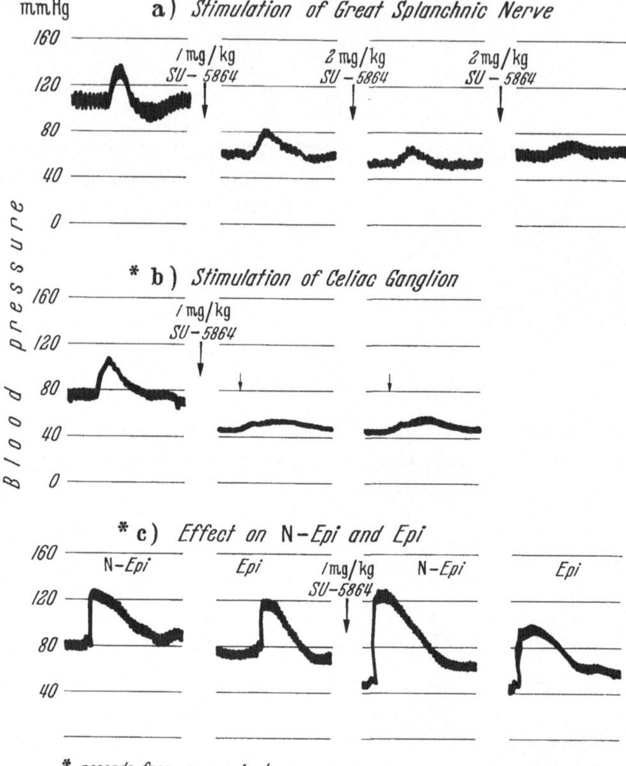

Fig. 3. Guanethidine-induced reduction of pressor effect following faradization of the splanchnic nerve and celiac ganglia, coupled with exaggerated pressor response to the injection of
norepinephrine

not affected. Finally, guanethidine also prevented the pressor
effect of the peripherally acting pressor amines, amphetamine and
ephedrine.

Recent biochemical studies by SHEPPARD (43) have established
that guanethidine reduces the catecholamine levels of the heart
(Fig. 4) and of the spleen gradually but that, in contrast to the

effects of reserpine, the brain and adrenal catecholamine contents
are not altered. The persistence of reduced levels of catecholamines in the heart and arteries of the dog up to two weeks after

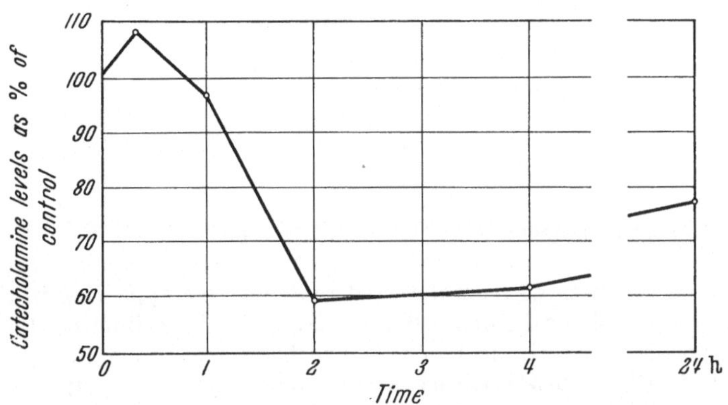

Fig. 4. Reduction of cardiac catecholamines by guanethidine in the rat

a single administration of the drug is consistent with the observed
prolonged circulatory effects of guanethidine; interestingly, the
reduced amine level tended to persist longer in the arteries than in
the heart. CASS, KUNTZMAN and BRODIE (44) made similar observations in rabbits and cats. On this basis the previously mentioned sensitivity of the blood vessels to intravenously administered
norepinephrine can be related to the partially "denervated" state
comparable to a diminution of the neurohumoral mediator; the
hypotension and diminished reactivity of the blood vessels to
splanchnic faradization are similarly explicable by this same mechanism. It is not yet known with certainty whether the binding or the
synthesis of norepinephrine by the tissues is primarily altered by
guanethidine.

Since guanethidine does not depress the parasympathetic
nervous system, it does not induce mydriasis, dryness of the mouth,
constipation or impotence, actions inseparably connected with the
use of the ganglionic blocking agents. Its potency is reflected in
a certain incidence of postural hypotension which is usually curbed
by proper dosage; some increased bowel activity, which diminishes
with continued treatment, appears to be due to a dampening action
on the inhibitory sympathetic innervation to the gastrointestinal
tract.

Bretylium. Within the past year another interesting compound known as bretylium has been proposed as an antihypertensive agent. Bretylium, which is a quaternary derivative, resulted from a search for a substance which would produce an exclusive block of sympathetic ganglia without influencing parasympathetid ganglia.

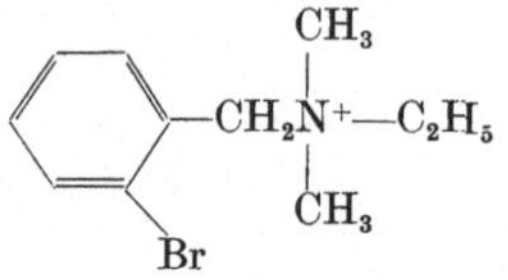

$$\text{C}_6\text{H}_4(\text{Br})-\text{CH}_2\overset{+}{\text{N}}(\text{CH}_3)_2-\text{C}_2\text{H}_5$$

Bretylium

Bretylium labeled with Carbon-14 has been shown by Boura et al. (*45*) to be concentrated in sympathetic ganglia and in adrenergic nerve fibers with no detected radioactivity appearing in the brain or spinal cord. The mechanism by which bretylium produces its specific sympathetic blockade has been ascribed to an interference with the usual release of norepinephrine by the sympathetic postganglionic nerves when these receive impulses which have traversed preganglionic fibers.

Since bretylium and guanethidine produce similar effects on the sympathetic nervous system by different actions, it is of some interest to compare their general pharmacological characteristics. They are entirely unrelated chemically. Both substances cause a fall, commonly preceded by a rise, in the blood pressure of the anesthetized dog. The onset of the hypotensive effect is more prompt in the case of a single effective intravenous dose of bretylium, while the duration of action following a comparable dose of guanethidine is much longer. A similar picture is seen in the case of the nictitating membrane, where each substance causes an initial retraction followed by a relaxation of the structure. The duration of effect of bretylium on both of these systems is measured in hours and that of guanethidine in days. Bradycardia appears to be more regularly associated with guanethidine than with bretylium administration in either the anesthetized or unanesthetized dog. Each substance potentiates the vasoconstrictor effect of injected norepinephrine. Guanethidine characteristically antagonizes the hypertensive effect of amphetamine and ephedrine, but bretylium lacks this action because of a fundamental difference in their modes of peripheral action. Both substances reduce the reflex hypertension caused by carotid occlusion. Bretylium exhibits good local anesthetic activity and moderate antihistaminic activity, while guanethidine has neither of these actions. Guanethidine decreases the pressor response in the cat following splanchnic faradization to a greater degree than does bretylium. This effect of guanethidine appears to be referable to a sympathetic inhibitory rather than an adrenal inhibitory influence, however, since guanethidine does not lower the catecholamine content of the adrenal medulla. Both substances have weak and transient ganglionic blocking properties at very high dosage, which probably play no part in the physiological range. Neither substance has any action referable to the central nervous or to the parasympathetic nervous system. Because of its quaternary nature, the oral absorption of bretylium, like that of the chemically related ganglionic blockers, is incomplete. In summary, then, in adequate dosage, each substance is capable of producing a pharmacological sympathectomy. The chief differentiating characteristics from a theoretical viewpoint are a fundamental difference in mechanism of action, and, from a more practical aspect, a significant difference in the duration and constancy of the pharmacological sympathectomies caused by these substances.

Sulfonamide diuretics. Within the last few years several compounds known as the sulfonamide diuretics have found a place as adjunctive agents in the therapeutic management of hypertension. These substances, of which the most thoroughly studied are chlorothiazide, prepared by SPRAGUE (*46*) and hydrochlorothiazide, prepared by DE STEVENS and WERNER (*47*), do not produce a "chemical sympathectomy", nor has it been possible to demonstrate that they possess any direct hypotensive action in the dog, even following large intravenous doses (*48*). Nevertheless, clinical reports (*49, 50, 51*) generally attribute antihypertensive properties to the sulfonamide diuretics. Such effects may be secondary to their diuretic and natriuretic actions, although HOLLANDER has provided persuasive evidence that sodium depletion may not be the sole or even the main cause of the antihypertensive action of hydrochlorothiazide.

Chlorothiazide

Hydrochlorothiazide

Supporting the importance of sodium depletion for the antihypertensive action of the thiazide derivatives was the recent observation by Gross (*52*) that hydrochlorothiazide retarded the hypertension induced in rats by the administration of desoxycorticosterone, since this steroid-induced hypertension is associated with a retention of sodium. Gross and Lichtlen (*53*) have also noted an intensified vasopressor reaction to epinephrine and norepinephrine in this experimental hypertension and have reasonably suggested that this may be due to an increased sensitivity of the arterioles to pressor stimuli resulting from a higher water and sodium content of the arterial wall. The sulfonamide diuretics accordingly would be presumed to obviate such a situation by preventing the accumulation of water and electrolytes within the arterial wall. In concert with this view is the further observation by Bock and Gross (*53a*) that the vasopressor effects of epinephrine, norepinephrine and hypertensin are clearly suppressed in the dog by hydrochlorothiazide pretreatment. It is significant for this thesis that hydrochlorothiazide does not prevent hydrocortisone or renal hypertension in the rat, since neither of these entities depends upon an increase in the sodium intake.

Raab (*54*) has shown a comparable mechanism to be operative in human physiology, for here as well, the administration of desoxycorticosterone and sodium chloride was followed by an augmentation of the pressor effects to catecholamines. The observation that hydrochlorothiazide is capable of suppressing the pressor effect of norepinephrine therefore assumes importance for the clinical situation as well, especially in view of the recent reports by Mendlowitz (*55*) and Barany (*56*) of an increased sensitivity displayed to norepinephrine-induced vasoconstriction by patients with essential hypertension. The further report by Mendlowitz (*57*) that such increased sensitivity to norepinephrine is reduced by hydrochlorothiazide is most interesting because of the obvious implications.

The weight of evidence indicates that the antihypertensive action of hydrochlorothiazide and related compounds in human essential hypertension is an indirect one which is secondary to their primary action of interfering with the tubular resorption of sodium. The enhancing action of these diuretics upon the action of the more potent antihypertensive agents such as reserpine, hydralazine and guanethidine in clinical situations may also be referable to this primary mechanism.

Summary

In the span of a few short years the therapeutic management of essential hypertension has been transformed from one of gross empiricism to that of a stable, rational approach based on established pharmacological principles. This success has required a close liaison among the disciplines of chemistry, of pharmacology, and of the clinic, for the niceties and fine nuances governing the relationship between chemical structure and type of biological activity of a compound are all too elusive for charting a reliable course through unfamiliar synthetic molecular configurations.

Although autonomic nervous overactivity had never been demonstrably implicated as an etiological factor in essential hypertension, it had been realized earlier that suppression of this system by pharmacological means offered potential therapeutic benefit. Unfortunately, early investigative work had not yielded specific potent autonomic blocking agents with sufficiently wide therapeutic indices to be suitable for human use. The initial successful surgical approach to the problem of sympathetic nervous dampening by means of a dorsal thoracolumbar sympathectomy established the validity of such a procedure and laid the groundwork for an ultimate pharmacological approach. Among the effective agents which have been discussed, an action either directly or indirectly upon the sympathetic nervous system or upon the neurohumors which it elaborates has been a common denominator. Such an occurrence inevitably poses the question as to whether such a common denominator has basic meaning or is merely coincidental with respect to the mode of action of the drug. If the relationship is truly basic, as can reasonably be inferred, the availability of these antihypertensive agents may serve not only to furnish treatment for essential hypertension but also to provide persuasive evidence that an altered vascular responsivity to sympathetic nervous stimulation may be a significant factor in the genesis of the hypertensive state.

Since a circulatory dysfunction of unknown causes and of varying severity was being attacked, it has been advantageous frequently to combine one or more of these specific agents in treatment until a salutary effect is obtained. This procedure has a rational experimental basis. For example, the blood pressure fall produced by the daily administration of hydralazine to the dog can be increased by the addition of reserpine or syrosingopine to the regime; the addition of the latter also has the desirable effect of eliminating any tendency to tachycardia which may have been produced by hydralazine. As mentioned earlier, the sulfonamide diuretics are capable of potentiating the action of the more specific antihypertensives and also of lessening the reactivity of the blood vessels to several vasoconstrictors occurring normally in the body.

The availability of more specific and potent sympathetic antihypertensives such as guanethidine provides the physician with an opportunity to control the ravages of essential hypertension in an ever increasing number of patients. In fact, guanethidine is capable of producing a more effective type of sympathectomy than could ever be managed surgically, since it affects all sympathetic pathways, including those beyond the reach of the surgeon. By its very nature also, the pharmacological sympathectomy provided by guanethidine is not an irreversible procedure and so affords the physician an opportunity to alter the degree and duration of the effect to the needs of the individual patient.

With the advantage of a decade of experience in the laboratories and of steadily improving pharmacological and biochemical methods for assessing potentially useful antihypertensive action, the hope for further life-enhancing drug therapy seems bright indeed.

Résumé

En l'espace de quelques années, le traitement de l'hypertension essentielle a évolué à partir d'une base empirique jusqu'à une thérapeutique solide, rationnelle, basée sur des données pharmacologiques. Cette évolution a exigé une liaison étroite entre la chimie, la pharmacologie et la clinique, car les relations entre la structure chimique d'un composé et son activité biologique sont trop aléatoires et nuancées pour qu'on puisse se fier à la seule exploration de la structure d'une molécule synthétique.

Bien qu'il n'ait jamais été démontré que l'hyperactivité du système nerveux autonome joue un rôle étiologique dans l'hypertension essentielle, on s'est rapidement rendu compte que l'inhibition de ce sytème par des moyens pharmacologiques pouvait constituer une thérapeutique adéquate. Malheureusement, les premières recherches n'avaient pas fourni d'inhibiteur spécifique puissant du système nerveux autonome et dont la marge thérapeutique fut suffisante pour permettre l'application clinique. Le succès des premières sympathectomies dorso-lombaires a établi la légitimité d'une intervention sur le sympathique et jeté les bases d'une approche analogue par des moyens pharmacologiques.

Les produits actifs qui ont été envisagés ont tous pour dénominateur commun une action directe ou indirecte sur le sympathique ou ses médiateurs chimiques. Un tel fait pose inévitablement la question de savoir si ce dénominateur commun a une signification fondamentale ou n'est qu'une pure coïncidence en rapport avec le mode d'action de la drogue. Si la relation est vraiment fondamentale, comme on peut raisonnablement le penser, l'existence de ces anti-hypertenseurs non seulement représente une acquisition dans le traitement de l'hypertension essentielle, mais aussi permet d'apporter la preuve qu'un trouble de la réactivité vasculaire aux stimulations sympathiques peut être un facteur important dans la genèse des états hypertensifs.

Puisqu'on s'est attaqué à un trouble circulatoire de gravité variable lié à des causes inconnues, il a été fréquemment avantageux d'associer deux ou plusieurs de ces agents spécifiques jusqu'à obtenir le résultat recherché. Cette manière de faire a une base expérimentale rationnelle. Par exemple, la chute de pression produite chez le chien par l'administration quotidienne d'hydralazine peut être augmentée par l'adjonction de réserpine ou de syrosingopine; l'addition de ces dernières a également pour effet de supprimer la tendance à la tachycardie que peut provoquer l'hydralazine. Comme il a été dit plus haut, les sulfamides diurétiques sont capables de potentialiser l'action d'anti-hypertenseurs plus spécifiques et aussi de diminuer la réactivité des vaisseaux sanguins à plusieurs vasoconstricteurs existant normalement dans l'organisme.

L'introduction récente d'agents anti-hypertenseurs plus puissants et plus spécifiques, comme la guanéthidine, donne au médecin l'occasion de contrôler les méfaits de l'hypertension essentielle chez un nombre toujours plus grand de malades. En effet, la guanéthidine est capable d'assurer une sympathectomie beaucoup plus efficace que ne pourrait jamais le faire une intervention chirurgicale, car elle bloque tous les filets sympathiques, y compris ceux inaccesibles au chirurgien. De par sa nature même, la «sympathectomie chimique» produite par la guanéthidine n'est pas un état irréversible et donne ainsi la possibilité au médecin de modifier le degré et la durée de l'effet selon les besoins individuels du malade.

Après dix ans d'expérience de laboratoire et grâce à l'amélioration constante des méthodes de détermination de l'action antihypertensive, les chances d'améliorer le pronostic vital par une thérapeutique adéquate semblent réellement bonnes.

Figs. 1, 3 and 4 are reproduced by permission of the Journal of Pharmacology and Experimental Therapeutics: MAXWELL, R. A., A. J. PLUMMER, F. SCHNEIDER, H. POVALSKI and A. I. DANIEL: J. Pharmacol. Exper. Therap. (U.S.A.) 128, 22 (1960). Fig. 2 is reproduced by permission of Schweiz. med. Wschr.: MAXWELL, R. A., A. J. PLUMMER, F. SCHNEIDER, H. POVALSKI and A. I. DANIEL: Schweiz. med. Wschr. 90, 109 (1960).

References

1. SMITHWICK, R. H.: Surgery (U.S.A.) 7, 1 (1940).
2. BARGER, G., F. H. CARR, and H. DALE: Brit. Med. J. 1906/II, 792.
3. HARTMANN, M., and H. ISLER: Naunyn-Schmiedebergs Arch. exper. Path. (G.) 192, 141 (1939).
4. MEIER, R., F. F. YONKMAN, B. N. CRAVER, and F. GROSS: Proc. Soc. Exper. Biol. Med. (U.S.A.) 71, 70 (1949).
5. LANGLEY, J. N., and W. L. DICKINSON: Proc. Roy. Soc. (G.B.) 46, 423 (1889).
6. ACHESON, G. H., and S. A. PEREIRA: J. Pharmacol. Exper. Therap. (U.S.A.) 87, 273 (1946).
7. PATON, W. D. M., and W. L. M. PERRY: J. Physiol. (G.B.) 119, 43 (1953).
8. BARLOW, R. B., and H. R. ING: Brit. J. Pharmacol. 3, 298 (1948).
9. PATON, W. D. M., and E. J. ZAIMIS: Brit. J. Pharmacol. 4, 381 (1949).
10. LEVINE, R. M., and B. B. CLARK: Fed. Proc. (U.S.A.) 13, 380 (1954).
11. PLUMMER, A. J., J. H. TRAPOLD, J. A. SCHNEIDER, R. A. MAXWELL, and A. E. EARL: J. Pharmacol. Exper. Therap. (U.S.A.) 115, 172 (1955).
12. STONE, C. A., M. L. TORCHINA, A. NAVARRO, and K. H. BEYER: J. Pharmacol. Exper. Therap. (U.S.A.) 117, 169 (1956).
13. SPINKS, A., and E. H. P. YOUNG: Nature (G.B.) 181, 1397 (1958).
14. GROSS, F., F. DRUEY, and R. MEIER: Experientia (Switz.) 6, 19 (1950).
15. MUELLER, J. M., E. SCHLITTLER, and H. J. BEIN: Experientia (Switz.) 8, 338 (1952).
16. CRAVER, B. N., W. BARRETT, A. CAMERON, and F. F. YONKMAN: J. Amer. Pharm. Ass. (Sc. Ed.) 40, 559 (1951).
17. REUBI, F.: Helvet. med. acta. 16, 297 (1949).
18. RENZI, A. A., and R. GAUNT: Amer. J. Physiol. 175, 313 (1953).
19. BEIN, H. J., F. GROSS, J. TRIPOD, and R. MEIER: Schweiz. med. Wschr. 83, 336 (1953).
20. BARRETT, W., W. REITZE, A. J. PLUMMER, and F. F. YONKMAN: Fed. Proc. (U.S.A.) 11, 320 (1952).
21. WILKINSON, E. L., H. BACKMAN, and H. H. HECHT: J. Clin. Invest. (U.S.A.) 31, 872 (1952).
22. SCHROEDER, H. A., and H. M. PERRY: J. Laborat. Clin. Med. (U.S.A.) 46, 416 (1955).
23. JAQUES, R., J. TRIPOD, and R. MEIER: Naunyn-Schmiedebergs Arch. exper. Path. (G.) 230, 26 (1957).
24. BEIN, H. J.: Experientia (Switz.) 9, 107 (1953).
25. BEIN, H. J.: Ann. N.Y. Acad. Sc. 61, 4 (1955).
26. TRAPOLD, J., A. J. PLUMMER, and F. F. YONKMAN: J. Pharmacol. Exper. Therap. (U.S.A.) 110, 205 (1954).
27. PLETSCHER, A., P. A. SHORE, and B. B. BRODIE: Science (U.S.A.) 122, 374 (1955).
28. HOLZBAUER, M., and M. VOGT: J. Neurochem. (U.S.A.) 1, 8 (1956).

29. BRODIE, B. B., J. S. OLIN, R. G. KUNTZMAN, and P. A. SHORE: Science (U.S.A.) **125**, 1293 (1957).
30. CARLSSON, A., E. ROSENGREN, A. BERTLER, and J.NILSSON: Psychotropic drugs. Amsterdam: Elsevier Publishing Co. 1957, pp. 363.
31. MUSCHOLL, E., and M. VOGT: J. Physiol. (G.B.) **141**, 132 (1958).
32. BURN, J. H., and M. J. RAND: Brit. Med. J. **1958/I**, 903.
33. PLUMMER, A. J., A. EARL, J. A. SCHNEIDER, J. TRAPOLD, and W. BARRETT: Ann. N.Y. Acad. Sc. **59**, 8 (1954).
34. KRAYER, O., and J. J. FUENTES: J. Pharmacol. Exper. Therap. (U.S.A.) **123**, 145 (1958).
35. IGGO, A., and M. VOGT: J. Physiol. (G.B.) **150**, 114 (1960).
36. LUCAS, R. A., M. J. KUEHNE, M. J. CEGLOWSKI, R. L. DZIEMIAN, and H. B. MACPHILLAMY: J. Amer. Chem. Soc. **81**, 1928 (1959).
37. PLUMMER, A. J., W. E. BARRETT, R. A. MAXWELL, D. FINOCCHIO, R. LUCAS, and A. E. EARL: Arch. internat. pharmacodyn. thérap. (Belg.) **119**, 245 (1959).
38. ORLANS, F., B. HUGHES, K. F. FINGER, and B. B. BRODIE: J. Pharmacol. Exper. Therap. (U.S.A.) **128**, 131 (1960).
39. GARATTINI, S., A. MORTARI, A. VOLSECCHI, and L. VALZELLI: Nature (G.B.) **183**, 1273 (1959).
40. MAXWELL, R. A., R. P. MULL, and A. J. PLUMMER: Experientia (Switz.) **15/7**, 267 (1959).
41. MAXWELL, R. A., A. J. PLUMMER, F. SCHNEIDER, H. POVALSKI and A. DANIEL: J. Pharmacol. Exper. Therap. (U.S.A.) **128**, 22 (1960).
42. BEIN, H. J.: Ciba Foundation Symposium, March 30 (1960).
43. SHEPPARD, H., and J. ZIMMERMAN: Pharmacologist (U.S.A.) **1**, 69 (1959).
44. CASS, R., R. KUNTZMAN, and B. B. BRODIE: Proc. Soc. Exper. Biol. Med. (U.S.A.) **103**, 871 (1960).
45. BOURA, A. L. A., A. F. GREEN, A. MCCOUBREY, D. R. LAURENCE, R. MOULTON, and M. L. ROSENHEIM: Lancet **1959/II**, 17.
46. SPRAGUE, J. M.: Ann. N.Y. Acad. Sc. **71**, 328 (1958).
47. DE STEVENS, G., L. H. WERNER, A. HALAMANDARIS, and S. RICCA JR.: Experientia (Switz.) **14**, 463 (1958).
48. BARRETT, W. E., R. A. RUTLEDGE, H. SHEPPARD, and A. J. PLUMMER: Toxicol. and Appl. Pharmacol. (U.S.A.) **1**, 333 (1959).
49. WILKINS, R. W., W. HOLLANDER, and A. V. CHOBANIAN: Ann. N.Y. Acad. Sc. **71**, 465 (1958).
50. FREIS, E.D., and I.M. WILSON: Med.Ann.District of Columbia **26**, 468 (1957).
51. HOLLANDER, W., A. V. CHOBANIAN, and R. W. WILKINS: Hypertension. Philadelphia: W. B. Saunders Company 1959, pp. 570.
52. GROSS, F., A. PLUMMER, and H. ZEUGIN: Bull. Schweiz. Akad. med. Wiss. **15**, 346 (1959).
53. GROSS, F., and P. LICHTLEN: Naunyn-Schmiedebergs Arch. exper. Path. (G.) **233**, 323 (1958).
53a. BOCK, K. D., and F. GROSS: Naunyn-Schmiedebergs Arch. exper. Path. (G.) **238**, 339 (1960).
54. RAAB, W., R. J. HUMPHREYS, and E. LEPESCHKIN: J. Clin. Invest. (U.S.A.) **29**, 1397 (1950).
55. MENDLOWITZ, M., and A. MEYER: Fed. Proc. (U.S.A.) **14**, 100 (1955).
56. BARANY, F. R., and P. JAMES: Clin. Sc. (G.B.) **18**, 543 (1959).
57. MENDLOWITZ, M., N. NAFTCHI, S. E. GITLOW, H. L. WEINREB, and R. L. WOLF: Presented at the Conference on New Diuretics and Antihypertensive Agents — New York Academy of Sciences, May 5—6 (1960).
58. PAGE, I. H., and H. P. DUSTAN: J. Amer. med. Ass. **170**, 1265 (1959).

Bretylium and Guanethidine

Clinical results

By

T. HILDEN

Since the pharmacology of the new adrenergic blockers has already been mentioned, I shall immediately proceed to submit our clinical results of treatment with these substances.

Our series consists of patients suffering from severe benign or malignant hypertension. Apart from a few of the first treated patients, the treatment was conducted on an out-patient basis. The doses of the drugs were gradually increased until response or prohibiting side-effects appeared.

By 'satisfactory effect' we understand a mean blood pressure below 140 mm Hg both in the lying and in the standing position and by 'fairly satisfactory effect' a mean blood pressure below 140 mm Hg in the standing position only. By 'mean blood pressure' is understood the diastolic pressure plus one-third of the pulse pressure.

Bretylium

The drug was given 4 times daily. The maintenance dose ranged between 600 and 5200 mg, on an average 2000 mg. The period of treatment was from 2 to 6 months, on an average 3 months.

A total of 20 patients were treated. 10 had not been treated previously, 10 patients were already receiving ganglion-blocking drugs, and these drugs were replaced by bretylium. (Several of the latter patients also received reserpine and/or hydralazine.)

The results of the first 10 patients are summarized in Table 1. A satisfactory effect was obtained in 1 patient, and a fairly satisfactory one in 6. Two patients did not respond to treatment; one of them was given a total dosage of up to 5200 mg. In 1 case the treatment had to be discontinued very quickly because of side-effects. The average fall in mean blood pressure was 10 mm Hg in the lying position and 34 mm Hg in the standing position.

The second group of patients is shown in Table 2. A satisfactory effect was found in 3 cases, and a fairly satisfactory one in 3. In

Table 1. *10 hypertensive patients treated with bretylium*

No.	Sex	Age	BP	F.H.	Dose (mg)	Mean blood pressure-supine		Mean blood pressure-erect	
						Before	Bre-tylium	Before	Bre-tylium
1	M	56	240/140	III	1600	173	145	173	115
2	M	43	205/130	III	800	155	128	150	108
3	M	52	215/120	III	2400	152	158	145	135
4	M	58	235/135	II	(400)	(168)	sep.	(172)	sep.
5	F	30	215/135	III	4000	162	143	180	115
6	F	36	180/130	—	2400	147	153	147	137
7	F	63	240/135	III	1200	170	150	170	113
8	F	47	230/125	II	2400	157	165	155	138
9	M	52	180/125	III	5200	143	157	142	140
10	M	38	200/130	II	1600	153	142	150	150
Mean	(9 patients)				2400	157	147	157	123

1 case the drug had to be withdrawn quickly owing to the occurrence of side-effects. After treatment with ganglion-blocking agents a satisfactory effect was obtained in 5 cases, and a fairly satisfactory one in 2.

Table 2. *10 hypertensive patients. Comparison between the effect of ganglionblocking drugs and of bretylium*

No.	Sex	Age	BP	F.H.	Dose (mg)	Mean blood pressure-supine			Mean blood pressure-erect		
						Be-fore	Gangl. block.	Bre-tylium	Be-fore	Gangl. block.	Bre-tylium
1	M	58	210/130	II	1600	157	138	133	153	132	112
2	M	69	250/130	III	1200	170	133	148	173	117	135
3	F	60	280/155	III	600	197	187	180	183	165	138
4	M	54	210/120	III	2000	150	133	157	157	142	142
5	F	25	240/190	III	3200	207	118	135	210	108	122
6	M	62	230/140	IV	800	170	140	163	163	127	120
7	F	54	240/165	III	1600	190	173	172	183	165	160
8	M	41	235/140	IV	1000	172	128	118	170	113	112
9	M	52	235/130	III	800	165	150	sep.	160	122	sep.
10	F	70	275/130	III	2200	178	160	157	168	140	150
Mean	(9 Patients)				1500	177	145	151	174	134	132

In Table 3 the average decreases in the mean blood pressure are compared. It seems as if bretylium brings about a greater orthostatic reduction of the blood pressure than the ganglion-blocking agents.

The side-effects connected with the use of bretylium are recorded in Table 4. A number of minor complaints were observed, such as lassitude, dizziness, ptosis, nasal congestion, and pains in the parotid glands. In none of the cases were these symptoms of decisive importance.

The predominant side-effect was exertional symptoms, which developed in 13 patients. In 4 cases the treatment had to be discontinued on account of these complaints. The patients described this complex of symptoms as a feeling of faintness, sometimes accompanied by dizziness and shortness of breath. It was provoked especially by climbing stairs, but also by walking on the level at a normal pace. The exertional symptoms do not seem to have any relation to the fall in blood pressure in the standing position which is observed at the ordinary blood pressure control (Table 5).

Table 3. *Changes in mean blood pressure after ganglionic blockers and after bretylium*

9 patients	Reduction in mean blood pressure	
	supine mm Hg	erect mm Hg
Ganglionic blockers .	32	40
Bretylium	26	42

Table 4. *Side-effects in 20 patients treated with bretylium*

Weakness	7
Dizziness	4
Ptosis	4
Nasal stuffiness	2
Parotid pains	4
Exertional symptoms	13

(Treatment discontinued in 4 cases)

Table 5. *Exertional symptoms in 20 patients treated with bretylium*

Exertional symptoms	Reduction in M.B.P. erect mm Hg	Mean blood pressure erect mm Hg	Fall in M.B.P. on exertion mm Hg
No sympt., 6 patients	36	130	—
Moderate symptoms, 9 patients	42	122	33
Severe symptoms, 4 patients .	23	147	58

In most of the patients who complained of exertional symptoms, blood pressure measurements were made before and immediately after climbing some flights of stairs, corresponding to two storeys (stair test). An extremely pronounced fall in mean blood pressure in the standing position was often observed immediately after climbing stairs. A marked fall was also found with this test, without it being possible to demonstrate an orthostatic fall by measuring the blood pressure at rest.

Apart from the aforementioned side-effects it should be pointed out that the effect of bretylium is very variable and that tolerance to the drug often develops.

The clinical reports on bretylium published so far will not be dealt with in detail, as I am sure that they are well known to the audience and that several of those present will comment on these reports. I shall only mention the following: The first communication by Boura and co-workers (*1*) in July 1959 was more promising than subsequent reports. Dollery and co-workers (2) found a questionable effect in the severe cases, while Turner and Lowther (*6*) emphasized the variable effect and the frequent incidence of tolerance.

Our results correspond mainly to the last-mentioned authors' observations. Furthermore, the incidence of exertional symptoms in our cases has caused considerable inconvenience.

Guanethidine

This drug was administered once daily. The maintenance dose ranged between 25 and 225 mg daily, on an average 90 mg. The period of treatment was 2 to 8 months, on an average 3.5 months.

As I did with bretylium, I shall first show a series of patients who had not been treated previously (Table 6). In 2 of these 14 cases the treatment had to be discontinued very soon on account

Table 6. *14 patients with hypertension treated with guanethidine*

No.	Sex	Age	BP	F.H.	Dose (mg)	Mean BP-supine		Mean BP-erect	
						Before	Guan.	Before	Guan.
1	F	56	180/105	I	(40)	130	sep.	132	sep.
2	M	62	235/135	III	75	168	148	162	143
3	M	50	210/135	III	50	160	150	160	138
4	M	55	270/160	III	225	197	147	197	132
5	F	35	205/125	II	150	152	123	158	112
6	M	47	180/115	II	100	136	126	133	117
7	M	46	200/125	II	175	146	143	147	125
8	M	25	200/145	II	125	163	117	163	102
9	F	66	225/120	III	(40)	155	sep.	153	sep.
10	M	41	280/150	III	120	193	185	187	163
11	F	37	200/130	II	50	153	137	153	114
12	F	19	165/115	II	75	132	113	137	105
13	M	38	210/125	II	75	153	142	153	128
14	M	50	190/120	II	50	143	122	143	108
Mean		(12 patients)			107	158	138	158	124

of side-effects. Otherwise, a satisfactory effect was observed in 6 patients and a fairly satisfactory one in 4. Two of the patients did not respond to guanethidine. The average fall in mean blood pressure was 20 mm Hg in the lying and 34 mm Hg in the standing position.

Table 7. *8 patients with hypertension. Comparison between ganglionic blockers and guanethidine*

No.	Sex	Age	BP	F.H.	Dose (mg)	Mean BP-supine			Mean BP-erect		
						Before	Gangl. bl.	Guan.	Before	Gangl. bl.	Guan.
1	M	59	230/140	II	(50)	170	141	sep.	170	126	sep.
2	F	67	240/130	III	(40)	166	155	sep.	163	143	sep.
3	M	42	220/145	III	125	170	150	121	163	148	96
4	M	55	225/130	III	50	161	146	130	165	145	120
5	F	45	245/135	II	25	172	127	130	162	118	120
6	M	49	230/180	IV	37.5	197	140	128	195	118	112
7	F	45	230/140	II	50	170	132	120	170	122	105
8	M	40	210/150	III	50	170	132	135	170	118	115
Mean	(6 patients)				56	173	138	127	171	128	111

The next group comprises 8 patients, who were given guanethidine in place of ganglion-blocking drugs (Table 7). In this group, too, treatment had to be discontinued in two cases. A satisfactory effect was observed in the remaining 6 patients. With ganglion-blocking agents a satisfactory effect was obtained in 3 cases, and a fairly satisfactory one in 2.

In Table 8 the decreases in mean blood pressure obtained in this group of patients are compared. The effect of guanethidine does not seem to be considerably more orthostatic than in the case of ganglion-blocking drugs.

Table 8. *Changes in mean blood pressure after ganglionic blockers and after guanethidine*

	Reduction of mean blood pressure	
	Supine mm Hg	Erect mm Hg
Ganglionic blockers .	35	43
Guanethidine . . .	46	60

The side-effects accompanying guanethidine are shown in Table 9. Pronounced water retention was found in 3 patients, and in all 3 cases it resulted in withdrawal of the drug. The water retention was accompanied by symptoms like those seen in congestive heart failure. The occurrence of this side-effect makes a combination with diuretics desirable, as will be mentioned later on.

Table 9. *Side-effects in 22 patients with hypertension treated with guanethidine*

Side-effect	Degree of severity			Number of side-effects	Decrease of side-effects	Treatment discontinued
	++	+	(+)			
Water retention .	3	1	—	4	—	3
Diarrhoea	3	3	7	13	6	—
Dizziness	3	9	1	13	7	1
Weakness	2	8	2	12	2	—
Exertional symptoms . . .	—	3	3	6	3	—
Failure of ejaculation . . .	1	1	—	2	—	1
Depression	—	2	—	2	1	1
22 patients				(52)	(19)	6

Diarrhoea occurred frequently, but abated in many cases spontaneously. In other cases the diarrhoea stopped after administration of atropine. On the whole, this complaint has not presented any serious difficulty. Dizziness and weakness, especially in the morning, have been annoying side-effects in many cases, but improved during treatment. In a few cases Ritalin produced a beneficial effect. We have only seen very mild cases of exertional symptoms resembling those described in connection with bretylium. Depression occurred in 2 cases, in one of which the drug had to be withdrawn. Failure of ejaculation was observed in 2 patients, and in one of these cases the treatment had to be given up in spite of favourable blood pressure response.

The effect of guanethidine is somewhat varying, but not so much as with bretylium. Development of tolerance appears fairly often, but when dosage was increased, a beneficial therapeutic effect was usually again achieved.

As yet, we are not able to submit methodical investigations into the combined effect of guanethidine and diuretics. In some cases we have observed a very favourable effect after administration of hydrochlorothiazide in addition to guanethidine. At present our primary therapeutic medium is hydrochlorothiazide, to which guanethidine is added according to requirement. By so doing, we hope to avoid water retention caused by guanethidine. The combination of a diuretic and guanethidine does not bring about any particularly pronounced orthostatic blood pressure effect.

The existing publications on the clinical effect of guanethidine show by and large concurrent results. PAGE and DUSTAN (5) did not find any development of tolerance, while LEISHMAN and co-workers (4) did; we, too, have observed this phenomenon in our material. JAQUEROD and SPÜHLER (*3*) state that in their opinion a combination with diuretics is beneficial; our experiences fit in with this theory and are in this respect inconsistent with those of LEISHMAN and co-workers (*4*). As regards dosage, PAGE and DUSTAN (*5*) have employed an average dose of 160 mg daily; the doses adopted by JAQUEROD and SPÜHLER (*3*) and our doses are almost identical, namely about 90 mg daily. LEISHMAN and co-workers (*4*) gave an average dose of 40 mg daily, and the decreases in blood pressure obtained were hardly satisfactory either.

On the whole, we are of the opinion that guanethidine is a suitable antihypertensive drug, especially when combined with a diuretic. The most troublesome side-effects are dizziness and weakness in the morning. The potential danger of psychic disturbances and ejaculation trouble should be borne in mind, as they are important complaints.

In conclusion, I shall make an attempt to drawn certain comparisons between the ganglion-blocking drugs, bretylium, and guanethidine (Table 10). Bretylium seems to cause a more

Table 10. *Comparison between ganglionic blocking and adrenergic blocking agents*

	No.	Clinical result		
		Satisfactory	Fair	Unsatisfactory
Bretylium	10	1	6	3
Guanethidine	14	6	4	4
Ganglionic blockers .) in comb.	18	8	4	6
Bretylium . . . . . } treat-	10	3	3	4
Guanethidine . . . .) ment	8	6	0	2

	No.	Reduction in mean blood pressure	
		Supine	Erect
Bretylium	9	10	34
Guanethidine	12	20	34
Ganglionic blockers .) in comb.	18	31	40
Bretylium . . . . . } treat-	9	26	42
Guanethidine . . . .) ment	6	46	60

	No. alone/ comb.	Ratio: $\dfrac{\text{Fall in M.B.P. erect}}{\text{Fall in M.B.P. supine}}$	
		Used alone	In combination
Ganglionic blockers	5/18	1.81	1.28
Bretylium	9/9	3.40	1.61
Guanethidine	12/6	1.70	1.31

pronounced orthostatic fall in blood pressure than the other drugs, and it will, therefore, be difficult to obtain a suitable fall in blood pressure in the lying position, and consequently, not so many quite satisfactory therapeutic results. According to our experiences, guanethidine seems to be easier to use. Both substances have the great advantage of not having a parasympathetic-blocking effect. To take a long-range view of the applicability of the substances is not easy; certain side-effects will sometimes not appear till the drugs have been used over a long period of time. At any rate, the new adrenergic blocking agents indicate a considerable theoretical gain, and they will in all probability introduce a new epoch in the medicamentous treatment of hypertension.

Summary

Clinical experiences with bretylium and with guanethidine are reported.

Bretylium mainly decreases the standing blood pressure. Consequently, it is difficult to obtain satisfactory lying blood pressure levels. Moreover, the action of bretylium is rather unpredictable and tolerance develops very frequently. The most important side effect is a characteristic syndrome consisting of weakness, dizziness, and dyspnoea during physical exercise. This side effect has often prohibited increase in dosage or enforced the withdrawal of the substance. Following guanethidine orthostatic hypotension also occurs, but in our experience is less pronounced than in response to bretylium. We have found guanethidine a suitable substance for the treatment of hypertension. A number of side effects are seen, including especially weakness, dizziness, diarrhoea, and failure of ejaculation. In many cases, however, these side effects subside during prolonged treatment. Fluid retention has been the most important side effect, being very pronounced in a few cases. The use of diuretics in combination with guanethidine will probably diminish this side effect considerably.

Résumé

Le brétylium a pour principale propriété de faire baisser la tension artérielle en position debout. Il est donc difficile d'obtenir avec cette drogue des niveaux tensionnels adéquats en position couchée. En outre, l'action du brétylium est quelque peu imprévisible et il apparaît fréquemment une accoutumance. L'effet secondaire le plus important est représenté par un syndrome caractéristique qui se traduit par une sensation de faiblesse, de vertige, et de dyspnée au cours d'efforts physiques. Cet effet secondaire empêche souvent d'augmenter la posologie, ce qui nous a incité à abandonner cette substance.

Avec la guanéthidine, la réduction de la tension artérielle est également orthostatique, mais d'après notre expérience, elle est moins prononcée qu'avec le brétylium. Nous avons trouvé que la guanéthidine convenait bien au traitement de l'hypertension. On a signalé un certain nombre d'effets secondaires, spécialement des sensations de faiblesse, de vertige, de la diarrhée et des troubles de l'éjaculation. Dans maints cas, toutefois, ces accidents secondaires ont diminué après une cure prolongée. La rétention liquidienne est apparue comme étant l'effet secondaire le plus important, et elle est parfois très prononcée. L'emploi combiné de diurétiques et de guanéthidine diminuera sans doute considérablement cet effet fâcheux.

References

1. BOURA, A. L. A., A. F. GREEN, A. McCOUBREY, D. R. LAURENCE, R. MOULTON, and M. L. ROSENHEIM. Lancet (G.B.) **1959/II**, 17.
2. DOLLERY, C. T., D. EMSLIE-SMITH, and J. McMICHAEL. Lancet (G.B.) **1960/I**, 296.
3. JAQUEROD, R., and O. SPÜHLER: Schweiz. med. Wschr. **90**, 113 (1960).
4. LEISHMAN, A. W. D., H. L. MATTHEWS, and A. J. SMITH: Lancet (G.B.) **1959/II**, 1044.
5. PAGE, I. H., and H. P. DUSTAN: J. Amer. Med. Ass. **170**, 1265 (1959).
6. TURNER, R., and C. LOWTHER: Lancet (G.B.) **1960/I**, 381.

Combined drug therapy of hypertension

By

S. W. Hoobler and **P. Lauwers**

Since current drug treatment of hypertension is primarily suppressive rather than curative, the prolonged maintenance of blood pressure reduction is as important as the ability to cause an early and marked depression of the blood pressure by acute treatment. Since such prolonged suppressive treatment has been demonstrated to diminish the incidence of major cerebro-vascular, cardiac and renal complications of patients with severe forms of the disease, it is presumed, although not proven, that asymptomatic hypertension will also be favorably influenced by reduction of the blood pressure. However, since all forms of drug treatment are attended by inconvenience and expense to the patient, one should attempt if possible to distinguish those persons whose prognosis is so benign that no drug treatment is necessary. In our current practice we identify four types of patients in whom treatment is not initiated but who are asked to return for a follow-up in the event their condition should worsen in later years. The following groups are recognized:

Group I. Patients with a labile blood pressure who frequently exhibit a normal reading but whose usual blood pressure[1] is at or near the upper normal level and in whom transient rises in blood pressure never exceed 200/110.

Group II. Women over 40 years of age with the recent onset of persistent hypertension never exceeding a usual level of 180/100.

Group III. Elderly subjects with usual systolic readings not in excess of 200 and diastolic readings below 105 mm Hg.

Group IV. Patients who exhibit substantial blood pressure elevations under usual conditions in the physician's office but who have no evidence of vascular complications of hypertension and whose home-recorded blood pressures are within the normal range. It is presumed that in these four groups no evidence of serious

---

[1] "Usual blood pressure" is hereafter taken to mean the average of five or six casual blood pressure readings taken on clinical examination. "Upper normal blood pressure" is defined as 150/100 in patients under the age of 50.

vascular lesions is apparent. Such patients should exhibit no evidence of left ventricular hypertrophy; no major renal functional impairments; and no history of focal neurologic disturbances or cardiac insufficiency.

Another four groups may be distinguished in which vigorous treatment is not justified but in which it is believed that milder forms of treatment, if they can be demonstrated to lower blood pressure, are considered to be beneficial. These include:

Group I. Younger persons of both sexes with usual and home recorded readings in excess of 160/100 mm.

Group II. Middle aged men with usual blood pressures of 160—180 over 100—110 mm Hg (because of the increased coronary risk in the male sex with moderately elevated blood pressure).

Group III. Women in middle life with usual clinic and home readings in excess of 180/100 mm Hg.

Group IV. All subjects with transient or established hypertension who present one or more of the vascular complications mentioned above.

Patients whose usual blood pressure exceeds 240/120 mm Hg should be candidates for more vigorous therapy if milder regimens do not lower the blood pressure and particularly if vascular complications have appeared. In these persons the risk of a serious accident or death from the disease takes precedence over the inconvenience to be expected from the use of more potent drugs. They need to be hospitalized and treated vigorously until the blood pressure falls below 160/100 mm Hg at least in the upright position, and effective suppressive treatment must thereafter be maintained. Since in this group of individuals readings recorded in the office may be falsely elevated when compared to home-recorded blood pressure, it is advised that these patients take their blood pressure in order to regulate the dosage of potent drugs, which may on occasion produce excessive hypotension. In this way they are able to achieve a more accurate control of dosage and assure themselves of protection against unregulated hypertension much as a diabetic is able to supervise the dosage of insulin by testing the urine repeatedly for the presence of sugar and acetone.

Such patients are frequently seen as a result of a serious hypertensive crisis, and prompt effective therapy sometimes of an emergency nature is necessary. Table I presents advantages and disadvantages of certain regimens for the rapid control of unregulated hypertension.

When the blood pressure has been reduced in the hospital to reasonable levels it is useful to begin prolonged suppressive treatment

Table 1

	Mode of Rx	Advantage	Disadvantage
Reserpine	2.5—5.0 mg i.m.	Rarely excess hypotension. Close supervision unnecessary	Mental confusion may follow. Delayed, often inadequate response
Ganglion blockers: pentolinium	(either) 0.5 mg min i.v. (or) 1—2—4—8 mgm s. c. given $^1/_2$ hourly until B. P. falls	Control rapid and effective	Needs close supervision. Bowel and bladder paralysis may occur in susceptible patients. Do not give in anuria
Trimethaphen	4—20 mg/min i. v.	Precise and rapid control at desired B. P. level including hypotension, as may be indicated in hemorrhage. If hypotensive effect adverse, effect wears off rapidly	Close supervision necessary. Prolonged infusion may cause ileus
Direct dilators: hydralazine	25 mg s.c.	Hypodynamic effect of other Rx avoided; cardiac output stimulated. Useful in anuria, toxemia, juvenile hypertension	Often ineffective. Headache and nausea may result
Sodium nitroprusside	200—400 mg/ min i.v.	Precise and rapid control. Effective in patients refractory to ganglion-blockers	No proprietary preparation available. Often ineffective or poorly sustained

with drugs having as few side effects as possible and affecting the recumbent as well as the upright pressure. The most widely used regimen includes the administration of rauwolfia alkaloids and oral diuretic agents. Our preference, so long as the blood pressure does not get out of control during the therapeutic trial, is to administer *chlorothiazide*[1] 500 mg twice daily (or a larger dose unless there is an initial weight loss of at least three pounds in the first 3—4 days), and to continue this program for 6—8 weeks before concluding that it is ineffective in controlling the blood

---

[1] Hydrochlorothiazide 50 mg, flumethiazide 500 mg, or benzhydroflumethiazide 5 mg may be substituted.

pressure. In at least one-half of the individuals so treated a reduction of 15 mm Hg in both standing and recumbent blood pressures is observed. It is not necessary to restrict the dietary salt intake;

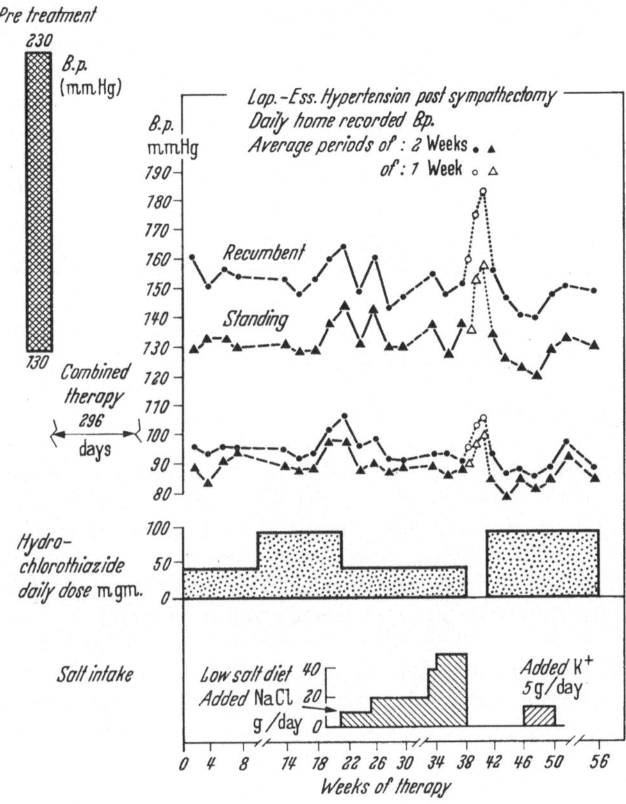

Fig. 1. Effect of treatment with hydrochlorothiazide as sole antihypertensive drug. Patient had been under continuous treatment for over one year. Addition of NaCl or K did not raise the blood pressure, while withdrawal of hydrochlorothiazide resulted in an immediate rise in blood pressure and return of hypertensive symptoms such as headache and nervousness

potassium supplementation is optional and depends on symptoms or serum potassium levels obtained after prolonged treatment. It is possible to prevent some potassium depletion by omitting drug therapy two days of each week, but it should be emphasized that even after several years of demonstrable blood pressure reduction a rise in blood pressure is encountered one or two weeks after withdrawal of a thiazide diuretic (Fig. 1).

Studies in our laboratory (*1, 2*) suggest the following mechanism of action of thiazide derivatives in hypertension: the immediate response to treatment is a decrease in plasma volume and cardiac output. This is followed in a few weeks by a restoration of these values to normal without a rise in blood pressure. Thus under chronic chlorothiazide treatment the total peripheral resistance of the hypertensive subject is reduced: total body water remains depressed (antipyrine space) and potassium depletion is evident in the chronically reduced serum potassium level with the associated increase in carbon dioxide combining power. Total exchangeable sodium is restored to normal possibly as the result of endogenous secretion of aldosterone in response to the chronic dehydration.

One might expect that such prolonged hypokalemia might be harmful. However, in patients treated for 2—3 years a diligent search for hypokalemic renal lesions, or adverse electrocardiographic changes has not indicated a serious effect. It is true that during the initial treatment phase many patients complain of weakness due to fluid depletion or hypokalemia, and rhythm disturbances particularly in association with digitalis administration may occur in patients with serious hypertensive heart disease. Hyperuricemia is observed in a few cases and gout has been precipitated; on the other hand a survey of serum uric acid in a number of individuals who have been treated for a long period with chlorothiazide has not yielded evidence of a consistent increase in uric acid levels which might be considered potentially toxic. In association with the early phase of plasma volume depletion, blood urea may rise in both patients with normal renal function and those with azotemia, but usually there is a restoration to pretreatment levels without precipitation of serious uremic intoxication. It is our custom to prescribe smaller doses of thiazide derivatives in patients with azotemia. Skin eruptions and thrombocytopenia sometimes occur and may be avoided by using an alternate thiazide derivative. Nausea and occasional dizziness seem to be related to one specific agent and can also be relieved without sacrificing therapeutic effect by changing to another of the derivatives now available.

When the blood pressure does not respond in one to two months of such treatment or if the hypertension is deemed too severe to allow such a delay in therapy, *reserpine* should be added to the chlorothiazide regimen in a dosage of .75 to 1 mg daily for six weeks, a dosage sufficient to deplete peripheral vascular stores of catechol amines; this is followed by a maintenance dose of .25 mg per day or less, which produces fewer of the well-known side effects of rauwolfia but is likely to maintain the therapeutic advantage.

In many patients rauwolfia derivatives are without effect on the
blood pressure and in others induce a marked fatigue, depression,
or agitation, which are so slow in onset as not to be identified by
the patient as caused by therapy. While prolonged treatment with
reserpine (Fig. 2) provides a great benefit in many cases, we

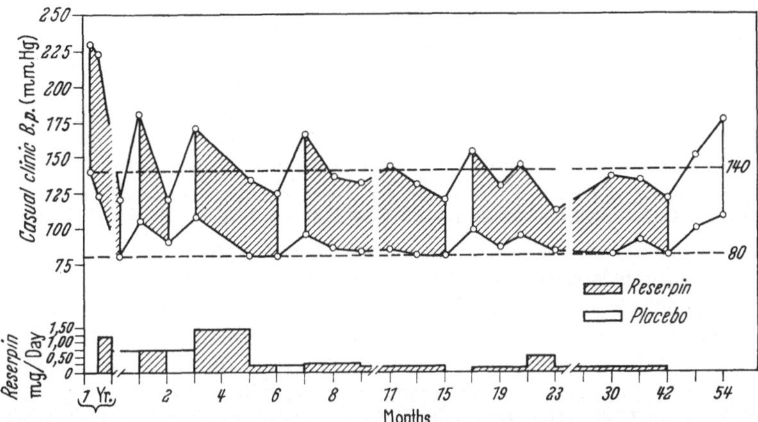

Fig. 2. Prolonged effect of reserpine as sole antihypertensive drug: Response to minute
daily dosage proven by treatment withdrawal. (Reprinted from MOYER: J: Hypertension: The
first HAHNEMANN Symposium on Hypertensive Disease. W. B. Saunders, Philadelphia and
London 1959, p. 385)

believe that no patient should continue therapy with this agent
unless it has been proven by careful observation of the effects
of addition or withdrawal of the drug that it is successful in
reducing the blood pressure.

The next drug of choice for therapeutic trial is *hydralazine*,
which like reserpine should be administered during background
therapy with thiazide derivatives. It is said that reserpine reduces
the frequency of hydralazine side effects and therefore this agent
should be continued if it is not in itself producing major side actions
such as fatigue and depression. Hydralazine may be prescribed
in doses of 10—25 mg four times daily, increasing gradually and
only as tolerated up to a total daily dose of 400 mg. In our experience, which differs sharply from that found in other laboratories (*3*), the drug may be initially effective and be followed
by the development of tolerance, or its full antihypertensive
effect may not appear until after the third month of treatment.
When the drug was prescribed to patients with long experience on
self-regulation of the blood pressure with ganglion-blocking agents

18*

our experience (*4*) was that approximately one-third of the patients were unable to achieve a significant dosage without developing unpleasant side effects. One-third exhibited no added depressor response after six months of combined therapy with hydralazine and ganglion-blocking agents, while another one-third showed a considerable reduction in the requirement for ganglion-blockade when hydralazine was administered for a six-month period. The drug is a cardiac stimulant and exhibits anti-histaminase actions; it is therefore contraindicated in angina pectoris, heart failure, and peptic ulceration, and anti-histaminics frequently relieve many of the side effects. The drug may be particularly useful in lowering the diastolic blood pressure in patients in whom there is a proportionally excessive elevation in this reading. Despite the many side effects such as headaches, urticaria, edema, palpitation, and gastro-intestinal upset, there is no doubt that certain patients respond consistently and continuously to this therapy, and so long as the dose is kept within the range of 200—400 mg a day the likelihood of a serious late reaction resembling lupus erythematosus (*5*) is so remote as not to justify concern. On the other hand, in patients with serious forms of hypertensive disease it is not wise to wait for several months for a beneficial effect from hydralazine to appear nor to prescribe it in cases of early renal insufficiency with the hope that the azotemia will be improved. In the first case much valuable time may be lost while the blood pressure is out of control and before it is decided to change to more potent therapy; in the latter instance prolonged renal circulatory improvement has not been demonstrated. Further, the early increases in renal blood flow are not associated with improvement in glomerular filtration rate and are in any event transient only (*6*). Other and more effective means of preserving minimal renal functional mass require the careful and graded reduction of the blood pressure with agents having a more certain but carefully controlled depressor action.

In patients with the more serious forms of hypertension who are not responsive to one of the above regimens or in whom time is not available to experiment with such treatment programs, as in the case of rapidly advancing malignant hypertension, it is necessary to proceed with more vigorous therapy even at the expense of producing more frequent side effects. Since the drugs to be recommended frequently result in serious hypotensive reactions and since dosage adjustment is critical, the authors prefer to achieve final adjustment of the dosage by means of the blood pressure recordings taken twice daily in the home in the standing position. In this way fluctuations in responsiveness can be detected and dizziness and blackout either prevented or their explanation made evident to the patient, who thereby gains more confidence in the management of his blood pressure than when the explanation for the symptoms is not immediately evident. In the past it has been necessary to use one of a variety of ganglionic blocking agents to suppress elevated blood pressure in these individuals, but it is now our preference to proceed with sympathetic blocking agents which act primarily to reduce the standing blood pressure and only secondarily to lower the recumbent readings and which probably have their effect chiefly by reducing cardiac output.

The new sympatholytic agents in current use include bretylium tosylate (*7, 8*) and guanethidine (*9, 10*).

The effects of *bretylium* last for a period of 6—8 hrs and the dose should be repeated two to three times daily. The blood pressure reduction is predominantly in the upright position, and in the event of over-absorption or excessive sensitivity as in the early morning hours postural syncope may occur. The drug should be given immediately after meals to insure more even absorption. We prefer to start with 200 mg three times daily, increasing by 100 mg three times daily every one to three days until the standing blood pressure reaches a level just above that which produces syncopal symptoms. After the proper dosage has been reached (this may vary between 300 or 3000 mg per day) some tolerance may develop, but this may be overcome by a further increase in dosage. Because of the relatively rapid onset and offset of action and the variation in daily response, it is strongly advised that the patient take his blood pressure in the standing position each morning just prior to the first dose, so that he may reduce or increase the amount taken depending upon the level recorded. Most side effects including severe early morning fatigue following bretylium are indirectly associated with orthostatic hypotension, which is greatest in the early morning and after exertion. Occasionally idiosyncrasies are noted; parotid swelling and conjunctival injection are sometimes prominent. The drug produces no parasympathetic blockade and potency is not disturbed. It is said to act by inhibiting the release of norepinephrine from the sympathetic transmitter; unlike adrenergic blocking agents such as dibenzyline it does not interfere with the receptor on the end organ and consequently hypotension from overdosage can be counteracted by administration of the usual pressor agents.

Guanethidine is reported to have a similar mode of action but differs in that the onset and offset of action are more prolonged

        S. W. Hoobler and P. Lauwers:

and because diarrhea may be a side effect, presumably of unopposed parasympathetic activity. A few patients exhibit profound brady-cardia with guanethidine. The prolonged blockade causes in many individuals no reduction in recumbent pressure but an exaggeration of the normal diurnal variation in orthostatic blood pressure, so that the early morning reading in the standing position is the

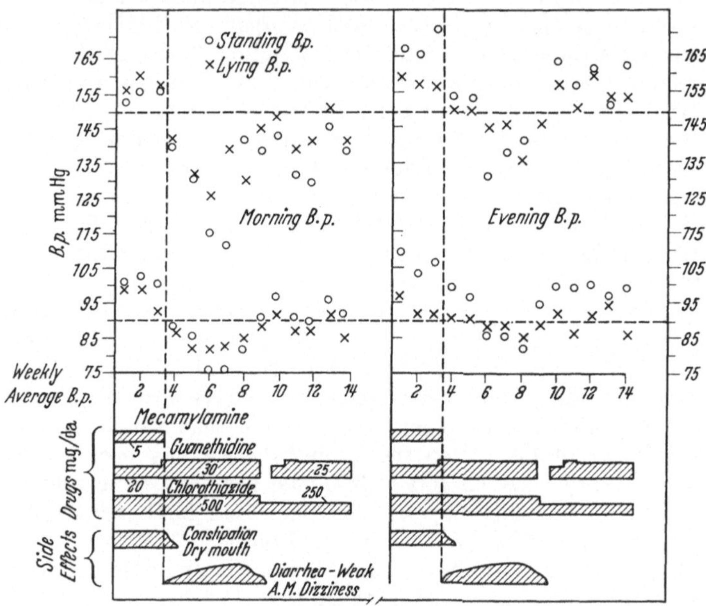

Fig. 3. Long-term effect of guanethidine on the blood pressure in essential hypertension. Note the greater reduction in standing blood pressure in the morning (left half of graphic) as opposed to the evening period (right side of figure). The same blood pressure reduction was achieved without the parasympatholytic side effects apparent with mecamylamine

lowest in the day and the most frequently associated with symp-toms of syncope or weakness. Toward the afternoon the standing blood pressure may rise toward pretreatment levels in some patients and thus the net reduction in blood pressure through the day is minimal. Unpredictably, in other subjects, evenly main-tained reduction in both recumbent and standing blood pressures has been observed (Fig. 3). It is to be emphasized that careful dosage adjustment, usually with the help of home-recorded blood pressures, is necessary for ideal control.

Treatment is usually initiated by the administration of 25 mg daily, increasing the dosage by $12^{1}/_{2}$ mg every one to three days until the morning standing blood pressure first shows a substantial reduction. Dosage should then be reduced or omitted for a few days until the maximum cumulative effect of preceding treatment has been reached, following which the drug is administered at such a rate that the early morning blood pressure in the standing position falls to levels just above syncope for the individual patient. The final dosage may vary from 25 to 250 mg and is occasionally associated with diarrhea requiring atropine-like drugs for its control. Occasionally some tolerance develops, but usually the greatest difficulty in management is to achieve successful blood pressure reduction in the afternoon without the cost of disabling postural or exertional hypotension in the morning hours. In about one-third of patients a substantial reduction in the recumbent blood pressure may be achieved without orthostatic disability. Chlorothiazide or its congeners should be administered simultaneously, as they enhance the effect of the sympathetic inhibitors.

At present the blood pressure of most patients can be regulated by combining one or the other of the sympathetic blocking agents with chlorothiazide or reserpine. Despite their similar mode of action patients may respond to only one of the two sympathetic blockers and therefore both should be tried. The seriously ill patient, as well as the patient refractory to these drugs, should undergo therapeutic trial of a *ganglion-blocking agent* in combination with thiazide derivatives. Reductions in blood pressure can be frequently achieved with only minor disabling symptoms. Pentolinium may be given by injection for the immediate control of blood pressure. For prolonged oral administration mecamylamine is preferred because of its total absorption from the gastro-intestinal tract and more consistent effect on the circulation from hour to hour. Chlorisondamine is a partially absorbed, long acting, quaternary blocking agent which has some advantages over oral pentolinium but has the disadvantage of affecting visual acuity more than either of the other two orally useful ganglion-blocking agents. With all such forms of treatment in which parasympathetic blockade is also produced, daily laxatives should be given to prevent the development of ileus.

If it is impractical to treat the patient effectively with these blocking agents and other regimens are unsuccessful, it is the authors' preference, in the absence of azotemia, to recommend sympathectomy particularly of the supradiaphragmatic variety. While this procedure carries the penalty of some degree of backache, the removal of the sympathetic innervation to the splanchnic area without interruption of the lumbar ganglia, in combination with maintained thiazide therapy, results in a highly significant number of patients who may be maintained at normal blood pressures with minimum side effects. Furthermore, if the lumbar sympathetic innervation is undisturbed, the blood pressure reduction which is achieved does not suffer a further decline when the patient stands upright as is more likely to be the case following lumbodorsal sympathectomy. Although we have had little experience with this procedure, since most patients are well controlled on drugs alone, it would appear that 60—80% of patients with hypertension generally refractory to drugs exhibit a satisfactory reduction of blood pressure when supradiaphragmatic sympathectomy is followed by chlorothiazide therapy. Moreover, it can be demonstrated that mortality rates from hypertensive disease are substantially reduced, particularly in patients who have had encephalopathic episodes prior to surgery. If the "good results" obtained in a former era with sympathectomy can be produced with increasing effectiveness by the addition of thiazide derivatives to sympathectomy this treatment should not remain in its present state of oblivion.

Each year sees major advances in the control of hypertension with the use of drugs. Unfortunately the more recent advances have resulted in the development of agents affecting the sympathetic reflexes and producing predominantly postural hypotension. While this effect should not be denied a seriously ill patient, it goes without saying that agents which will lower both recumbent and standing blood pressure and which act at the site of increased peripheral resistance are greatly to be preferred. For this reason we have not been inclined to give *amine oxidase inhibitors*, of which a great variety are available, for prolonged therapeutic trial. Even the most enthusiastic proponents admit that only orthostatic hypotension is secured. These drugs vary in their toxicity, but most of them have been known to produce serious hepatic lesions and some in addition have a cerebral excitatory action which may or may not be beneficial.

For theoretical and practical reasons drugs of the *spironolactone* series are of great interest. Because of the considerable expense in prescribing these agents and their relatively recent availability in sufficient quantities for clinical trial, few extensive studies have been completed. Our own experience confirms in part that reported by Hollander (*11*). Spironolactone has been observed to lower recumbent and standing blood pressures occasionally in three classes of patients: 1) In those who likewise respond to thiazide diuretics; 2) When given in addition to thiazide diuretics; and 3) When administered as the sole antihypertensive agent. In the latter category may fall some forms of primary aldosteronism not recognized by the usual criteria (Fig. 4). If further investigation proves that this is the case, a preliminary trial with spironolactone therapy may be an empiric way of identifying patients with

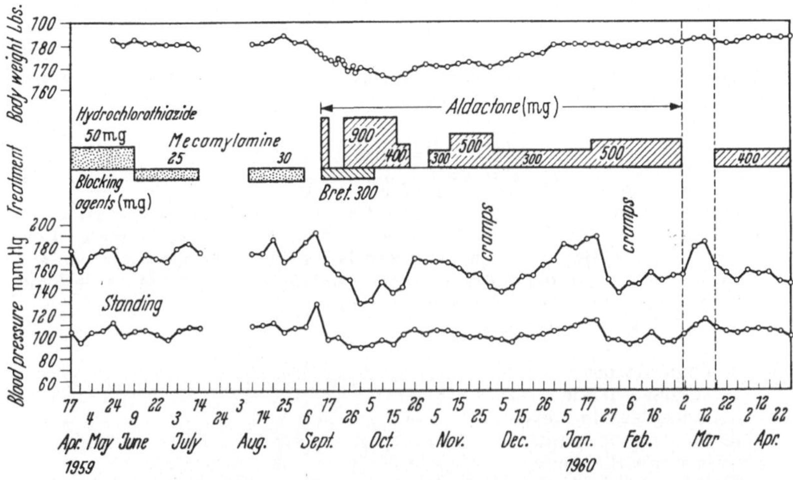

Fig. 4. Effect of spironolactone on blood pressure in patient with elevated aldosterone excretion and intermittent hypokalemia. At a dosage in excess of 300 mg daily a definite effect on the blood pressure was observed together with a rise on withdrawal of treatment

hyperaldosteronism. At the present writing it would appear that Aldactone may also exert diuretic action independent of or synergistic with the thiazide diuretics and be valuable as adjunctive therapy in patients refractory to the diuretic agents. In our clinical trials a dosage of 600 mg per day for a period of four to six weeks has been used, but it is probable that a smaller dosage and a lesser duration of therapeutic trial would be effective in identifying those individuals likely to respond to spironolactone either alone or in combination with diuretic agents. Because this agent, like chlorothiazide, hydralazine, and reserpine, affects the recumbent as well as the standing blood pressure and is well tolerated when carefully administered, it is surely to be preferred over more potent drugs causing orthostatic hypotension or producing more severe side actions. The future of antihypertensive therapy surely lies with such types of clinical response.

Conclusions

Patients with hypertension are divided into three groups, according to whether reduction of blood pressure is unnecessary, elective, or mandatory. Acute treatment of the hypertensive crisis is discussed. Long-acting agents which reduce recumbent as well as standing blood pressure are listed in order of effectiveness and infrequency of side effects in the following order: 1) thiazide diuretics, 2) reserpine, 3) hydralazine, 4) guanethidine, 5) bretylium tosylate, 6) ganglion-blocking agents, 7) sympathectomy. The place of amine oxidase inhibitors and of spironolactones is also briefly discussed.

The authors wish to express their appreciation to Dr. F. J. Conway, established investigator of the American Heart Association, for his assistance in the collection of the data herewith presented and in the hemodynamic investigations quoted in this report.

Résumé

Les hypertendus peuvent être divisés en trois groupes thérapeutiques selon que la réduction de leur tension artérielle est superflue, facultative ou indispensable. Le traitement des poussées hypertensives est discuté. Les produits d'action prolongée qui réduisent la tension artérielle aussi bien en position couchée que debout sont classés comme suit selon l'ordre de leur efficacité et la rareté de leurs effets secondaires:

1. les thiazides diurétiques
2. la réserpine
3. l'hydralazine
4. la guanéthidine
5. le tosylate de bretylium
6. les ganglioplégiques
7. la sympathectomie.

La place des inhibiteurs de l'amino-oxydase et des spirolactones est également brièvement discutée.

References

1. Conway, J., and P. Lauwers: Circulation (U.S.A.) **21**, 21 (1960).
2. Lauwers, P., and J. Conway: J. Laborat. Clin. Med. (U.S.A.) (To be published).
3. Taylor, R. D., H. P. Dustan, A. C. Corcoran, and I. H. Page: A. M. A. Arch. Int. Med. **90**, 2734 (1952).
4. Blaquier, P., and S. W. Hoobler: Amer. J. Med. Sc. **238**, 740 (1959).
5. Dustan, H. P., R. D. Taylor, A. C. Corcoran, and I. H. Page: J. Amer. Med. Ass. **154**, 23 (1954).
6. Vanderkolk, K., A. S. Dontas, and S. W. Hoobler: Amer. Heart J. **48**, 95 (1954).
7. Boura, A. O. A., A. F. Green, A. McCoubrey, D. R. Lawrence, R. Moulton, and M. Rosenheim: Lancet **1959/II**, 17.
8. Conway, J., P. Lauwers, and S. W. Hoobler: J. Laborat. Clin. Med. (U.S.A.) **56**, December 1960 (in press).
9. Page, I. H., and H. P. Dustan: J. Amer. Med. Ass. **170**, 1265 (1959).
10. Frohlich, E. D., and E. D. Freis: Med. Ann. District of Columbia **28**, 419 (1959).
11. Hollander, W., and A. V. Chobanian: Circulation (U.S.A.) **20**, 713 (1959).

Effects of the administration of saluretic drugs in the treatment of arterial hypertension

By

C. Bartorelli

It is already more than two years since saluretic drugs were first tested in the treatment of arterial hypertension, and the time seems now to have come when not only the pharmacodynamic approach followed so far, but also a critical clinical evaluation of the overall effectiveness of these drugs in the long run has become possible. Since we are dealing with a chronic, enduring disease, a long follow-up period is required before the real value of a new procedure or of a new drug in the management of arterial hypertension can be assessed.

There is a general consensus of opinion that decreasing blood pressure values improve conditions and prolong life expectancy in hypertensive patients (*1, 5, 24, 27, 28, 29, 30, 31*). It matters little whether pressure control is achieved by surgery or drug administration, provided that care is taken to avoid severe depression of renal function. We do not propose to dwell upon this general problem, but would rather discuss the more limited issue of the effectiveness of saluretic drugs in inducing and maintaining lasting decrease in blood pressure, and the consequences of a prolonged administration of saluretic compounds on electrolyte metabolism and, broadly speaking, on the patient's welfare. A few physiological considerations, suggested by the clinical trials, will also be discussed.

Our presentation is based upon a series of 122 hypertensive patients, who in the last two years have been treated with saluretic drugs, either as the sole hypotensive medication or in association with various antihypertensive agents. Most of these subjects were observed for a period of time while in the hospital, and were afterwards followed up at close intervals as out-patients. A number of subjects were studied as out-patients from the beginning. Blood pressure was always measured with the patient in both the lying and standing positions; the serum electrolytes were measured periodically in all cases; a few patients were kept for some time on a diet with a constant electrolyte content, and studied with particular regard to their sodium and potassium balances. Patients with hypertensive disease of all degrees, from mild to malignant, came under our observation. Although the therapeutic approach often had to be adapted to the needs of the individual subject, we have striven to adopt a rather uniform schedule of treatment, so as to arrive at a correct assessment of short and long-term effectiveness, side-effects, advantages, and complications of each drug and of combinations of drugs. According to this schedule, medication was initiated by administering a saluretic drug, which was subsequently combined, when necessary, with reserpine, hydralazine, and mecamylamine, in that order. Of course, in each patient we adhered to the first effective combination, i. e. saluretic plus reserpine, or saluretic plus reserpine and hydralazine; mecamylamine was added only in the severest cases of hypertension.

1. Results of administration of saluretic drugs alone

Conway and Lauwers have recently published a careful study of the hypotensive effects of long-term therapy with chlorothiazide in 83 hypertensive patients. A significant fall in blood pressure was found to occur in 66% of patients, the average reduction in pressure being 27/17 mm Hg. This confirms previous reports of Heider et al. (*11*), Gifford (*9*), Hoobler et al. (*17*), and others (*23*). Our personal experience is in substantial agreement with that of the preceding authors, although the effectiveness of chlorothiazide and hydrochlorothiazide, as the sole antihypertensive agents, appears limited to those patients with only milder forms of hypertension (see also *6*). In these subjects it is frequently possible to lower blood pressure to approximately normal values, provided that adequate doses (0.5 g chlorothiazide twice daily, or 25 mg hydrochlorothiazide twice daily) are maintained without interruption. Fig. 1 shows the successful treatment of one of these cases of fairly mild hypertension. Lowering of arterial pressure lasts as long as saluretic administration is continued. Upon interruption of saluretic administration, the blood pressure returns slowly, and with some delay, to the initial values. Studies of the sodium and potassium balances carried out in patients maintained on a fixed diet demonstrate that decrease in arterial pressure initially parallels sodium depletion, but later pressure values remain lowered, although sodium excretion becomes progressively smaller and the sodium balance returns to pre-treatment levels or even becomes positive. It is noteworthy that increase in potassium elimination lasts as long as treatment is carried on, so that the potassium balance becomes progressively negative. These observations will be commented upon later. Also patients having severer

forms of hypertension have often shown, in our experience, some
arterial pressure decrease following priming with a saluretic drug
only. In most of them, however, the consequent antihypertensive

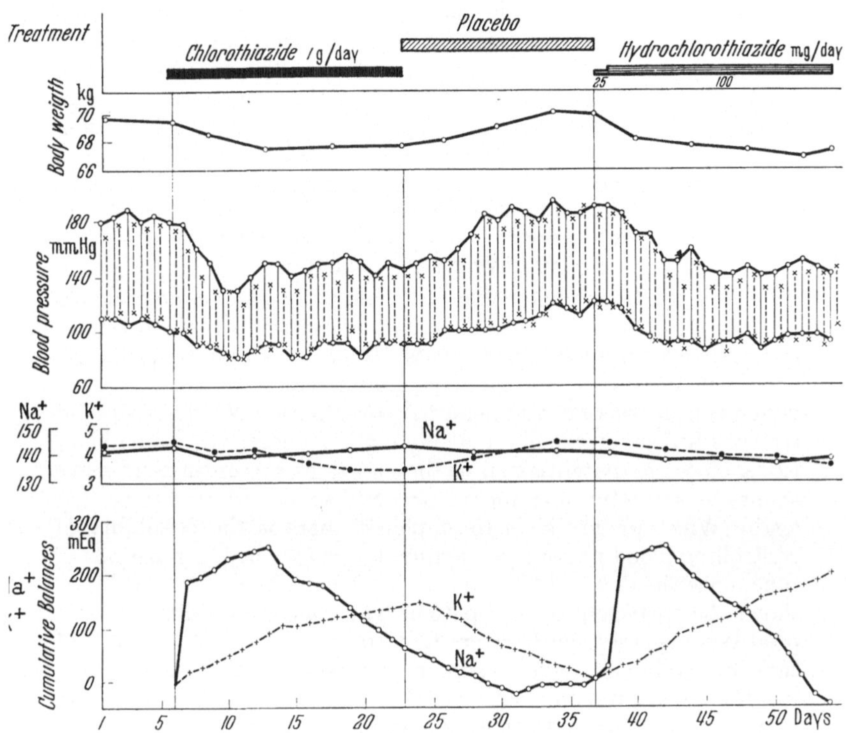

Fig. 1. Effects of the administration of chlorothiazide or hydrochlorothiazide as the sole
hypotensive medication in a moderately hypertensive patient. Note persistence of hypotensive
effect when cumulative sodium balance has reverted to normal or has become positive.
During treatment potassium balance is increasingly negative

effect was small, say, from 10 to 20 mm Hg, and insufficient to
bring the blood pressure to reasonable levels. This is in complete
agreement with recent data of FINNERTY et al. (6). The better
results of CONWAY and LAUWERS (2), as compared with ours and
with those reported by previous authors, can be explained by the
fact that a number of patients in CONWAY and LAUWERS's series had
undergone splanchnicectomy, so that the hypotension observed in

these subjects was presumably the combined result of saluretic administration and partial sympathetic blockade. Finally, let us recall certain hemodynamic data. Conway and Lauwers (2) have shown that the hypotensive effects of chlorothiazide are associated with a decreased plasma volume and cardiac output only during the first one or two weeks of therapy, while after one month or more of continued treatment the plasma volume and cardiac output are restored to pre-treatment values, the persisting hypotension resulting from a decrease in total vascular resistance. The modifications of plasma volume and their correlation with the hypotensive effect of saluretic administration are in keeping with the changes in sodium balance which previous authors and we ourselves have observed in earlier and later phases of saluretic treatment.

2. Results of the combined administration of saluretic drugs and antihypertensive agents

When treatment with chlorothiazide or hydrochlorothiazide is ineffective, or insufficiently effective, we resort to the addition of alternative antihypertensive agents. Reserpine and hydralazine are used first, while mecamylamine is administered only in those cases which appear resistant to the former combination. We do not intend to dwell further on the pharmacodynamic aspects of these combinations, since the potentiation of the effects of the antihypertensive agents by saluretic substances is too well known to need reviewing again. What we are keen to emphasize here is the possibility of controlling blood pressure at definite levels for very long periods of time, once the doses of the various drugs have been titrated. Fig. 2 shows the treatment of one patient who was admitted to our hospital two years ago with severe hypertension of long standing and signs of cerebral vascular disorder. It was impossible then to control the blood pressure satisfactorily with chlorothiazide and oral reserpine; therefore, 5 mg mecamylamine twice daily was combined with 0.5 g chlorothiazide twice daily. In a few days, lying arterial pressure levels were brought down to 150 mm Hg systolic and 90 mm Hg diastolic, while the standing values were 130 and 90 mm Hg. These values were thereafter maintained smoothly by carefully continuing this therapy for 17 months. More recently, the improved condition of the patient and at the same time some slight but annoying side-effects of mecamylamine suggested a return to reserpine, which this time was very successful. Since then, i.e. for the past nine months, the blood pressure of this patient has been controlled adequately with 1 mg reserpine and 1 g chlorothiazide daily. There is no doubt that most patients with severe or even

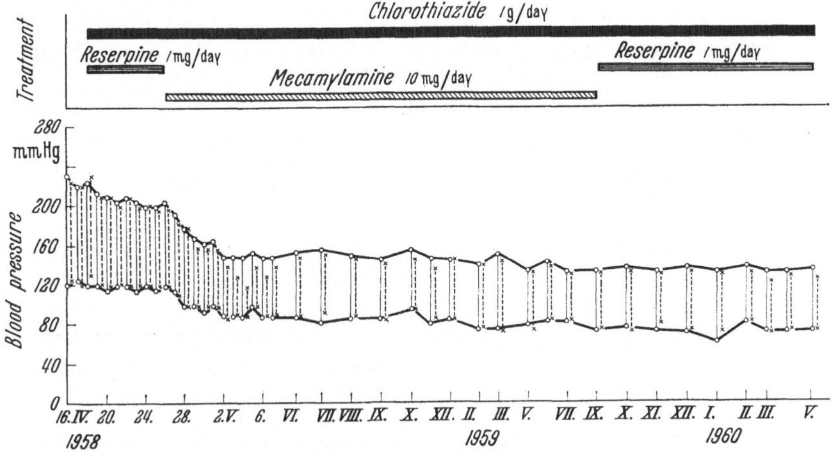

Fig. 2. Prolonged treatment of a severely hypertensive patient with chlorothiazide combined with other antihypertensive agents

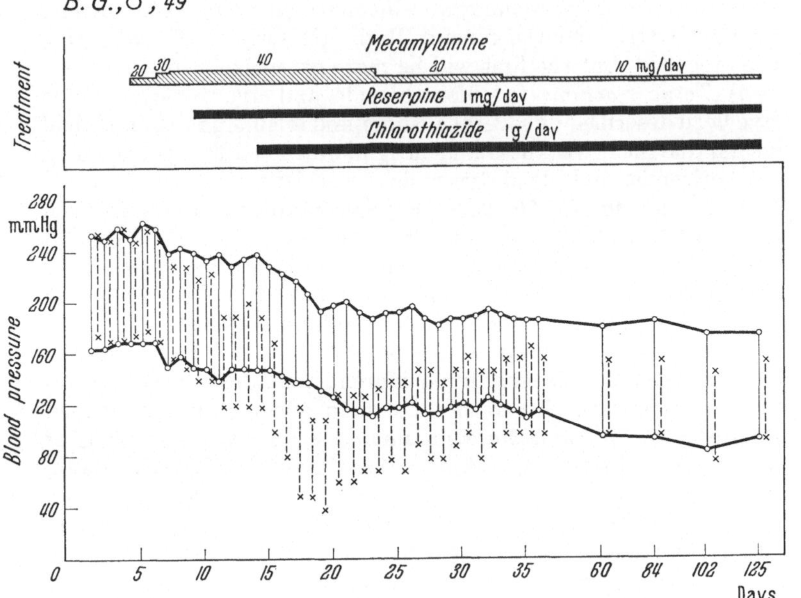

Fig. 3. Raised blood pressure in a malignant hypertensive patient successfully controlled only when chlorothiazide is given in addition to mecamylamine and reserpine

malignant hypertension can be maintained at reasonable arterial pressure levels when antihypertensive drugs are combined with a saluretic compound. It has to be emphasized that the usefulness of these substances is not limited merely to reducing side-effects of the other hypotensive drugs. In some subjects with severe hypertension blood pressure cannot be reduced to adequate levels by any clinically safe amount of reserpine, hydralazine or even mecamylamine, but the addition of chlorothiazide or hydrochlorothiazide changes ineffective into satisfactory treatment. Fig. 3 shows one of these cases.

In recent months we have also tried to combine hydrochlorothiazide with the newly synthesized drug, guanethidine. The results have been quite good, at least from the pharmacodynamic standpoint. However, since other speakers on the program will be dealing with the effects of this drug, our experiences with this substance will be referred to later.

3. Limitations to the effective treatment of arterial hypertension with drugs including saluretic compounds

These limitations include inconveniences arising from saluretic administration in particular, and inconveniences involved in any hypotensive treatment in general. Both categories of effects deserve to be recalled, but the first will be more extensively discussed.

a) *Toxic reactions* to chlorothiazide and hydrochlorothiazide have been described by several authors, and include gastro-intestinal upsets, diarrhea, weakness and fatigue unrelated to hypokalemia, hyperuricemia, and blood dyscrasias, especially thrombocytopenia (*4, 8, 12, 13, 16, 18, 20, 26, 33*). Some fatalities have also been reported (*7*). However, in our extensive series of patients treated with thiazide derivatives not one case of serious toxic reaction has been noticed. Of course, the very possibility of any such reaction represents a contra-indication to be carefully watched.

b) *Metabolic disturbances*, mainly troubles in the electrolyte balance, viz. hyponatremia, hypochloremia, alkalosis, and hypokalemia, are considered a rather common effect of the prolonged administration of saluretic compounds. In our extensive group of patients, who have been taking 0.5 g chlorothiazide twice daily, or 25 mg hydrochlorothiazide twice daily for one or two years, we have not noticed any case of severe or lasting hyponatremia, hypochloremia, or alkalosis, provided that the diet was sufficiently rich in electrolytes. A decrease in the plasma concentration of sodium and chloride is often observed during the first few days of saluretic administration, but usually rights itself as treatment is continued. Hypokalemia is quite another matter. Plasma potassium levels show a tendency towards a slight but continuous decrease, and values below 3.0 mEq/l can occasionally be recorded. This untoward effect, however, has satisfactorily been controlled in our patients by using a diet containing approximately 70 mEq of potassium with addition of 10 to 20 mEq in the form of coated potassium tartrate tablets. It is true, however, that concentrations of electrolytes give a very rough index of their real balance, and it is quite possible that some electrolyte disturbance may underlie apparently normal plasma concentrations. To evaluate this problem better, we are at present studying total exchangeable sodium and potassium in our hypertensive subjects before and during treatment with saluretic drugs. Unfortunately, our study is too recent to have any bearing yet on the problem of the consequences of a very prolonged treatment. However, although pre-treatment values are unknown, it can at least be stated that hypertensive patients taking saluretic drugs for one or two years have total exchangeable sodium values which are within the normal range. Of course, this research is being complemented by other measurements in order to determine whether chronic saluretic administration induces some peculiar change in the distribution of electrolyte and water in the extracellular and intracellular phases. This is a problem of great importance, since it cannot be ruled out with certainty that even slight disturbances in electrolyte metabolism, e. g. an extracellular shift of potassium ions or sodium entry into cells, might have untoward effects in the long run which are as yet unsuspected.

c) *Severe hypotension on standing* with collapse is rather common, especially in subjects with severe hypertension, when ganglionic blocking drugs are potentiated by saluretic administration. However, this cannot be considered as a side-effect characteristic of saluretic compounds, since it simply represents a result of the more effective hypotension obtained by combining diuretic therapy with antihypertensive drugs. Be that as it may, orthostatic hypotension is an important limiting factor in the treatment of patients with severe hypertension.

d) *The side-effects of the antihypertensive drugs* represent a limiting factor only when saluretic administration does not make it possible to reduce basic antihypertensive medication to a dose free of significant collateral disturbances. In this respect, the addition of thiazide drugs helps patients to bear prolonged hypotensive treatment. Indeed, in our series of hypertensive subjects, we have not observed any intolerance to reserpine or hydralazine when the doses of these drugs could be reduced by associating hydrochlorothiazide.

The side-effects of mecamylamine are observed more frequently: dryness of the mouth and persistent constipation are significantly reduced, but they are far from being abolished when thiazide drugs are added.

e) *Severe impairment of renal function*, with or without hyperazotemia, is an important limitation to any kind of hypotensive treatment. We have recently confirmed with clearance studies the

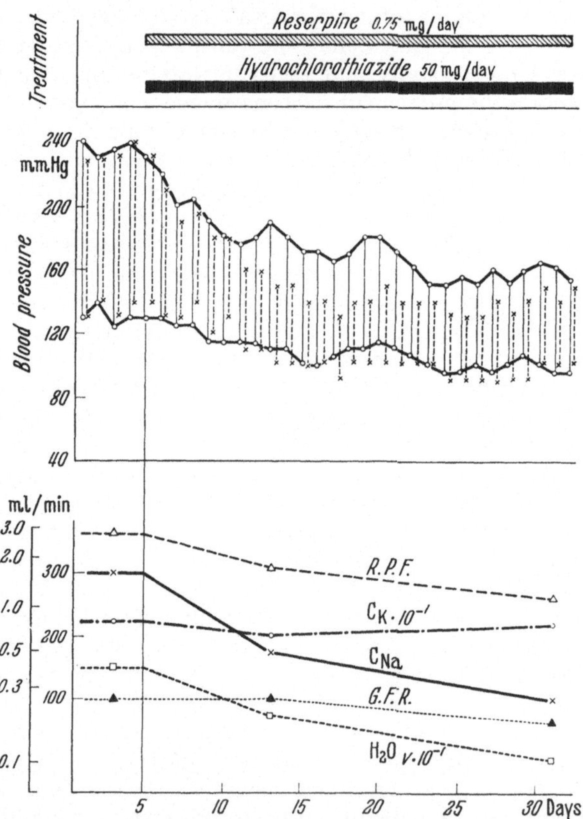

Fig. 4. Effects of blood pressure reduction on renal function. Severely hypertensive patient. R.P.F.: renal plasma flow; G.F.R.: glomerular filtration rate; C_{Na}: sodium clearance; C_K: potassium clearance; H_2O v: water excretion. Left row of values refers to sodium, potassium and water excretion; right row to renal plasma flow and glomerular filtration rate. For C_K and H_2O v, multiply the values indicated by 10. Note that hypotension affects Na and water excretion more severely than R.P.F. and G.F.R.

previous observation (*21, 25*) that lowering of arterial pressure in hypertensive patients definitely decreases the glomerular filtration rate and renal plasma flow, and impairs water and electrolyte excretion to a quite considerable extent (Fig. 4). If kidney function is already reduced before treatment is started, further reduction may produce an augmentation of blood urea nitrogen far beyond normal levels. Hyperazotemia represents a more specific, although by no means an absolute, contra-indication to saluretic treatment.Increase in blood urea nitrogen concentration can be induced by chlorothiazide or its derivatives not only via an arterial hypotension such as to reduce renal function below critical levels, but also via a more direct reduction of glomerular filtration rate and, possibly, through an increase in urea reabsorption (*3*). Of course, in hypertensive patients with severe kidney impairment, even with hyperazotemia, moderate hypotensive treatment must not be abandoned without a careful trial. Arterial pressure has to be slightly and progressively decreased, an attentive eye being kept on blood urea nitrogen, and the hypotensive treatment being adapted to the BUN values, though there is no need to be excessively apprehensive about some slight transient increase in azotemia. However, pressure levels should be raised if progressive increase in blood urea nitrogen concentration is observed. At any rate, in hyperazotemic patients it is advisable to try to control blood pressure without the use of saluretic drugs, but these substances might be administered cautiously when antihypertensive drugs alone are ineffective in managing hypertension.

f) The most important limiting factor in the therapy of arterial hypertension is *cooperation* on the part of the patient, i.e. his willingness to endure the discomforts of a treatment lasting indefinitely, and the severe restraints imposed upon him by a uniform daily regimen. Unfortunately, this factor plays an unfavorable role especially in those patients in the earlier stages of hypertensive disease, who are usually more distressed by the inconveniences of antihypertensive treatment than by the subjective disturbances of the ailment itself. Addition of saluretic drugs to antihypertensive medication is likely to make it easier for the patient to collaborate. Indeed, not only does it decrease the frequency and intensity of the annoying side-effects of, say, hydralazine, mecamylamine or guanethidine, but it also helps appreciably to avoid or at least mitigate the discomfort of a strict dietary regimen. There has been some dicussion (*10, 16, 22*) as to whether a low salt diet improves the hypotensive effects of saluretic drugs. This discussion is likely to have some significance in countries, such as the United States, where the daily intake of salt is exceptionally high, around 12 to

19*

15 g, but has little value in Italy or, we think, in most European countries, where the salt content in the diet is no more than 6 to 7 g. We have found that this sodium intake does not significantly hinder the hypotensive effect of the usual doses of chlorothiazide and hydrochlorothiazide, that it avoids the dangers of hyponatremia and hypochloremia, and, last but not least, that it tremendously increases the effectiveness of antihypertensive treatment by stimulating the essential spirit of cooperation in the patients.

4. Physiological considerations

As usual, clinical observations prompt several physiological considerations. A number of authors have become interested in the mechanism of the hypotensive action of thiazide derivatives, and

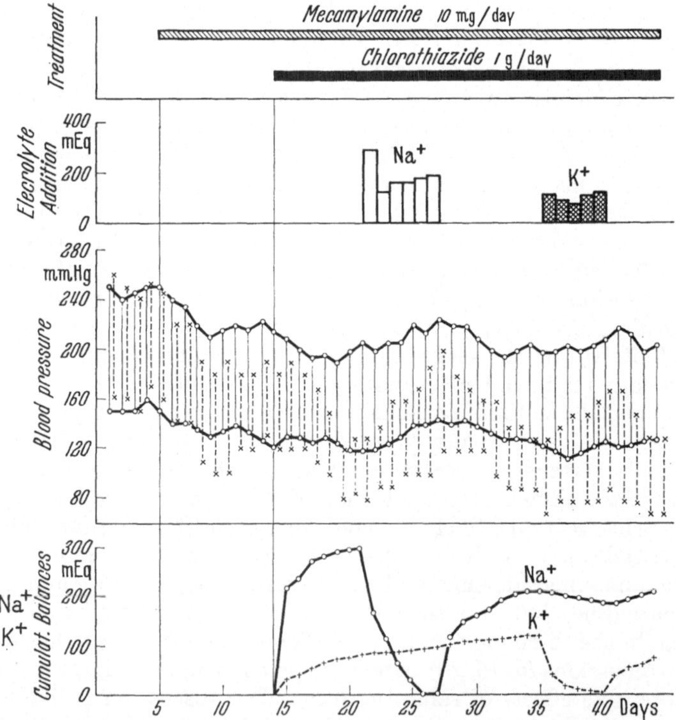

Fig. 5. Relationship of the hypotensive action of chlorothiazide to cumulative sodium and potassium balances. Effects of sodium and potassium repletion. For further details, see text

Dr. FREIS has just reviewed the different opinions and his own most recent results on this interesting problem. We are also studying some aspects of this question. Our research is still in too early a stage to permit us to take up any definite position on some of the issues debated. However, certain preliminary suggestions can be made.

Fig. 5 shows one patient with severe hypertension who was kept throughout the entire experimental period on a diet containing 120 mEq sodium, 90 mEq chloride and 60 mEq potassium. Administration of 10 mg mecamylamine daily induced a definite lowering of arterial pressure, and a further decrease, mainly on standing, followed addition of 1 g chlorothiazide daily. Sodium and potassium excretion were calculated from urine. By the eighth day, and for four more days, the sodium balance was gradually restored to normal by repeated infusions based on the excretion of the preceding hours. Blood pressure progressively returned to the pre-chlorothiazide levels, but it promptly reverted to lower levels when sodium addition was stopped. However, a few days later, when potassium acetate was infused to re-equilibrate the potassium balance, a slower but progressive increase of arterial pressure toward the levels recorded before chlorothiazide was observed, in spite of the fact that the sodium balance had reverted to negative. There is no doubt that sodium depletion plays a fundamental role in mediating the hypotensive effect of chlorothiazide, as has been demonstrated by a number of authors (*15, 16, 19, 32*), but our results, incomplete as they are as yet, hint that potassium depletion may also have some importance in producing, or perhaps maintaining, the hypotensive phenomenon. It might well be that, in later stages of saluretic treatment, when sodium balance and body fluids return spontaneously to normal, potassium depletion, known to be maintained throughout treatment, comes to assume a more direct importance in lowering arterial pressure.

5. Conclusions

Approximately two years of experience in the administration of saluretic drugs to hypertensive patients enable a few conclusions to be drawn. In patients with mild hypertension chlorothiazide and hydrochlorothiazide are often capable of lowering blood pressure to satisfactory values, even when administered as the sole antihypertensive medication. Patients with severe hypertension need a combination of saluretic drugs with other antihypertensive agents, in order to reduce arterial pressure to sufficiently safe values. The hypotensive action of saluretic compounds, either alone or in combination, is maintained even when treatment is prolonged for at least two years, although the sodium balance reverts to normal. There are obvious limitations to any kind of antihypertensive therapy, which are shared by treatment with saluretic drugs, but in none of our patients have important alterations in electrolyte equilibrium been observed which might suggest potential dangers inherent in prolonged saluretic administration. Some physiological implications have been discussed.

Résumé

Chez les malades atteints d'hypertension labile, le chlorothiazide et l'hydrochlorothiazide se sont souvent montrés, selon notre expérience, suffisants pour faire baisser la tension artérielle, même sans autre adjonction médicamenteuse. Chez les patients présentant une hypertension grave, la combinaison de salurétiques avec d'autres agents anti-hypertenseurs a amené une réduction suffisante et sûre de la pression artérielle.

L'action hypotensive des composés salurétiques, utilisés seuls ou en combinaison, reste soutenue, bien qu'après un traitement prolongé le taux du sodium tende de nouveau vers la normale. Il n'existe pas de limitation valable du traitement de l'hypertension par les salurétiques. Bien que chez aucun de nos malades il n'ait été observé d'altération importante de l'équilibre des électrolytes, cette possibilité existe lors d'une administration prolongée de ces médicaments.

References

1. Beem, J. R.: In Moyer (23), p. 106.
2. Conway, J., and P. Lauwers: Circulation (U.S.A.) **21**, 22 (1960).
3. Corcoran, A. C., C. McLeod, H. P. Dustan, and H. Page: Circulation (U.S.A.) **19**, 355 (1959).
4. Dinon, L. R., Y. S. Kim, and J. B. V. Veer: Amer. J. Med. Sc. **236**, 533 (1958).
5. Dustan, H. P., R. E. Schneckloth, A. C. Corcoran, and I. H. Page: Circulation (U.S.A.) **18**, 644 (1958).
6. Finnerty, F. A. Jr., J. H. Buchholz, J. Tuckman, G. T. Hajjar, and G. De Carlo Massaro: Circulation (U.S.A.) **20**, 1037 (1959).
7. Fitzgerald, E. W. Jr.: A. M. A. Arch. Int. Med. **105**, 305 (1960).
8. Friedberg, C. K.: In Diuresis and Diuretics. An International Symposium. Ed.: E. Buchborn and K. D. Bock. Berlin: Springer Verlag 1959, p. 221.
9. Gifford, R. W.: In Moyer (23), p. 561.
10. Grollman, A.: In Moyer (23), p. 510.
11. Heider, C., E. Dennis, and J. H. Moyer: Ann. N. Y. Acad. Sc. **71**, 456 (1958).
12. Herrmann, G. R., M. R. Hejtmancik, R. N. Grahan, and R. C. Margurger: Texas J. Med. **54**, 639 (1958).
13. Holboth, N., K. Thomsen, P. F. Haagensen, and N. Presnik: Uskr. Laeger (Den.) **120**, 1585 (1958).
14. Hollander, W., A. V. Chobanian, and R. W. Wilkins: Circulation (U.S.A.) **19**, 827 (1959).
15. Hollander, W., A. V. Chobanian, and R. W. Wilkins: In Diuresis and Diuretics. An International Symposium. Ed.: E. Buchborn and K. D. Bock. Berlin: Springer Verlag 1959, p. 297.
16. Hollander, W., and R. W. Wilkins: Boston Med. Quart. 8, 69 (1957).
17. Hoobler, S. W., J. M. Weller, and P. Blaquier: In Moyer (23), p. 581.
18. Jaffé, M. O., and R. R. Kierland: J. Amer. Med. Ass. **168**, 2264 (1959).

19. LOSSE, H., and H. WEHMEYER: In Diuresis and Diuretics. An International Symposium. Ed.: F. BUCHBORN and K. D. BOCK. Berlin: Springer Verlag 1959, p. 313.
20. MAGID, G. J., and P. H. FORSHAM: Metabolism (U.S.A.) **7**, 589 (1958).
21. MILLS, L. C., and J. H. MOYER: Amer. J. Med. Sc. **226**, 1 (1953).
22. MOSER, M.: In MOYER (*23*), p. 512.
23. MOYER, J.H. (Ed.): Hypertension. The First Hahnemann Symposium on Hypertensive Disease. Philadelphia: W. B. Saunders Co. 1959.
24. MOYER, J. H., C. HEIDER, K. PEVEY, and R. V. FORD: Amer. J. Med. **24**, 177 (1958).
25. MOYER, J. H., and L. C. MILLS: J. Clin. Invest. (U.S.A.) **32**, 172 (1953).
26. NORDQVIST, P., G. CRAMER, and P. BJÖRNTROP: Lancet (G.B.) **1959/I**, 271.
27. PERRY, H. M.: In MOYER (*23*), p. 112.
28. SCHROEDER, H. A.: Amer. J. Med. **17**, 540 (1954).
29. SCHROEDER, H. A.: Circulation (U.S.A.) **10**, 321 (1954).
30. SMITH, K. S., and P. B. S. FOWLER: Lancet (G.B.) **1955/I**, 417.
31. SMITHWICK, R. H.: In MOYER (*23*), p. 681.
32. WILKINS, R. W., W. HOLLANDER, and A. V. CHOBANIAN: Ann. N. Y. Acad. Sc. **71**, 465 (1958).
33. ZUCKERMAN, A. J., and A. A. CHAZAN: Brit. Med. J. **1958/II**, 1338.

Discussion

Reubi: I would suggest that we discuss first the pharmacology of new hypotensive drugs and the technique of hypotensive treatment. The results are going to be discussed later. I think it would be nice if Dr. Page, whose group had been doing the first studies on guanethidine, would make some comment.

Page: We believe that the treatment of hypertension is not satisfactory unless the blood pressure is about normal in the supine position. Therefore we do not believe that postural hypotension is always a bad thing or a "side effect". In the use of guanethidine we are inclined to give enough to elicit postural hypotension and keep the patients in bed for a week or more until they have more or less adjusted to this state. In some cases it may then be necessary to cut the dosage a little until a tolerable state has been reached. I think most people undertreat rather than overtreat, that is if you are treating severe hypertension. In a clinic like ours we are apt to see mostly very severe hypertensives and therefore the treatment must be fairly drastic. Enough guanethidine should, in our opinion, be given to insure significant reduction in supine pressure. We are not content with orthostatic hypotension only. We also believe that most patients do much better when they are started on the drug in the hospital. Incidentally, we have developed a padded bathroom which has much merit. I know there has been much talk of fur-lined bathtubs, but this is not what I mean. Many people when they feel ill head for the bathroom, they grab for anything when they feel faint and often end up on a cement floor, having hit a number of protruding objects on the way down. This can be extremely dangerous. So we now have specially padded bathrooms, even with plastic bottles for urine samples, to make the life of the patient with orthostatic hypotension bearable if not altogether delightful. So the principle of the "fur-lined bathtub" is a useful one and I commend it to you. If you keep blondes out of them and your hypotensive patients in them, you will avoid legal complications.

As regards guanethidine, we came to the conclusion from our pharmacological studies that part of its peripheral action was to cause the discharge of norepinephrine from the blood vessels. In the perfused dog's leg guanethidine caused the same pressor response blocked by phentolamine as in the intact animal. We are not so sure it does not have some central effects. But I will not take more of your time to discuss our views on the pharmacology of this drug, because Dr. Plummer has done it so adequately from his own studies. In general, I think I can say that our observations agree with his.

We have given up the use of bretylium, because of the development of tolerance and because of the severe parotid pain, which has often lasted several months after discontinuing the drug. In a few of our patients abdominal pain simulating pancreatitis was present. I am afraid this is the best I can contribute to the "break through" mentioned by the Lancet. But the basic principles involved in both bretylium and guanethidine seem to be new and important.

Genest: I would like to make a few comments. The first one concerns the significant water retention described in 4 patients as a side effect of guanethidine. From our experience in 30 hypertensive patients receiving this drug, we have not noticed such side effect and neither was it mentioned by other investigators at the Conference on Guanethidine last April 1960, in Memphis, U.S.A. The second one concerns the intravenous use of bretylium tosylate and guanethidine. We have given intravenous guanethidine to a patient with pheochromocytoma. Aware of the experimental findings concerning norepinephrine release, the intravenous administration of guanethidine was done through a three-way stopcock, to the side-arm of which was already connected a syringe containing phentolamine. As you can see (Fig. 1), there

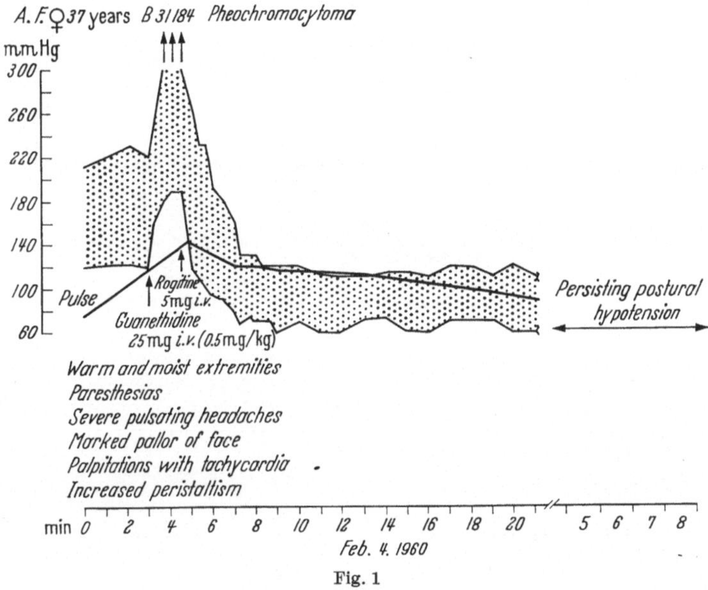

Fig. 1

is immediately after the injection of guanethidine a most severe rise in blood pressure above 300 mm Hg systolic and at 190 diastolic. This rise was accompanied by the signs and symptoms described, which are manifestations of the increased liberation of catechol amines. After a stormy period of some 90 sec, rapid injection of phentolamine brought the blood pressure rapidly down to normal or subnormal levels. A control experiment was done after operation. No rise was noted and the blood pressure fell to hypotensive levels with the patient in the upright position. In the next slide (Fig. 2) there is an illustration of the frequent occurrence of a short but severe rise in blood pressure in patients with essential hypertension. These sudden rises may be quite dangerous in patients with long-standing hypertension and signs of vascular degeneration or left ventricular failure. Dr. ROSENHEIM has mentioned the same dangerous blood pressure rise following the intravenous use of bretylium tosylate in a patient with pheochromocytoma.

The third comment concerns sympathectomy. I agree with Dr. HOOBLER that, at the present time, sympathectomy may have been discarded too quickly. There are still a few indications for this procedure, since patients

following this operation are much more sensitive to hypotensive drugs and
can often be well controlled with natriuretic agents. Some indications are:

a) resistance to the antihypertensive drugs,

b) reluctance to take so many pills, since we all know that the present
management of patients with severe hypertension with combined therapy may
sometimes involve the ingestion of 20 to 25 pills a day,

c) financial inability to afford the cost of anti-hypertensive drugs.

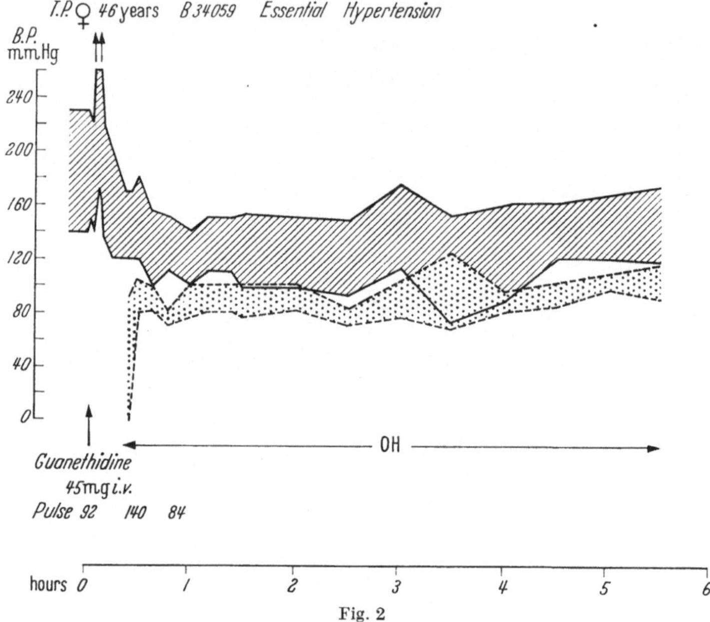

Fig. 2

As to my last comment, I would like to ask Dr. HOOBLER whether he has
forgotten to mention the use of protoveratrine? I remember reading only
a few years ago most enthusiastic papers of Dr. HOOBLER on the potency
and effectiveness of protoveratrine and Veratrum alkaloids. I did not agree
with this point of view, but I am wondering now if his ideas have changed
concerning these drugs?

HOOBLER: I think every investigator should have a few mistakes to
confess in his past. At least I hope so.

We studied protoveratrine at the time that ganglion blocking agents
were not available, at least to our laboratory. At the moment it seemed like
the most successful oral antihypertensive treatment. I think Dr. FREIS will
agree with me that we still do not know how Veratrum acts to lower the
blood pressure. If we knew how, we might have something useful, but at the
moment, in non-emetic doses it is not effective enough, so I would just as
soon forget about using it to treat hypertension.

REUBI: At this point in the discussion I think it would be useful to have
a comment by one of our British colleagues on Darenthin (bretylium tosylate).

WILSON: My experience is so small, and like Dr. PAGE I always confined my use of these hypotensive drugs to patients with malignant hypertension or severe benign essential or renal hypertension. I think there are several reasons why we should be dissatisfied with the present state of hypotensive drug therapy. Firstly, the practical difficulties of treating patients with three or four different kinds of pills over long periods of time are very serious in a crowded urban community. This is particularly the case when symptoms are few or absent. Secondly, even with a co-operative patient, supervision of the present drug therapy by general practitioners is extremely difficult. Thirdly, when severe hypertension is treated by ganglion blocking drugs and even by guanethidine, large fluctuations in blood pressure occur, either with changes in posture, severe exercise or straining. I think such changes may be responsible for some of the cerebral vascular accidents which may occur even while patients are under observation in hospital. In my view, there is no evidence that by giving adrenergic blocking drugs we are correcting the fundamental fault of hypertension. What is needed is further work on factors controlling basal arteriolar tone and on drugs which reduce this. Although the drugs at present available have great symptomatic value and may diminish morbidity and mortality, I think we should regard them as transitional until some more rational therapy is available.

PEART: As another English colleague, may I disagree with this last statement. I think this is a very pessimistic attitude and, looking at the cases of malignant hypertension alone, I do not think anybody can subscribe to that view. Everybody realises that the control of the high blood pressure is not perfect; it never will be at the moment; but I think that does not stop us assessing the results of the present and available therapies. I think that is what our job is surely to do at the moment. We all know the difficulties. I think it is fair to say after speaking to a lot of people in England that many are looking at Darenthin in particular (bretylium), and thinking that this is not quite such a good drug. I have largely personally given up using it, because of the high degree of tolerance which seems to occur, if not because of the side effects. And then I think with guanethidine I find that that has not been such a problem, as has been emphasized by various speakers.

SCHROEDER: I must disagree with Dr. WILSON. In St. Louis there has been a drastic reduction in the number of cases of malignant hypertension admitted to hospital. In 1951 we saw 83 cases and a few less in 1952. By 1953 chemotherapy was in use in the Central States surrounding St. Louis. The number dropped progressively year by year until in 1956 we only could find four, in spite of the fact that our clinic was well known and many severe cases were referred to us. A biochemical study on untreated malignant hypertension was given up for lack of cases. The explanation is, I think, that hypertension is being so widely, if inadequately, treated that the malignant stage no longer develops very often.

I must also say a word about hydralazine, although Dr. GROSS could do it better than I. Dr. HOOBLER did not give it too good a reputation. This is a unique drug acting on an area different from any of the other anti-hypertensive drugs. A few of its basic qualities are: Anti-enzyme (histaminase, dopa decarboxylase or what is now thought of as 1-aromatic amino acid decarboxylase, sometimes monoamine oxidase). Action of this nature should lead to interference with metabolism of aromatic vasoactive amines. Antiangiotensin and anti-pherentasin, both on the isolated aortic strip and the latter in man. A good chelating agent, opposing coronary constriction caused by copper in minute doses. Reducing agent for Fe^{+++} and V^{4+} (V may be the metallic cofactor for monoamine oxidase, as proposed by us and found by the Russians recently). Direct peripheral dilator of long action, sort of long-acting nitrate. The only drug increasing renal plasma flow in the face of a lowered blood pressure.

A third point. I am convinced that if you take enough measurements of blood pressure, say at two or four hourly intervals, you cannot obtain even control of blood pressure with ganglionic blocking agents alone in severe hypertension. These agents are excreted rapidly and frequent doses are essential at least every four hours. Furthermore, it is necessary to change the dose frequently, sometimes at each interval, in order to avoid peaks of hypertension and nadirs of hypotension.

FREIS: Our experiences are in good agreement with Dr. HILDEN's, with a few exceptions. One of the most important differences is that we have not as yet observed the mental depressions that occur with Rauwolfia. This would seem to be a very important point clinically. I wonder whether anyone else in this group has seen true depression develop in patients who were taking guanethidine. It is unfortunate, Dr. HILDEN, that Dr. FROHLICH and I may have given the impression in our paper that the postural hypotension was more profound with guanethidine than with ganglionic blocking agents. I do not believe this is so. The point we were trying to emphasize was that because of the long duration of action of guanethidine of 5—7 days, the dosages should be adjusted with great care in out-patients, since if the doses are increased too rapidly, one may precipitate disabling orthostatic hypotension that might last for several days.

With regard to Dr. HOOBLER's paper: I believe the study you mentioned on survival rates and blood pressure was based on clinic blood pressures. Is that right?

HOOBLER: Yes.

FREIS: You pointed out that vascular damage rather than blood pressure level is the important differential. Don't you think it is possible that the patients with similar elevations of blood pressure but without vascular damage may in reality have lower home blood pressures than those with the vascular damage? In our experience we find that there is better correlation of vascular damage with basal blood pressure levels and poor correlation of vascular damage with casual blood pressure levels. Your emphasis on home blood pressure recordings is in excellent agreement with our experience and is a procedure we have been applying for the past 9 years. We can confirm your observation that the hypokalaemia caused by chlorothiazide or other diuretics did not produce renal damage. This would seem to be an important clinical point. Since you do not believe in the plasma volume-reduction hypothesis to explain the fall of blood pressure after chlorothiazide, nor do you think that there is any moderation of the hypertension during prolonged treatment, I would like to ask you what you believe is the mechanism?

I might add a word about Dr. WILSON's comment. If you believe, Dr. WILSON, that hypertension in itself may produce vascular damage, is it not reasonable to try to treat the hypertension before rather than after the damage has occurred? Our experience would indicate that the treatment of hypertension before vascular damage is a simpler procedure than in the advanced cases and will not precipitate strokes. In fact, side effects are not very prevalent because thiazides and hydralazine will control many early cases without resorting to blocking agents or resorting to them only for initial treatment.

REUBI: Dr. HOOBLER, can you perhaps answer Dr. FREIS's question?

HOOBLER: In reply to Dr. FREIS's comments, I would entirely agree that a better correlation would exist between "usual" blood pressure levels, as taken in the home, and prognosis for death in hypertension. However, it is obviously impractical in a large series of subjects to take home blood pressure readings, so we must be content with the clinic readings in determining prognosis. Sometimes when a patient appears to have tolerated very high blood pressure for a long time, we find that his readings at home are so much lower than in the clinic as to explain the apparently benign prognosis. On the other hand, an element of vascular vulnerability surely exists. All of us have had patients with similar blood pressure readings but with a widely varying tendency to develop the vascular complications of the disease. Regarding the question of how chlorothiazide lowers peripheral resistance, I surely do not pretend to know. However, the prolonged depletion of total body water, associated with the restoration of normal blood and extracellular fluid volume and total exchangeable sodium in a patient under long-term treatment emphasizes the possible rôle of body water, particularly intracellular water, in the decreased peripheral vascular resistance.

Concerning Dr. FREIS's claim to priority in insisting on the value of blood pressure determinations in the home, I would certainly agree, and only say that our practice was learned from him and reinforces his views.

GROSS: Also in pharmacology there are problems of definition. Dr. HILDEN classified these new drugs, Darenthin and guanethidine, as adrenergic blocking agents. I think in order to avoid confusion we should not use this term, which has to be reserved for substances which either diminish blood pressure response to injected nor-adrenaline or reverse adrenaline. The term for the new compounds should be sympathetic inhibitors, perhaps adrenergic depletors, but we have to avoid a term which might give a wrong impression.

A second point: One of the most interesting side effects of guanethidine in my opinion is the oedema formation. It is not observed in experimental animals, as the animal in general is not prone to develop oedema. I wonder if oedema formation has something to do with the liberation of serotonin or similar amines. You may remember that occasionally a similar oedema formation is seen in patients under reserpine treatment, but the factors responsible never became established. It might be that the oedema which develops during reserpine therapy is comparable to that which is seen in patients treated with guanethidine.

HOOD: The hydralazine question: We have been using the drug for 9 years in a joint programme of two departments. We have about 800 patients in whom we have tried the drug. There is one special experience which I would like to mention and that is in the very severe type of case, where you have got a very high degree of control — let us say at diastolic levels continuously around 100 mm Hg or less — in malignant or grade three if we use the KEITH and WAGENER classification. If then as a late thing you get hydralazine disease and are forced to omit the drug, there is no amount of juggling around with any combinations of any amounts of other drugs in this very serious situation which will in our experience prevent a slow progressive rise in diastolic blood pressure level. This is a constant experience. The number of patients in whom we have been forced to omit the drug due to these particular reasons is now, I would say as a rough guess, 30.

BROD: I would like only to ask two questions. One is: It was mentioned repeatedly that the new drugs guanethidine and Darenthin have possibly unfavourable renal effects. My question is, what happens to the heart, or to the coronaries and to the brain, because this is equally important ? Have Dr. HILDEN and others seen any complications from these sides ?

About hydralazine: I did not hear anybody mention Dr. LEWIS from Glasgow, who maintained that this drug interferes with carbohydrate metabolism of the smooth muscle in the vessel wall. If this were so, this would be a drug which to a certain extent would correspond to what Dr. WILSON has been asking for. Now can this possibility be ruled out or shall we calculate with this effect ?

REUBI: Any answer to that question ?

SCHROEDER: All available evidence points to the idea that the hydralazine drugs act very fundamentally on the metabolism of vascular smooth muscle, interfering with constriction caused by a variety of stimuli. There is as yet no certain proof of just how and where they act.

BARTORELLI: I should like to report the results of our experiences with guanethidine. Our observations cover some 50 patients suffering from essential hypertension, and I have here a slide (Fig. 1) illustrating the effectiveness

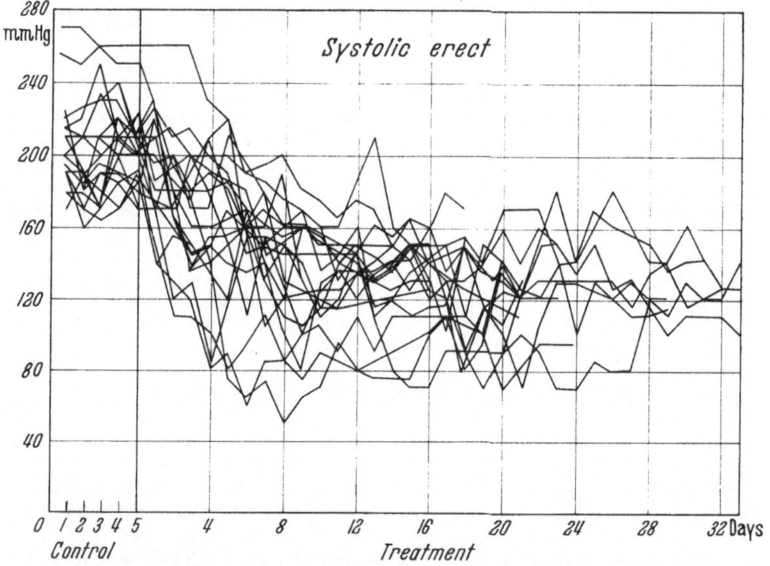

Fig. 1. *Effect of guanethidine on systolic pressure in the standing position.* Figures recorded in 22 hospitalised hypertensives for 5 days prior to treatment (control) and during administration of guanethidine (treatment). The figures recorded after the 32nd day have been omitted. The doses vary from patient to patient and are not indicated here. (BARTORELLI, GARGANO, REGOLI, and ZANCHETTI, to be published shortly)

of this drug. The figure shows that, in all our patients without exception, guanethidine exerted a hypotensive action which is reflected particularly clearly in the systolic levels recorded in the standing position. The incidence of very low systolic figures, i. e. below 80 mm Hg, indicates the frequency with which orthostatic collapse was observed. The following slide shows that the diastolic pressure was also affected, especially in the standing position (Fig. 2). However, I should like to emphasise that we found it difficult to prevent orthostatic collapse in the course of prolonged guanethidine treatment, particularly on account of the drug's tendency to exert a progressive

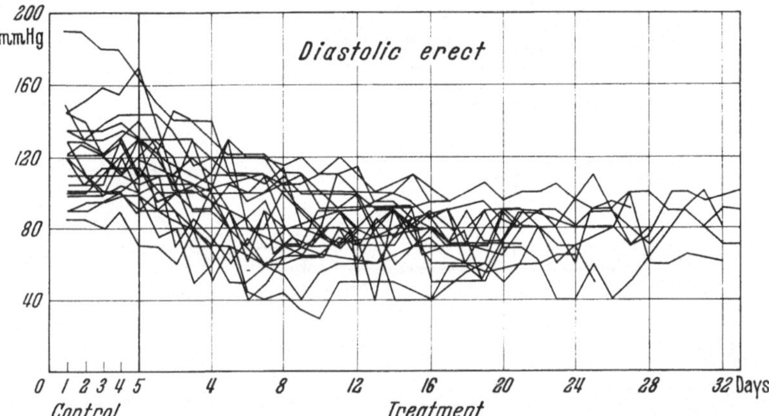

Fig. 2. *Effect of guanethidine on diastolic pressure in the standing position.* For further details, see Fig. 1. (BARTORELLI, GARGANO, REGOLI, and ZANCHETTI, to be published shortly)

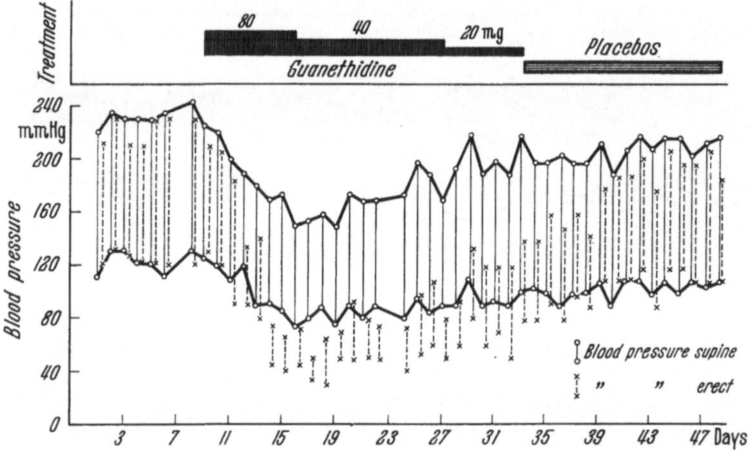

Fig. 3. *Effect of guanethidine, administered in diminishing doses.* Hospitalised patient. (BARTORELLI, GARGANO, REGOLI, and ZANCHETTI, to be published shortly)

cumulative effect. At the beginning of our study, we thought that as an initial tentative approach to treatment, we could administer large priming doses for a few days, followed by smaller maintenance doses once a satisfactory hypotensive effect had been achieved. Unfortunately, we soon discovered that this method was not without its snags. As the following slide (Fig. 3) shows, with this dosage schedule we encountered very marked postural hypotension.

Better results were obtained using the opposite approach, i. e. initiating treatment cautiously with small doses and then progressively raising the

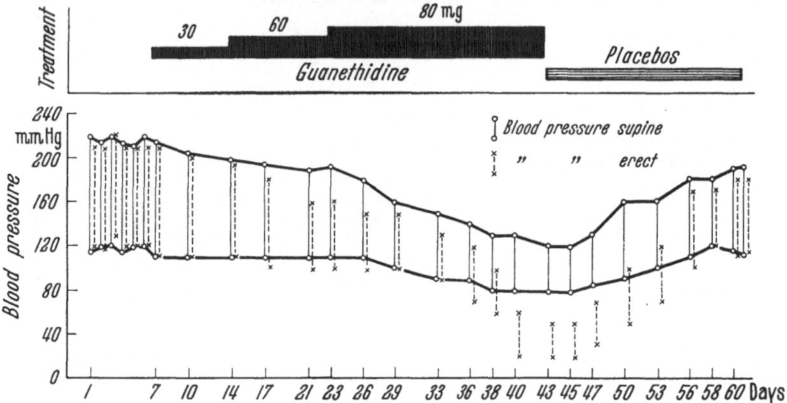

Fig. 4. *Effect of guanethidine, administered in increasing doses.* Ambulant patient. (BARTORELLI, GARGANO, REGOLI, and ZANCHETTI, to be published shortly)

dosage in the light of the hypotensive effect obtained. But this method, too, has serious drawbacks, especially where treatment is being given on an

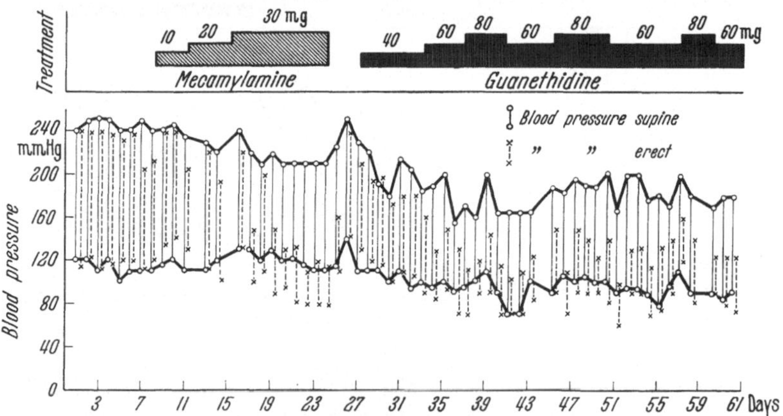

Fig. 5. *Effect of guanethidine, administered in alternating doses.* Hospitalised patient. (BARTORELLI, GARGANO, REGOLI, and ZANCHETTI, to be published shortly)

ambulatory basis. The fact is that guanethidine has a prolonged duration of action, so that, if one adheres to what was initially an effective dose, the drug ultimately exerts a cumulative effect in most cases, leading to marked hypotension (Fig. 4). Recently we have experimented with a new dosage schedule which has proved more satisfactory and enables one to keep the blood pressure at a fairly uniform level: we initiate treatment with a rather small dose (generally 20—40 mg daily), which is administered for 5 to 7 days; we then progressively increase the daily dose by 20 mg every 4 or 5 days until the desired anti-hypertensive response is elicited. Then, in order to prevent excessive hypotension, we reduce the daily dose for a few days to below the minimum effective level, i. e. to a "subliminal" dose of 20 mg. As a rule, we find it advisable to alternate the two doses — in other words, the "liminal" and the "subliminal" — every 4 or 5 days (Fig. 5). Finally, we have also carried out trials using a combination of guanethidine with hydrochlorothiazide and reserpine. The effect of guanethidine has invariably been greatly reinforced by the addition of the sali-diuretic and the reserpine.

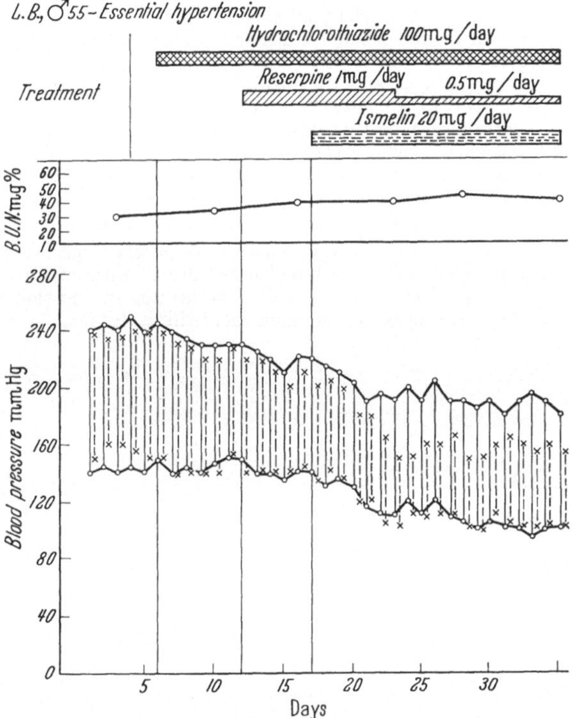

Fig. 6. *Effect of combined treatment with guanethidine, reserpine, and hydrochlorothiazide.*
Hospitalised patient

The last slide (Fig. 6) shows that, by administering combined treatment of this kind, it is possible to bring the blood pressure under control with small doses of guanethidine, even in severe cases of hypertension. We have found that such doses have a negligible cumulative action and that hence it is no longer necessary to alternate liminal with subliminal doses.

REUBI: Thank you. I quite agree with you. We also make it a practice to begin with 30 mg and to increase the dose by 10 mg every 3 days until the desired effect is obtained. Often we observe after some weeks or months of treatment that one can reduce the dose progressively.

HILDEN: I would like to say a few words about the use of diuretics in hypertension. We have been very influenced along these lines during the last two years and, like some of the other speakers we have heard, we decided that we would make diuretics our first choice in the treatment of hypertension. Now the problem of hypokalaemia has troubled us a great deal. I was interested to hear that Dr. BARTORELLI has not so far found any reduction of exchangeable potassium and that Dr. HOOBLER found no renal changes. Nevertheless, I think it is not advisable to produce hypokalaemia and to allow it to persist for months or years. I would therefore be interested to find out how much potassium one should give to these patients in order to make sure that they do not get hypokalaemia. I would like to show you one slide. These are our results where we gave hydrochlorothiazide. In one series we added 0.5 g of potassium chloride, and in the other series, 1 g of potassium chloride per 25 mg of hydrochlorothiazide. In the last series the e are very small changes in the range between the figures recorded before treatment and during treatment. A few go down and few go up, and not too much. These are all patients in whom renal function was not severely diminished, because this has to be considered. Now if you have patients with kidney function so seriously impaired that they cannot excrete potassium, then these are very very bad cases, in which you may not be able to do anything.

REUBI: Thank you. In my experience, the amounts of potassium needed are quite variable and the fall in blood potassium is unpredictable in most cases. For that reason I do not like tablets containing in addition to chlorothiazide a small amount of potassium chloride. I think this is a very dangerous practice.

Survival rates in severe hypertension intensively treated with hydralazine and ganglionic blockade

By

H. A. Schroeder and H. M. Perry, jr.

Introduction

When a new therapeutic tool is developed for control of a serious or fatal disease, it must be tested against the more severe forms of that disease in order that its limits of effectiveness be found. In fatal diseases, the criterion for effectiveness is survival. In diseases with fatality rates varying with time, the problem of evaluating a regimen becomes complicated. Arterial hypertension is such a disorder.

Hydralazine became available to us in August 1949. Reubi was the first to use it in man, showing its well-known and unique renal vasodilating property (1). It was the best of more than a hundred agents tested in hypertensive dogs; therefore, it was given to human patients continuously.

While effective in more than two-thirds of patients, significantly lowering blood pressure, it soon became obvious that this agent acted on only one of the factors contributing to chronic vasospasm. Many others were tried in combination; none was additive in effect.

In July 1951, oral hexamethonium chloride became available. The addition of an oral ganglionic blocking agent to oral hydralazine caused remarkable results, results which I (Schroeder) had never before observed in my experience with about two thousand patients during 15 years. To watch the miracle of hypertensive heart failure regressing overnight, hemorrhagic and exudative lesions in ocular fundi disappearing in days or weeks, and totally incapacitated persons returning to active lives within a few months, was a new experience which happens only once in a lifetime.

We decided at that time (August 1951) that we had found a regimen extremely effective against severe arterial hypertension, and that it should be tried to its limits. Therefore, we excluded cases from treatment when blood pressure fell considerably after admission to the hospital, and treated every case of intractable hypertension regardless of the severity of secondary signs such as the presence of heart failure, apoplexy, renal insufficiency, angina pectoris, hemorrhagic and exudative retinitis and the like. We included cases of hypertension associated with disseminated lupus erythematosus, polyarteritis nodosa, dissecting aortic aneurysm, pyelonephritis, Cushing's syndrome, polycystic kidneys, thrombosis of renal artery, severe atherosclerosis, chronic glomerulonephritis, toxemia of pregnancy and the like, and we treated vigorously such secondary hypertensive phenomena as hypertensive encephalopathy (wet brain). We believed that the regimen affected the hypertensive process, *per se,* and that the only criterion for treatment was intractable hypertension.

No case was too severe for us; many were too mild and were excluded.

It now lacks but a month or two of nine years since the first patient was treated; aged 48, she had been in severe intractable heart failure for six months and her ocular fundi showed hemorrhages, exudates and papilledema. She has been working regularly since October 1951. This discourse, therefore, summarizes the mortality and survival rates of a large number of patients, most of whom were started on therapy from 1951 to 1955 and continued, as need be, until the present.

Method

The method has been previously described (*2, 3, 4, 5, 6*). Briefly, it consisted of giving gradually increasing doses of a ganglionic blocking agent orally at four-hour intervals until swings of blood pressure in the supine position reached normal levels (less than 140 mm Hg systolic). Hydralazine was then added in increasing doses at four-hourly intervals until the blood pressure was normal, or a dose of 600 mg per day was reached. Each dose of ganglionic blocking agent was adjusted at each four-hour interval so that a full dose was given for a systolic pressure over 140 mm, a half dose for one between 140 and 130 mm, a quarter dose for one between 130 and 120 mm, and none for one below 120 mm Hg. All blood pressures were taken by nurses. After a suitable interval, recordings were made in the sitting position; doses of blocking agents thus readjusted themselves downward. Patients took their own readings on discharge from the hospital, omitting the night (2 A. M.) dose. By this method, changes in doses of ganglionic blocking agents were self-adjusting; changes in doses of hydralazine were controlled by us.

We have been unable to satisfy ourselves that adequate control of severe hypertension could be achieved by us on ganglionic blocking agents alone in patients coming to us in St. Louis, Missouri, when blood pressures were measured in the supine position by nurses, at four-hourly intervals. Except for relatively minor qualities, we have been unable to satisfy ourselves that one ganglionic blocking agent was superior to another. Hexamethonium chloride, pentolinium bitartrate, chlorisondamine and mecamylamine were used in this study as each became available, but patients were not given a new drug if the action of the older one was satisfactory.

It must be reemphasized that the aim of therapy was strict normotension, not merely a modification of hypertension. By normotension is meant a diastolic blood pressure averaging below 90 mm Hg in any 35 consecutive determinations (1 week's observations).

The series represents a total of 388 patients vigorously treated as outlined. Nineteen have been lost to follow-up; therefore, 369 will be considered in detail. Of these, about one-half (178) were in malignant stages; one-half (88) of those were azotemic and 13 had non-protein nitrogen (N.P.N.) levels of more than 100 mg per 100 ml plasma. Males and females, Negro and White, are grouped together. There were 165 white men and 159 white women, 21 Negro men and 43 Negro women. All but one 6-year old child were over 18 years of age. Those discontinuing drugs did so on their own volition or upon the advice of a physician not a member of our team.

Results

We will discuss the mortalities of the various groups from the most to the least severe forms of the disease (Table 1).

Malignant hypertension with azotemia. Eleven formerly azotemic patients are living, 6 for four to seven years and 5 for seven to nine years. All still require drugs. None had plasma N.P.N. levels of 100 mg per 100 ml or more. The remainder are dead. Twenty-seven died within less than six months of beginning therapy and 15 within less than one year. Fourteen lived one to four years (2 with levels of N.P.N. more than 100 mg per 100 ml), and 7, four to seven years.

In 14, drugs were discontinued for one reason or another. Eight died in less than six months, and 6 in less than a year.

Thus, the gross survival rate in those continuing drugs is 14.9% and in those discontinuing drugs 0%. Of the 32 who survived more than one year (42.1%), the survival rate to date is 34.4%.

Table 1. *Survival rates of hypertensive patients treated with hydralazine and ganglionic blockade*

Type	No Patients	% Living	Dead. Years survived				Living. Years		
			< 1	1—4	4—7	7—9	1—4	4—7	7—9
Malignant hypertension with azotemia									
Continued	74	14.9	42	14	7			6	5
Discontinued . . .	14	0	14						
Malignant hypertension without azotemia									
Continued	72	72.2	5	9	5	1	2	20	30
Discontinued . . .	18	11.1	9	6	1		2		
Benign hypertension[1]									
Continued (total) . .	161	75.8	5	21	12	1	2	16	104
Grade 4	43	65.1	2	6	7			2	26
Grade 3	73	83.6	2	6	3	1			61
Grade 2	20	80.0	1	2	1				16
ungraded	25	68.0		7	1		2	14	1
Discontinued (total)	30	40.0	4	10	3	1		2	10
Grade 4	11	9.1	3	6		1			1
Grade 3	10	50.0	1	2	2				5
Grade 2	5	60.0		1	1				3
ungraded	4	75.0		1				2	1
Summary									
With azotemia . . .	369								
Continued	307	59.6	52	44	24		2	42	139
Per cent[2]			16.9	14.3	7.8		0.6	13.7	45.3
Discontinued . .	62	22.6	27	16	4	1	2	2	10
Per cent			43.5	25.8	6.5	1.6	3.2	3.2	16.1
Without azotemia .	281								
Continued	233	74.7	10	30	17	2	4	36	134
Per cent[2]			4.3	12.9	7.3	0.9	1.7	15.5	57.5
Discontinued . .	48	29.2	13	16	4	1	2	2	10
Per cent			27.1	33.3	8.3	2.1	4.2	4.2	20.8

One may conclude that this form of therapy is justified in malignant hypertension with azotemia if azotemia is not too severe. If such a patient survives for one year, he has one chance in three of surviving several more. In another study we have shown that patients with azotemia at levels of N.P.N. of less than 60 to 80 mg per 100 ml have reasonable chances of survival for four years or more, while those with higher levels have little (7). The results in this group clearly indicate the limits of therapeutic efficacy of the combined form of treatment.

---

[1] SMITHWICK grade.
[2] Living or dead.

Malignant hypertension without azotemia. There were 90 patients in this group. In order to assess, by means of a standard technique, the degree of secondary hypertensive and atherosclerotic degeneration, most cases were graded according to the criteria of SMITHWICK (8). All but 4 were in SMITHWICK's grade 4 and all showed diminution of renal function (none was able to excrete more than 22% of an injected dose of phenolsulphonephthalein in 15 minutes and only 5 were able to excrete more than 15%). Eighteen discontinued treatment for one reason or another after achieving successful control of elevated blood pressure; 9 died within less than one year (most within a few weeks), 6 died one to four years later and 1, four to seven years later. Two are living for one to four years. The survival rate without drugs in this group is therefore 11%.

Seventy-two continued treatment. Fifty-two are living, 2 for one to four years, 20 for four to seven, and 30 for seven to nine years. The survival rate for this group is therefore 72.2%. Signs of the malignant stage have uniformly disappeared.

Of the 20 who died, 5 survived less than one year, 9 one to four years, 5 four to seven years, and one seven to nine. One may conclude that the use of this form of therapy is indicated in malignant hypertension without azotemia, and that a reasonable chance of survival is assured in this formerly rapidly progressive and fatal disorder.

Benign hypertension. While severe forms of this type of hypertension are not "benign" in the true sense of the word, usually ending in heart failure or apoplexy, drugs might be expected to be more effective in this than in the malignant form. They are not. Patients in this group totaled 191.

Thirty discontinued using the drugs; 12 are living and 18 are dead; ten of the living have survived for seven to nine years, 2 for four to seven. Of the dead, 4 survived less than one year, 10 for one to four, 3 for four to seven and 1 for seven to nine. The gross survival rate in this group is therefore 40%.

Of the 161 who continued using the drugs, 39 are dead, a survival rate of 75.8%, which is approximately that for malignant hypertension without azotemia. Five died in less than one year, 21 in one to four, 12 in four to seven, and one after more than seven years of therapy.

Of the 122 living patients continuing therapy, 104 have survived for seven to nine years, 16 for four to seven years, and 2 for three to four years. The severity of the secondary manifestations of hypertension and atherosclerosis in this group is evidenced by the SMITHWICK grades found: 43 were in grade 4, 73 in grade 3,

20 in grade 2, and 25 were not graded. All but 2 of those graded lived for seven to nine years.

The dead patients continuing treatment were graded as follows: 15 in grade 4, 12 in grade 3, 4 in grade 2, 8 ungraded. Of the dead discontinuing treatment, 10 were in grade 4, 5 in grade 3, 2 in grade 2, and 1 ungraded. Of the 12 living, 1 was in grade 4, 5 in grade 3, 3 in grade 2, and 3 ungraded.

Survival rates for treated patients according to grade are as follows: grade 4, 65.1%; grade 3, 83.6%; grade 2, 80%; ungraded, 68%. Survival rates for patients discontinuing treatment are: grade 4, 9.1%; grade 3, 50%, grade 2, 60%. These survival rates cover the period seven to nine years.

"Cures". The most interesting group from a therapeutic viewpoint are the so-called cures, e.g. patients who have no longer needed any drugs for four years or more (Table 2). They make up 29 individuals, or 13.1% of all continuing treatment, excluding those with azotemia. Two are dead of sudden coronary occlusion, a survival rate of 93.1%. The remainder continue to take their blood pressures from time to time, knowing that drugs will be required should they become elevated, as has happened to several in the past for a few months. Five of these were in malignant stages, or 8.3% of the group; one is dead. Of the remaining 24, 7 were in Smithwick grade 4 (one is dead), 9 in grade 3, and 8 in grade 2. Regression of signs secondary to hypertension, with the exception of electrocardiographic findings of old infarctions or residua of apoplexy, has occurred slowly. These individuals are to all outward signs well and healthy, and many have passed physical examinations for employment or life insurance. These so-called "cures" have occurred only after three or more years of slowly diminishing therapy, and only after diastolic pressure had been controlled at levels below

Table 2. *So-called "cures" in hypertensive patients formerly requiring treatment but maintaining normotension three to seven years without drugs*

Stage[1]	Surviving (Years)		
	1—4	4—7	7—9
Living . . .			27
Malignant .			4
Benign . .			23
Grade 4 .			6
Grade 3 .			9
Grade 2 .			8
Dead			
Malignant .		1	
Grade 4 . .	1		

---

[1] At onset of therapy.

90 mm Hg for these periods of time. Time without drugs has varied from three to seven years.

Drug toxicity. Serious toxicity to three agents occurred, hydralazine, hexamethonium ion and mecamylamine ion. None was detected as caused by pentolinium or chlorisondamine.

Hydralazine. Toxicity resulting in signs suggestive of or positive findings of disseminated lupus erythematosus occurred in 49 patients (15.8% of those continuing treatment). Azotemia was present in 9, malignant hypertension without azotemia in 12, benign hypertension, grade 4 in 10, grade 3 in 12, grade 2 in 2, and secondary manifestations were ungraded in 4. Survival and mortality rates are shown in Table 3. Seventeen are dead, 10 living four to seven years, 6 one to four, and 1 less than a year.

Table 3. *Serious drug toxicity in hypertensive patients with hydralazine and ganglionic blocking agents, survival rates*

Toxicity from:	No. Patients	% Living	Dead—survived (years)			Living for (years)		
			< 1	1—4	4—7	1—4	4—7	7+
Hexamethonium ion . .	9	*11.1*						
Malignant with azotemia	6	*0*	6					
Malignant without azotemia	2	*0*	2					
Benign, grade 4	1							1
Mecamylamine ion . . .	8	*25.0*						
Malignant with azotemia	6	*33.3*	3	1			2	
Malignant without azotemia	2	*0*		1	1			
Hydralazine	49							
Malignant with azotemia	9	*44.4*		1	4		2	2
Malignant without azotemia	12	*58.3*	1	2	2		1	6
Benign, grade 4	10	*70.0*		1	2			7
Benign, grade 3	12	*75.0*		1	2			9
Benign, grade 2	2	*100.0*						2
Benign, ungraded . . .	4	*75.0*		1			2	1

Thirty-two are living, 27 for seven to nine years, and 5 for four to seven. Toxicity was always preceded by diastolic normotension and usually by hypotension. In no case was disseminated lupus a cause of death; in every case, stopping administration of the drug resulted in reversal of all signs and symptoms except for the rare instance of mild renal insufficiency.

Hexamethonium ion. Nine patients showed signs during life or at post mortem examination of the "hexamethonium lung" or acute interstitial fibrous pneumonitis. Eight died in less than one year, 6 being azotemic and 2 in malignant stages without azotemia. The course was often rapidly downhill, lasting one to two weeks. In one azotemic individual, pulmonary lesions and symptoms temporarily regressed with the use of hydrocortisone. One patient in benign stages, apparently with the disease, survived.

Mecamylamine. Flapping tremor and mental disturbances including hallucinations appeared in 8 individuals in malignant stages, 6 of whom were azotemic. Two with azotemia have survived from four to seven years while taking other ganglionic blocking agents. After appearance of the tremor, death often occurred within a month or more. Discontinuation of all ganglionic blockade in 3 cases was followed by early death.

Comment

As we are aware of no other study comparable to this one, where doses of drugs were large enough to achieve diastolic normotension in most (79%) cases (7) and where half the cases represented malignant stages of the disease, it would be unrewarding to compare these results with those of other studies of chemotherapy, using smaller doses or different combinations of drugs. Some reference point, however, can be established as to the value of this particular form of chemotherapy by comparing these survival rates with those of patients subjected to lumbodorsal sympathectomy (9) (Table 4). Azotemia has usually been a contraindication for sympathectomy; therefore azotemic patients were omitted.

Table 4. *Comparison of survival rates of non-azotemic patients treated by ganglionic blockade and hydralazine, by lumbodorsal sympathectomy and by older forms of "medical management", for 7 to 9 years*

Smithwick's group	"Medical"		Surgical		Chemotherapy	
	No. cases	%	No. cases	%	No. cases	%
4	119	3	157	35	89	63
3	149	30	344	70	73	84
2	293	50+	1077	83	20	80

"Cooperation" of the patient is secured after surgery, while drugs can be discontinued at will; therefore, patients discontinuing drugs were excluded. The results are better with drugs in groups 4 and 3 and about the same in group 2 when compared with lumbodorsal sympathectomy. Others using single agents, smaller doses or other methods of measuring blood pressure have not, to our knowledge, caused results comparable to ours. Survival in patients who have not achieved strict normotension has not been as high as in those who have (7).

We have been unable to differentiate on purely physical grounds between patients who continued therapy and those who discontinued it. Withdrawal of drugs was either done on the orders of another physician sceptical of their potencies, or by the patient because of side effects or bother. Having seen sudden deaths from cerebral hemorrhage and heart failure and rapid worsening of renal insufficiency shortly after withdrawal or the substitution of placebos, and the almost consistent development of drug resistance requiring very much larger doses later on, we were careful not to discontinue drugs except rarely in milder stages of the disease. The group discontinuing drugs, therefore, serves as a control, differing from the treated group perhaps only in innate psychological characteristics.

It is possible that some of the basic causes of hypertension differ in persons from different areas of the world. Therefore, the results here reported apply only to patients native to St. Louis, Missouri, and to most mid-western and some eastern and southern states from which our patients came. We have not subdivided our results for males and females, various age groups, or white and Negro races in the interests of simplicity; Negroes, on the whole, had almost twice the white mortality rates, while patients older than age 50 fared almost as well as those under 50; men did almost as well as women and ward patients almost as well as private (7).

Summary and conclusion

By the use of doses of ganglionic blocking agents and hydralazine sufficient to achieve sustained normotension, 369 patients were treated for periods of up to nine years. Half were in malignant stages and one-fourth showed azotemia. Drugs were discontinued in the case of 62 who served as a form of control. Cases were selected on the basis of the severity of disease, milder stages being excluded.

Survival rates were: Malignant hypertension with azotemia, 14.9%; malignant hypertension without azotemia, 72.2%; "benign" hypertension, grade 4 (Smithwick) 65.1%; grade 3, 83.6%; grade 2, 80%. In patients discontinuing therapy, survival rates were: Azotemia, 0%; malignant hypertension, 11.1%; grade 4 benign, 9.1%; grade 3, 50%; grade 2, 60%.

29 patients, 5 of whom had malignant hypertension, have maintained normotension for three or more years' treatment during which time necessary drug doses gradually diminished to the vanishing point. In these cases normotension without further drug therapy has been observed for periods of 3—7 years. Two have died of coronary occlusion. The other 27 can be regarded as "cured" for the time being.

This form of intense chemotherapy or a similar regimen is indicated in all severe forms of the hypertensive diseases. Control of blood pressure at normotensive levels is associated with increased life span in an otherwise fatal disorder. The limits of effectiveness of chemotherapy for survival lie in severe azotemic states, but even at these stages life can often be prolonged for several years.

Résumé

369 malades ont été traités pendant des périodes allant jusqu'à 9 ans par les doses de gangiloplégiques et d'hydralazine nécessaires à maintenir une tension artérielle normale. La moitié d'entre eux était au stade de malignité et un quart présentait de l'hyperazotémie. Les médicaments ne purent être administrés de façon adéquate dans 62 cas qui servirent ainsi de témoins. Les cas ont été sélectionnés en raison de la gravité de la maladie, les stades moins avancés ayant été exclus.

Les pourcentages de survie ont été les suivants:

hypertension maligne avec hyperazotémie	14,9%
hypertension maligne sans hyperazotémie	72,2%
hypertension «bénigne», stade 4 (Smithwick)	65,1%
stade 3	83,6%
stade 2	80 %

Chez les témoins, les taux de survie furent les suivants:

hyperazotémie	0 %
hypertension maligne	11,1%
hypertension «bénigne», stade 4	9,1%
stade 3	50 %
stade 2	60 %

Cette forme de chimiothérapie intensive ou tout autre traitement analogue sont indiqués dans toutes les formes graves de la maladie hypertensive. Le retour de la tension artérielle à des chiffres normaux ~'accompagne d'une amélioration du pronostic vital d'une maladie qui serait autrement mortelle. Les limites de l'efficacité de la chimiothérapie en ce qui concerne la survie de tels malades sont constituées par les états hyperazotémiques graves, mais même à ce stade, la vie peut encore souvent être prolongée de plusieurs années.

References

1. Reubi, F. C.: Proc. Soc. Exper. Biol. Med. (U.S.A.) **73**, 102 (1950).
2. Schroeder, H. A.: A.M.A. Arch. Int. Med. **89**, 523 (1952).
3. Schroeder, H. A., and J. D. Morrow: Med. Clin. North America **37**, 991 (1953).
4. Schroeder, H. A., J. D. Morrow, and H. M. Perry jr.: Circulation (U.S.A.) **8**, 672 (1953).
5. Schroeder, H. A.: Amer. J. Med. **17**, 540 (1954).
6. Schroeder, H. A.: J. Chron. Dis. (U.S.A.) **1**, 497 (1955).
7. Perry, H. M., jr., and H. A. Schroeder: A.M.A. Arch. Int. Med. **102**, 418 (1958).
8. Smithwick, R. H.: J. Chron. Dis. (U.S.A.) **1**, 477 (1955).
9a. Smithwick, R. H.: Splanchnicectomy in the treatment of essential hypertension. In: Hypertension. The first Hahnemann symposium on hypertensive disease. Ed.: J. Moyer, p. 681. Philadelphia: W. B. Saunders Co. 1959.
9b. Smithwick, R. H.: The role of the sympathetic nervous system in essential hypertension in man. In: A Symposium on essential hypertension, p. 284. Boston: Wright & Potter Printing Company 1951.

The late effects of hypotensive drug therapy on renal functions of patients with essential hypertension

By

F. C. REUBI

Introduction

It has been well established that the renal functions of patients with essential hypertension may be essentially normal during the initial stage of the illness (*6, 14*). As the disease progresses, however, they become gradually impaired. This functional impairment may result from organic changes (arteriolar sclerosis, arteriolar necrosis or superimposed pyelonephritis) and/or from purely hemodynamic factors (arteriolar spasms, congestive heart failure). The degree of functional impairment, the rate of renal deterioration, and the significance of the etiological factors are extremely variable in different patients.

Experimental work in rats has suggested that the basic lesion of malignant hypertension, the arteriolar necrosis, is dependent on the level of arterial pressure (*1, 8*). On the other hand, dogs appear to be more resistant to the nephrosclerotic effects of experimental hypertension than are rats (*5, 7*). In man, the controversy as to the primacy of high blood pressure in the pathogenesis of arterial changes, especially nephrosclerosis, has not yet been resolved. There is, however, a considerable body of evidence to indicate that high arterial pressure participates to some extent in the causation of vascular lesions, at least in malignant cases (*12*). Since it is now possible not only to achieve a significant reduction of blood pressure in many hypertensive patients, but also to measure the glomerular filtration rate and the renal plasma flow in man (*6*), it would appear that a new approach has been made to this problem.

During such a study, however, several difficulties may be encountered and have to be considered here briefly.

The first question which arises concerns the reliability of clearance methods in hypertensive patients. As the glomerular filtration rate is usually less reduced than is the PAH-clearance, it seems that the main problem is to ascertain the validity of the latter. This can be achieved by determining the extraction ratio of PAH, using renal vein catheterization and employing the following equations:

$$\text{True renal plasma flow} = \frac{C_{PAH}}{E_{PAH}} = \frac{U_{PAH}\,V}{P_{PAH} - R_{PAH}}$$

where C_{PAH} = PAH-clearance

E_{PAH} = PAH-extraction ratio

P_{PAH}, R_{PAH} and U_{PAH} = PAH-concentrations in arterial blood, renal venous blood, and urine

V = urine volume per minute.

We determined C_{PAH} and E_{PAH} simultaneously in 30 hypertensive patients with various degrees of renal impairment. In normal subjects the extraction ratio usually lies between 0.95 and 0.83 (15). We found it to be within the normal range in 22 (73%) hypertensive subjects, averaging for the whole group 0.84 (15). In only 8 cases, most of them having a PAH-clearance below 300 ml/min, was the extraction ratio somewhat reduced, ranging from 0.61 to 0.81. Therefore, we can consider that in most hypertensive patients the PAH-clearance is a good approximation of the renal plasma flow.

The acute effects of hypotensive drugs upon renal hemodynamics have been studied extensively by numerous investigators. However, if our purpose is to examine whether hypotensive drug therapy is effective in preventing the development of renal lesions, only long-term observations can be used. Short-term investigations are inadequate for several reasons:

1. In patients with nephrosclerosis an acute drop in blood pressure will generally produce a marked impairment of the glomerular filtration rate, and to a lesser extent of the renal plasma flow. In many cases it can be shown that the changes observed in renal hemodynamics are related to a corresponding reduction of the cardiac output (10). But if the blood pressure is maintained at the same level for weeks or months, a progressive adjustment of the arteriolar tone will take place. This will result in a lowering of the peripheral resistance accompanied by an increase in cardiac output and renal functions as well (4).

2. In acute experiments, various hypotensive drugs may influence renal hemodynamics in a different manner. It has been shown, for instance, that hydralazine can produce a significant increase in renal blood flow (13), while other drugs usually reduce the PAH-clearance. On the other hand, chlorothiazide may reduce the glomerular filtration rate, even when it does not change the blood pressure (16). These differences are, however, much less

significant when the renal functions are measured again after the patient has been treated continuously for 4 weeks (Table 1) (*13*). Furthermore, it is seldom possible to achieve effective hypotensive therapy with only one drug, so that in most cases successfully treated the renal changes observed will result from the combination of several effects.

Table 1. *Per cent changes from control values in mean blood pressure and renal functions of hypertensive patients after 4 weeks of hypotensive treatment*

	Mean blood pressure	$C_{In}(C_T)$	C_{PAH}
Rauwolfia (10 cases)	$- 3.7$	$- 2.4$	-2.8
	$(+10/-29)$	$(+42/-28)$	$(+12/-14)$
Chlorothiazide (11 cases) . . .	-11.6	$- 7.5$	-0.8
	$(+ 1/-33)$	$(+31/-33)$	$(+22/-17)$
Ganglionic blocking agent (15 cases)	$- 7.0$	-12.5	-6.5
	$(+ 4/-15)$	$(+8/-43)$	$(+16/-38)$
Hydralazine (12 cases)	$- 7.3$	$+ 3.9$	$- 0.5$
	$(+ 8/-22)$	$(+20/-19)$	$(+ 8/-13)$

But even during the course of long-term studies, there are several pitfalls to be avoided:

1. Another kidney disease, for instance chronic pyelonephritis, may develop or become exacerbated in hypertensive patients under treatment. We should like to report briefly 2 examples:

Case I (Table 2) — P. G., 1907. — This patient suffered from severe essential hypertension for many years. Until 1958, no effective treatment had been given. The patient then received chlorothiazide and showed an excellent blood pressure response. But simultaneously, signs of urinary tract infection were noticed and renal functions became progressively impaired. The patient died in renal failure $1^{1}/_{2}$ years later. Post-mortem examination showed vascular nephrosclerosis and superimposed pyelonephritis with papillary necrosis.

Table 2. *Serial observations of renal clearances in a patient with hypertension and pyelonephritis (P. G., 1907)*

Date	B.P. mm Hg	C_T ml/min	C_{PAH} ml/min	FF	NPN mg.-%	Hypotensive treatment
1956	200/130	50.5	239	0.212	26	none
3/1958	210/140	42	133	0.315	36	none
5/1958	170/115	31	110	0.28	31	chlorothiazide
6/1958	165/110	13	70	0.186	44	chlorothiazide
2/1959	200/100	14.5	53	0.27	47	chlorothiazide
5/1959	170/100	—	—	—	120	none
5/1959	160/110	—	—	—	142	none
6/1959	Died of uremia					

Case II (Table 3) — E. B., 1905. — In this patient, suffering for many years from essential hypertension, serial clearance measurements were performed between 1955 and 1960. Until 1958, there was only a very slow impairment of renal functions. At this time, the patient was placed on chlorothiazide, hydralazine and mecamylamine. The blood pressure response was satisfactory. However, his general condition seemed to deteriorate progressively. At the end of 1959, a diagnosis of hypernephroma with metastases was made. In the meanwhile clearances had dropped markedly. The patient died of cachexia several months later. Post-mortem examination showed functional exclusion of one kidney through tumor compression of the ureter and a large metastasis in the contralateral kidney. There was only moderate vascular nephrosclerosis.

Table 3. *Serial observations of renal clearances in a patient with hypertension and hypernephroma* (E. B., 1905)

Date	B.P. mm Hg	c_T ml/min	c_{PAH} ml/min	FF	Hypotensive treatment
1955	200/115	142	623	0.228	none
1956	180/115	116	453	0.256	none
2/1958	210/130	121	472	0.256	none
3/1958	200/120	103	446	0.230	chlorothiazide
4/1958 to 12/1959	180/115 to 190/100	—	—	—	chlorothiazide, hydralazine, mecamylamine
1/1960	175/90	25	83	0.307	none
3/1960	Died of cachexia (hypernephroma)				

In these 2 cases, the rapid deterioration of the kidney functions might have led to the erroneous conclusion that extensive arteriolar necrosis had developed during hypotensive treatment.

2. In hypertensive patients with congestive heart failure, the clearances values may be markedly depressed. This reduction is

Table 4. *Influence of heart failure on renal hemodynamics in a patient with hypertension* (A. A., 1895)

Date	B.P. mm Hg	c_T ml/min	c_{PAH} ml/min	FF	Condition	Treatment
1/1957	200/125	109	343	0.317	fair; no heart failure	none
5/1959	230/130	76	178	0.426	congestive heart failure	none
6/1959	215/110	110	255	0.421	fair; heart failure markedly improved	digitalisation, hydrochlorothiazide, hydralazine, reserpine

only partly due to the organic changes in the kidneys. Under bed rest, digitalisation and hypotensive therapy, renal clearances may improve markedly. But of course this improvement does not imply a regression of the nephrosclerotic changes. This aspect of the problem is demonstrated by the course in patient A. A., 1895 (Table 4).

3. As already stressed by CORCORAN and PAGE (2), the renal deterioration tends more often to be episodic rather than steadily progressive, at least in moderate essential hypertension. The rate of progression, therefore, in treated and untreated cases has to be estimated with great caution and only over long periods of time or in large groups of patients.

4. It is important that patients should only be assigned to the "treated group" if their blood pressure has been significantly reduced for a long period of time. While today most patients will receive some therapy, many of them are not treated in an adequate manner and cannot, therefore, be considered in comparative studies.

The present study has been performed with these considerations in mind.

Material and methods

72 patients with moderate to very severe essential hypertension have been followed over 1 to 5 years. 33 cases had no effective treatment during this period. In the remaining 39, the blood pressure had been significantly reduced. All patients were under ambulatory medical supervision; on certain occasions they were hospitalised for a short time. The renal functions were controlled repeatedly in every patient during the follow-up period, using the clearance technique (204 determinations of the sodium thiosulphate [or inulin] and PAH-clearance).

These patients have been divided into 3 groups according to the severity of the hypertension.

Group I: Diastolic blood pressure < 120 mm Hg, retinal changes of grade I to II (KEITH-WAGENER);

Group II: Diastolic blood pressure between 120—150 mm Hg, retinal changes of grade II;

Group III: Diastolic blood pressure > 130 mm Hg, retinal changes of grade III to IV.

In each group the renal functions of the treated and untreated patients have been compared (Table 5). The average changes at the end of the follow-up period have been calculated per year in percent of the control values. The t-test has been used to determine the significance of the differences.

Table 5. *Renal functional status in 72 treated and untreated hypertensive patients over a follow-up period of 1—5 years*

Group I. Diastolic B. P.: <120 mm Hg — Retinal changes: Grade I—II

No. of cases: 25	Untreated (10 cases)		Treated (15 cases)	
	Control	End of follow-up	Control	End of follow-up
Range of blood pressure (mm Hg)	150/100—205/120	170/85—200/110	165/105—230/120	155/90—200/105
Range of glomerular filtration rate (ml/min)	74—119	68—119	69—124	58—128
Range of PAH-clearance (ml/min)	299—538	292—614	237—575	213—538
Average follow-up time	$2^3/_4$ years (1—$4^1/_2$)		$2^1/_2$ years (1—5)	
Average changes per year in percent of control values				
Glomerular filtration rate . . .	—1.6 (+14/—23)		—3.1 (+28/—25)	
PAH-clearance	—1.3 (+ 7/— 7)		+1.2 (+28/—14)	

Group II. Diastolic B. P.: 120—150 mm Hg — Retinal changes: Grade II

No. of cases: 26	Untreated (15 cases)		Treated (11 cases)	
	Control	End of follow-up	Control	End of follow-up
Range of blood pressure (mm Hg)	165/120—260/150	160/115—230/150	180/120—250/150	155/90—215/130
Range of glomerular filtration rate (ml/min)	56—142	54—128	55— 96	51—102
Range of PAH-clearance (ml/min)	221—623	152—590	233—480	189—455
Average follow-up time	$2^3/_4$ years (1—5)		$2^1/_4$ years (1—5)	
Average changes per year in percent of control values				
Glomerular filtration rate . . .	—1.7 (+6/—10)		—3.6 (+8/—16)	
PAH-clearance	—5.0 (+4/—14)		—1.5 (+7/—16)	

Group III. Diastolic B. P.: > 130 mm Hg — Retinal changes: Grade III—IV

No. of cases: 21	Untreated (8 cases)		Treated (13 cases)	
	Control	End of follow-up	Control	End of follow-up
Range of blood pressure (mm Hg)	200/130—250/160	230/100—280/175	210/130—280/175	135/95—200/130
Range of glomerular filtration rate (ml/min)	25—127	11—119	26—119	15— 98
Range of PAH-clearance (ml/min) . . .	93—515	55—450	118—450	71—466
Average follow-up time	18 months (3 months—5 years)		2 years (1—4)	
Average changes per year in percent of control values				
Glomerular filtration rate . . .	—28.6 (+10/—100)		—7.4 (+18/—42)	
PAH-clearance	—36.5 (— 2/—100)		—2.7 (+42/—30)	

Results

(Table 5 and Fig. 1)

Group I: In the untreated patients the mean duration of follow-up was $2^3/_4$ years. There was an average decrease of 1.6% per year in C_T and 1.3% in C_{PAH}.

In the treated patients the mean duration of follow-up was $2^1/_2$ years. There was an average decrease of 3.1% per year in C_T and an increase of 1.2% in C_{PAH}. The differences observed between untreated and treated patients are not significant (p > 0.1).

Group II: In the untreated patients the mean duration of follow-up was $2^3/_4$ years. There was an average decrease of 1.7% per year in C_T and 5.0% in C_{PAH}.

In the treated patients the mean duration of follow-up was $2^1/_2$ years. There was an average decrease of 3.6% per year in C_T and 1.5% in C_{PAH}.

The differences between untreated and treated patients are not significant (p> 0.1).

Group III: In the untreated patients the mean duration of follow-up was 18 months. On the average there was a decrease of 28.6% per year in C_T and 36.5% in C_{PAH}.

One patient who died after 3 months has been included in this group. In this subject the decrease in C_T and C_{PAH} during the follow-up period was 64% and 68%, so that we arbitrarily assumed a decrease of 100% per year. If this case is left out, the average decrease in C_T and C_{PAH} for the remaining patients is 18.5% and 27.5% respectively.

In the treated patients the mean duration of follow-up was 2 years. On the average there was a decrease of 7.4% per year in C_T and 2.7% in C_{PAH}.

21*

The differences observed between untreated and treated patients are significant ($p < 0.05$ for C_T and $p < 0.01$ for C_{PAH}).

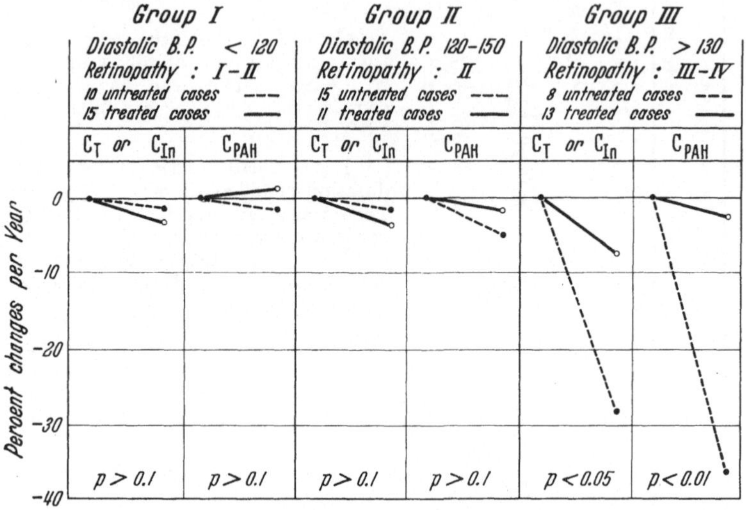

Fig. 1. Changes in renal functions of treated and untreated hypertensive patients during a follow-up period of 1—5 years. The 72 cases have been divided into 3 groups according to the severity of the disease. The changes are expressed in percent of control values per year

Discussion

So far, only a few studies have been concerned with the comparison of renal functions in treated and untreated patients with essential hypertension. Some years ago, CORCORAN and PAGE (2) reported serial observations in 3 cases with malignant hypertension. Each was treated with hydralazine or hexamethonium. All showed some improvement in the degree of renal vasoconstriction during therapy. PERRY and SCHROEDER (11) found an arrest of the renal vascular deterioration in patients with malignant hypertension submitted to hypotensive treatment. An extensive study has been published recently by MOYER et al. (9), who report serial clearance determinations in 64 patients. These patients were divided into 2 groups according to their diastolic blood pressure (more or less than 130 mm Hg). 45 were treated and 19 were not. From their results, the authors conclude that in malignant, severe, and moderately severe hypertension renal deterioration can be arrested by effective treatment, whereas in mild and moderate hypertension there is no difference in renal status between treated and untreated patients.

From our own results, it would appear that only in very severe or malignant cases is hypertensive therapy capable of slowing down the progressive decline in renal functions known to occur in untreated hypertensive patients. In group I the average decrease per year observed in untreated patients is very small and does not differ significantly from the figures obtained by WATKIN and SHOCK (*17*) for the agewise decrement in normal individuals. Treated patients of this group behave similarly. In group II the changes in glomerular filtration rate are quite comparable to the corresponding figures in group I. With respect to C_{PAH}, untreated patients show a somewhat greater decrease than treated subjects. The difference, however, is not statistically significant ($p > 0.1$).

If the individual case is considered rather than the mean, it appears that appreciable variations may be encountered within the same group (Table 6). While in some untreated patients, the kidney functions remain relatively stable over a long period of

Table 6. *Serial observations of renal functions in a few treated and untreated cases of moderate to severe hypertension*

Date	B.P. mm Hg	C_T ml/min	C_{PAH} ml/min	FF	Treatment
a) Stable renal functions in untreated case of group I (E. P., 1891)					
2/1955	200/115	74	310	0.240	none
3/1956	205/105	64	303	0.210	none
7/1959	195/105	68	294	0.232	none
b) Stable renal functions in treated case of group I (F. K., 1900)					
9/1955	205/120	110	540	0.204	none
5/1956	190/100	119	527	0.226	Ecolid
2/1958	190/105	119	473	0.261	chlorothiazide
2/1960	210/95	101	538	0.188	chlorothiazide, reserpine
c) Stable renal functions in treated and untreated case of group II (E. W., 1906)					
10/1955	240/140	67	261	0.256	none
1/1959	230/125	73	264	0.278	none; therapy started
2/1960	200/100	62	290	0.214	hydrochlorothiazide, hydralazine
d) Slow deterioration in untreated case of group II (V. E., 1922)					
10/1955	160/130	151	517	0.290	none
6/1957	160/125	120	502	0.238	none
9/1959	170/125	118	418	0.283	none

time, or even improve slightly, in other untreated cases of quite comparable severity there is a slow but definite decrease in both C_T and C_{PAH}. The same trends are also seen in the 2 treated subgroups.

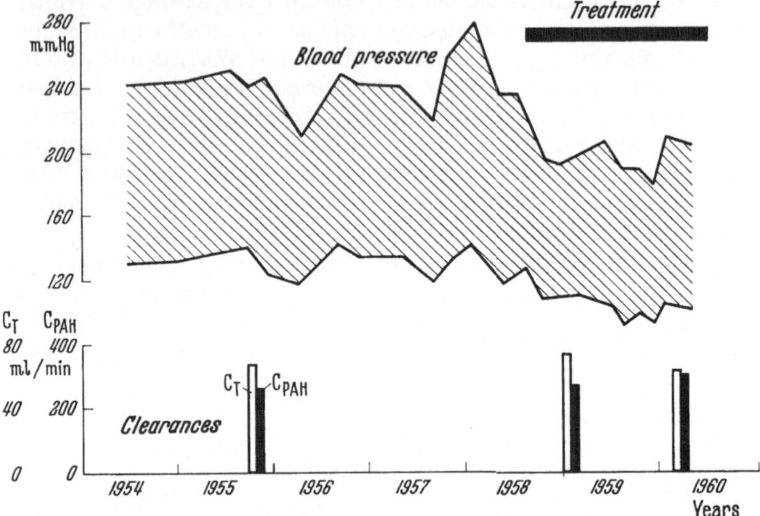

Fig. 2. Blood pressure and renal functions in a patient with moderately severe hypertension (Group II, case E.W.). Renal clearances remain stable over the whole follow-up period, before and under hypotensive treatment

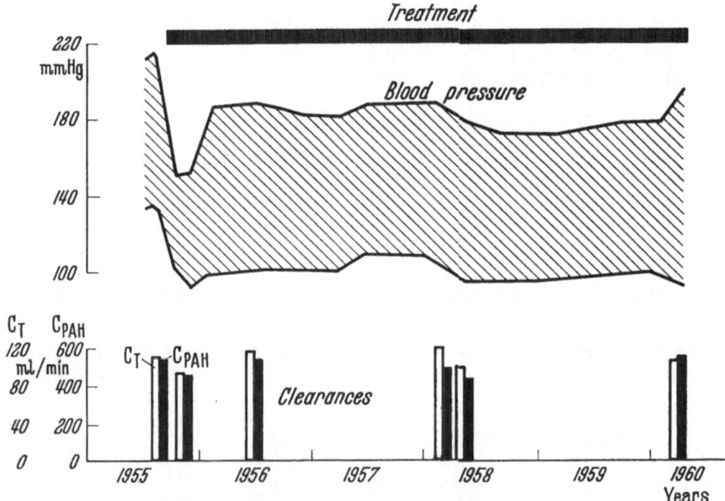

Fig. 3. Stable renal functions in a treated case of Group I (Case F.K.)

While in certain patients the improvement observed seems to be due to hypotensive treatment, it would appear that in others drug therapy is without influence on the renal functions (Figs. 2 and 3).

In group III, however, the differences between treated and untreated patients become significant. In untreated cases, the

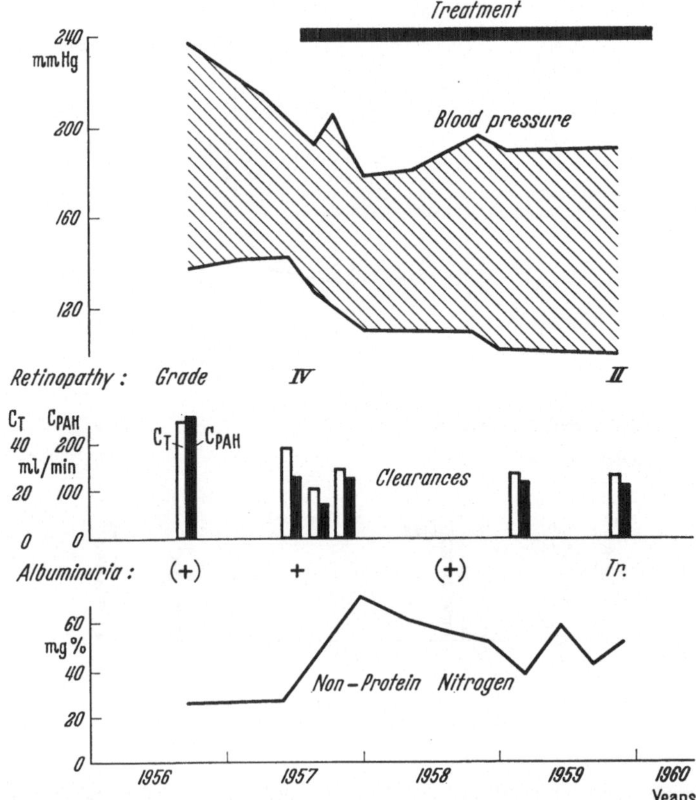

Fig. 4. Clinical course in a patient with malignant hypertension (Case A. M.). Marked deterioration of renal functions before therapy. Under hypotensive treatment there is first a further drop in thiosulphate and PAH clearances. Later on, renal functions remain stabilized at a low level

renal deterioration is obvious, but its rate is variable. It is most rapid in patients with high diastolic pressure together with grade IV retinal changes, and may be slower in less severe cases. If such patients receive adequate hypotensive drug therapy, there is, as a rule, an arrest of the renal deterioration (Figs. 4 and 5); at the beginning of the treatment, however, a further decrease in C_T and C_{PAH} is usually observed. Later on, the renal functions may remain at this level for months or years (Figs. 4), or they may improve gradually (Fig. 5); on rare occasions they will increase beyond the control values. In some severe cases, the progression is only partly inhibited (Table 7).

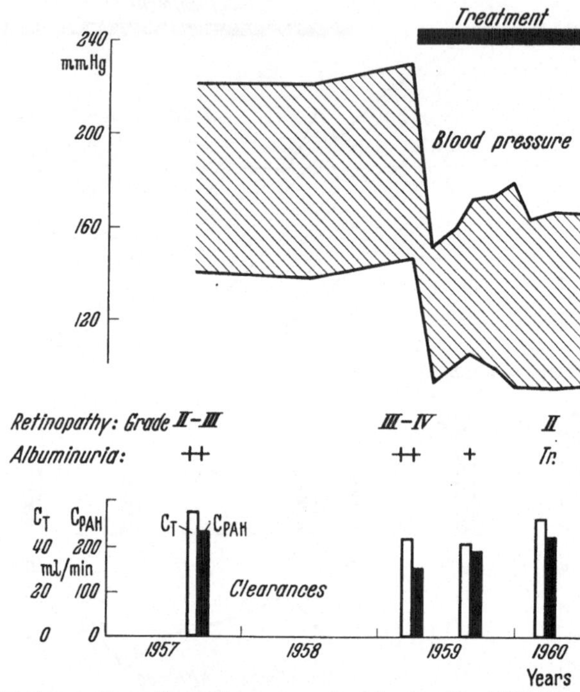

Fig. 5. Clinical course in a patient with very severe hypertension (Case M.B.). Renal functions show a marked deterioration before therapy and improve gradually under treatment

If the values for C_T and C_{PAH} are considered separately, it appears that the effects of therapy on C_{PAH} are very striking ($p < 0.01$), while the effects on C_T are somewhat less conspicuous ($p < 0.05$). In untreated cases, both C_T and C_{PAH} decrease at a rapid rate. In treated cases, C_T still shows a significant decrease of 7.4%. However, this reduction might be due to the drug therapy itself, as most of our cases were placed on chlorothiazide or hydrochlorothiazide, and these salidiuretics are known to depress the glomerular filtration rate, even in normotensive individuals (16). In treated cases, the decrease in C_{PAH} does not differ significantly from the values obtained in the other groups.

Table 7. *Serial observations of renal functions in 5 treated and untreated cases with very severe or malignant hypertension*

Date	B.P. mm Hg	C_T ml/min	C_{PAH} ml/min	FF	NPN mg %	Treatment
			a) Improvement in a treated case (R. N., 1914)			
1/1958	230/140	50	144	0.347	—	none, therapy started
8/1958	180/105	40	181	0.221	—	mecamylamine, hydralazine, hydrochlorothiazide
2/1960	170/95	53	194	0.274	—	hydralazine, hydrochlorothiazide
			b) Deterioration before therapy; gradual improvement under treatment (M. B., 1900)			
10/1957	220/140	55	233	0.236	—	none, or not effective
5/1959	230/145	44	156	0.281	—	none, effective therapy started
7/1959	180/90	42	193	0.217	—	hydralazine, hydrochlorothiazide, Singoserp
4/1960	165/90	52	222	0.235	—	hydralazine, hydrochlorothiazide, Singoserp
			c) Deterioration before therapy; stabilization under treatment (A. M., 1905)			
11/1956	230/130	51	260	0.196	23	none
7/1957	200/135	39	118	0.331	25	none, therapy started
8/1957	190/120	21	72	0.289	72	mecamylamine
9/1957	200/120	30	125	0.236	61	mecamylamine, hydralazine, chlorothiazide
3/1959	190/100	28	120	0.236	47	mecamylamine, hydralazine, chlorothiazide
10/1959	190/100	27	110	0.241	53	mecamylamine, hydralazine, chlorothiazide
			d) Abrupt decrease under therapy; later on, stabilization (G. J., 1904)			
1/1959	240/144	26	101	0.259	30	none, therapy started
2/1959	180/110	—	—	—	82	mecamylamine, hydrochlorothiazide
3/1959	180/120	12.5	62	0.204	60	mecamylamine, hydrochlorothiazide
9/1959	170/110	14.5	71	0.202	59	guanethidine, hydrochlorothiazide
4/1960	165/110	—	—	—	62	guanethidine, hydrochlorothiazide
			e) Stabilization under therapy; acute deterioration after arrest of treatment (M. M., 1898)			
1/1953	250/140	53.5	181	0.295	—	none, therapy started
6/1953	200/120	51	186	0.275	—	hexamethonium, hydralazine
11/1953	190/115	51	173	0.295	—	hexamethonium, hydralazine therapy discontinued
2/1954	280/175	18	56	0.321	—	none, died 5 days later

In cases with severely impaired renal function and very high diastolic pressure, the acute depression of renal hemodynamics produced by hypotensive therapy usually results in an increase in blood urea nitrogen or non-protein nitrogen (Fig. 4). This nitrogen retention may subside gradually after a couple of weeks, but in certain cases slight azotemia persists for months. We do not feel, however, that this symptom is of significance if at the same time the general condition improves and the proteinuria disappears.

Our observations seem to demonstrate the value of hypotensive treatment in arresting the renal deterioration associated with very severe or malignant hypertension. Even patients with a marked impairment of kidney functions may respond well to therapy. There is little doubt that excellent therapeutic results may be observed in most cases, if not in all.

In less severe cases, however, we found no conclusive evidence that hypotensive drug therapy would prevent renal deterioration or lead to an improvement of the renal status. But even in untreated patients of this type, the decrease in renal clearances is very slow. Observations should perhaps be extended over a longer follow-up period before the value of such therapy can be demonstrated. Nevertheless, we do not feel that this point is of great practical significance. There are many good reasons for treating hypertensive patients early, before they come into the malignant stage of the disease. In patients with moderate to severe hypertension, therapy is not primarily directed against renal lesions. But it is not unlikely that any kind of therapy intended for relief of other vascular symptoms may also be beneficial to the kidneys.

Summary

Serial observations of renal functions (glomerular filtration rate and PAH-clearance) have been performed in 72 hypertensive patients over a follow-up period extending from 1 to 5 years. 33 cases had no effective treatment during this period, while in 39 the blood pressure could be significantly reduced.

Our patients have been divided into 3 groups according to the severity of the disease:

Group I: Diastolic blood pressure: < 120 mm Hg. Retinal changes: grade I—II.

Group II: Diastolic blood pressure: between 120 and 150 mm Hg. Retinal changes: grade II.

Group III: Diastolic blood pressure: > 130 mm Hg. Retinal changes: grade III—IV.

Our observations show that in groups I and II the renal deterioration per year is very slow and does not differ significantly in treated and untreated patients. In group III the average decrease per year in untreated patients was —28.6% for the glomerular filtration rate and —36.5% for the PAH-clearance. In treated cases these values were —7.4% and —2.7% respectively.

The differences between treated and untreated patients are statistically significant.

These findings strongly suggest that in very severe and malignant hypertension, hypotensive therapy is of great value in arresting renal deterioration.

Résumé

Des déterminations de la fonction rénale (filtration glomérulaire et clearance du PAH) ont été faites à plusieurs reprises chez 72 hypertendus au cours d'une période d'observation de 1—5 ans. 33 cas ne bénéficiaient d'aucun traitement efficace, tandis que chez 39 la tension artérielle pouvait être réduite de façon significative.

Ces 72 patients ont été divisés en 3 groupes cliniques:

Groupe I: tension artérielle minima < 120 mm Hg; lésions rétiniennes du ler-2e degré.

Groupe II: tension artérielle minima entre 120—150 mm Hg; lésions rétiniennes du 2e degré.

Groupe III: tension artérielle minima > 130 mm Hg; lésions rétiniennes du 3e—4e degré.

Nos observations montrent que dans les groupes I et II, la détérioration rénale est très lente et ne diffère pas statistiquement chez les sujets traités et les témoins. Dans le groupe III, la diminution moyenne par année est de —28.6% pour la filtration glomérulaire et de —36.5% pour la clearance du PAH chez les sujets non traités; elle n'est que de —7.4% et —2.7% respectivement chez les sujets traités. Ces différences sont statistiquement significatives.

Nos résultats suggèrement fortement que chez les sujets souffrant d'hypertension très sévère ou maligne, le traitement hypotenseur est capable de stopper la progression des lésions rénales.

References

1. Byrom, F. B., and L. F. Dodson: Clin. Sc. (G.B.) 8, 1 (1949).
2. Corcoran, A. C., and I. H. Page: Med. Clin. North America, July 1955, p. 1027.
3. Cottier, P.: Helvet. med. acta, Suppl. 39 (1960).
4. Freis, E. D., J. C. Rose, E. A. Partenope et al.: J. Clin. Invest. (U.S.A.) 32, 1285 (1953).
5. Goldman, M. L., H. A. Schroeder, G. J. Dammin: Amer. J. Med. 14, 751 (1953).
6. Goldring, W., and H. Chasis: Hypertension and hypertensive disease. New York: The Commonwealth Fund. 1944.
7. Hermann, H.: J. méd. Lyon 31, 811 (1950).
8. Masson, G. M. C., A. C. Corcoran, and I. H. Page: Cleveland Clin. Quart. 26, 24 (1959).
9. Moyer, J. H., C. Heider, K. Pevey, and R. V. Ford: Amer. J. Med. 24, 177 (1958).
10. Notter, B., F. Wüthrich, A. Schmid et al.: Helvet. med. acta 23, 509 (1956).
11. Perry, H. M., and H. A. Schroeder: Circulation (U.S.A.) 14, 105 (1956).
12. Pickering, G. W.: High blood pressure. London: Churchill 1955.
13. Reubi, F.: Proc. Soc. Exper. Biol. Med. (U.S.A.) 73, 102 (1950).
14. Reubi, F.: Helvet. med. acta, Suppl. 26 (1950); Bruxelles-méd. 33, 1909 (1953).
15. Reubi, F., Nierenkrankheiten. Berne and Stuttgart: Huber 1960.
16. Reubi, F., E. Schmid, and P. Cottier: Circulation (U.S.A.) (in press).
17. Watkin, D. M., and N. W. Shock: J. Clin. Invest. (U.S.A.) 34, 969 (1955).

Late results of surgical therapy
(sympathectomy and adrenalectomy)

By

H. Sarre

The fact that medical therapy often yielded unsatisfactory results in severe cases of hypertension, especially among younger patients suffering from malignant hypertension, led already some decades ago to attempts at surgical treatment in the form of neurosurgery. Brüning, in 1923, was the first to advocate resection of the splanchnic nerves. In America, Adson (1925) performed lumbar sympathectomy on hypertensive patients; later, together with Craig, he developed a method consisting of bilateral sub-diaphragmatic resection of the splanchnic nerves and of the superior lumbar sympathetic chain (1935). In France, Leriche and Fontaine supplemented this procedure by unilateral adrenalectomy — in some cases together with renal decapsulation.

Since subdiaphragmatic sympathectomy produced unsatisfactory results, the trend of subsequent developments was towards resection of more extensive portions of the sympathetic system — a trend in which American surgeons took the lead. Thanks to the skilful technique they employed, Peet (1933) and Smithwick (1938) rendered the operation safer, and by resorting to more extensive sympathetic and splanchnic resection they also achieved a very considerable improvement in the results obtained (Peet performs bilateral supradiaphragmatic splanchnicectomy and sympathectomy from T 10 to T 12; Smithwick resects from T 9 to L 2).

In 1948, Peet reported on 2,000 cases operated on in this way, which had been observed over a period of 15 years; Smithwick et al. published figures of comparable magnitude. The statistics revealed that the patients who had undergone surgery survived much longer than those receiving conservative treatment. Smithwick classified his cases according to the severity of their hypertension by reference to a combination of the most important criteria, such as diastolic blood pressure, eyegrounds, and cardiac, cerebral, and renal complications. The percentage of survivors rose as follows:

	Group	1	2	3	4
	Survivors %				
(non-operated)	from	70	46	17	0%
(operated)	to	87	74	57	32%
	Difference	17	28	40	32%

In all four groups, the improvement in life expectancy of the patients operated on is clear-cut and statistically significant. This applies particularly to groups 2, 3 and 4, i. e. to the cases with severe to very severe malignant hypertension.

In Germany during the last 15 years, ZENKER in particular — in collaboration with VOLHARD, SARRE, KAMPMANN, and PFEFFER — has operated on quite a large number of hypertensives using the methods of PEET or SMITHWICK. The patients were classified not on the basis of the eyeground findings, the blood-pressure levels, or the renal findings, but according to whether the disease was still in a stage characterised by purely functional disorders or already involved organic complications such as coronary artery sclerosis and infarction, cerebrosclerosis, nephrosclerosis, etc. A distinction was accordingly drawn between 2 main groups (cf. Table 1).

Table 1

Group I: Functional disorders only

a) Diastolic blood pressure below 120 mm Hg, eyegrounds grade 1 or 2, no complications (benign, non-progressive hypertension).
b) Greater elevation of diastolic blood pressure (over 120 mm Hg), angiospastic retinopathy grade 3, headache, dizziness, disease progressive (incipient malignant hypertension). But still no organic complications.

Group II: With organic disorders

a) Diastolic blood pressure below 120 mm Hg, eyegrounds grade 1 or 2, but with cardiac or cerebral complications (infarction or apoplexy).
b) Diastolic blood pressure over 120 mm Hg, angiospastic retinitis (grade 3), complications as in a). Disease progressive (frank malignant hypertension).
c) Diastolic blood pressure over 130 mm Hg, severe angiospastic retinitis (grade 4), renal insufficiency and other complications (terminal stage of malignant hypertension).

Thus, the general criterion on which this classification is based is the absence or presence of organic manifestations of hypertension.

Following a preliminary report by us (ZENKER, SARRE, PFEFFER and collaborators, Ergebnisse der Inn. Med. 1952) on 176 patients operated on using the methods of PEET and SMITHWICK, there appeared a few years later a detailed account by PFEFFER, NIETH, and SCHNEIDER (1955) based on 206 cases of hypertension in which, after sympathectomy had been performed by ZENKER, the observation period amounted to at least 5 years. 306 hypertensive patients treated by conservative methods (low-salt diet, sedatives, anti-hypertensive drugs) were used as controls.

Fig. 1 shows the survival rates among the operated and non-operated cases in each group.

In the 6th year of the observation period, the percentage of survivors rose as follows

		Group			
Survivors %		Ib	IIa	IIb	IIc
(non-operated)	from	57.1	62.1	17.0	0%
(operated)	to	92.2	62.5	34.3	12%
Difference		35.1	0.4	17.3	12%

Group Ia is not included here, since among these cases of benign hypertension it was rightly concluded that hardly any patients were suitable for surgery; hence very few were operated on.

Group Ib (incipient malignant hypertension), consisting of patients with progressive disease, angiospastic retinitis, and severe subjective symptoms but no organic complications, bore the most impressive testimony to the superiority of sympathectomy over conservative therapy. Here, of 56 patients (100%) only 32 (57.1%) were still alive after 5 years of conservative treatment, whereas of 39 sympathectomised patients 36 (92.2%) survived over the same period. The difference is statistically significant ($\chi^2 = 11.9$; $p = $ greather than 99%).

In group IIa, comprising patients with organic disorders, coronary artery sclerosis, infarction or apoplexy, the results of surgery were no better and no worse than those obtained by conservative methods. After 5 years, the percentage of survivors receiving conservative treatment was 62.1% as compared with 62.5% in the case of those who underwent surgery.

In group IIb, i. e. patients with angiospastic retinitis and cerebral or cardiac complications, the prognosis was of course a poor one. Nevertheless, here the patients operated on had a distinctly better life expectancy. Of 67 hypertensives who underwent surgery, 23 (34.3%) were still alive after 5 years, as compared with only 11 (17%) of the 65 patients given conservative treatment. The difference is statistically significant ($\chi^2 = 4.31$, $p = $ greater than 95%).

Finally, in group IIc, made up of patients in the terminal stage of malignant hypertension, the life expectancy was extremely short; even in these cases, however, there is a marked difference between the figures for operated and non-operated patients. Of 48 patients receiving conservative therapy none was still alive after 5 years, whereas 12% of the sympathectomised patients had survived. In view of the small number of cases involved, however, this difference is not significant.

Of the hypertensives receiving conservative treatment, 29.6% died from uraemia, 17.4% from apoplexy, and 15% from heart failure. The figures for the sympathectomised cases are similar,

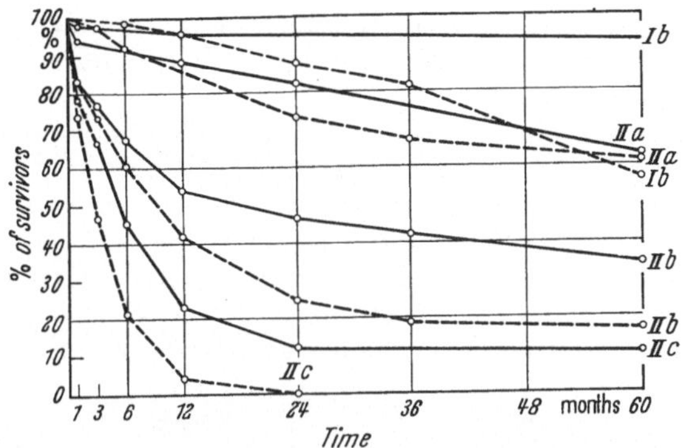

Fig. 1. Survivalrate of: ——— sympathectomised hypertensives; - - - hypertensives receiving conservative therapy followed up over 5 years. (For classification see text)

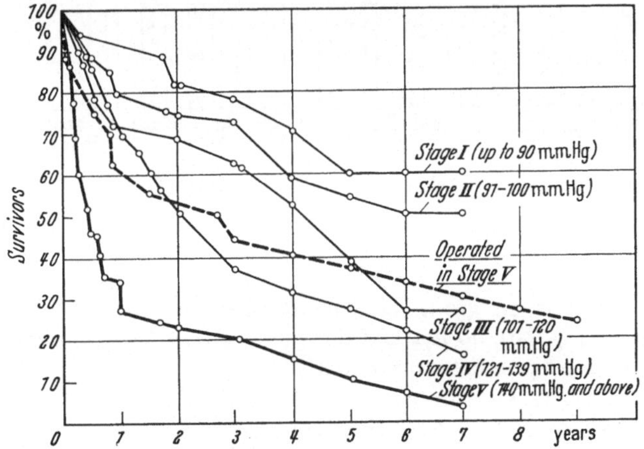

Fig. 2. Number of surviving hypertensives followed up over a period of 7—9 years and divided into 5 groups according to the height of their diastolic blood pressure. (The classification of the various stages according to diastolic pressure does not correspond to that adopted in the other diagrams). For comparison, the survival curve of sympathectomised hypertensives in Stage V is included. Note the appreciably better survival rate of the operated patients with malignant hypertension (diastolic pressure: 140 mm Hg and above)

except that, interestingly enough, the incidence of uraemia as the cause of death was lower. From this comparison it may be concluded that *sympathectomy improves the patient's life expectancy to a greater extent than conservative measures: this applies particularly to the first group (patients presenting functional disorders only)*, i. e. to cases where there are as yet no organic disorders (coronary artery sclerosis, cerebrosclerosis, nephrosclerosis) although the highly elevated blood pressure, the fact that the disease is worsening, and the serious state of the eyegrounds already indicate that the hypertension is of a progressive and malignant type. On the other hand, in group II the differences in life expectancy are only slight.

The improvement in life expectancy is only partly attributable to *a reduction in the systolic and diastolic blood pressure*. In group I (cf. Fig. 3a), the blood-pressure curves prior to operation show peaks at a level of 220—235 mm Hg systolic and 115—120 mm Hg diastolic. After operation, the systolic levels are concentrated around 160—175 mm Hg, i. e. 60 mm Hg lower, whereas the diastolic levels undergo little or no change; in other words, the decline in

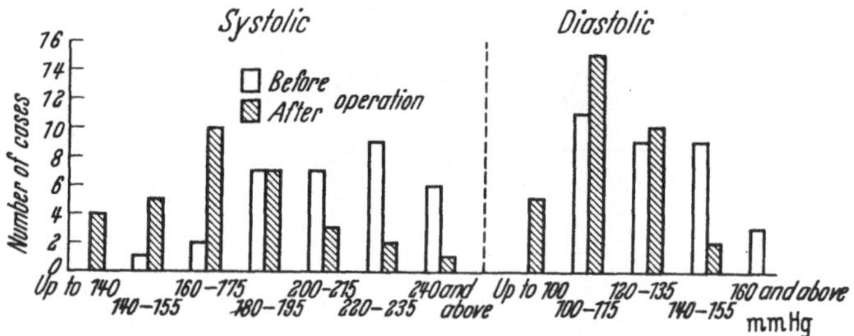

Fig. 3a. Blood-pressure levels before and after operation in group I: a) systolic, b) diastolic

blood pressure is considerable, but chiefly confined to the systolic levels.

By contrast, in group II, consisting of patients with organic lesions (cf. Fig. 3b), no marked decline in either the systolic or the diastolic blood pressures occurred.

Among 77 cases of hypertension treated by Peet in which there were no symptoms or complications, a very favourable effect on the blood pressure was achieved, 80.5% of the patients responding with a pronounced fall in pressure. Of 206 cases involving complications, however, only 34% showed notable reductions in blood pressure following sympathectomy.

Peet's experiences are thus closely matched by our own, which indicate that in the presence of organic complications no significant decline in blood pressure can be elicited by sympathectomy.

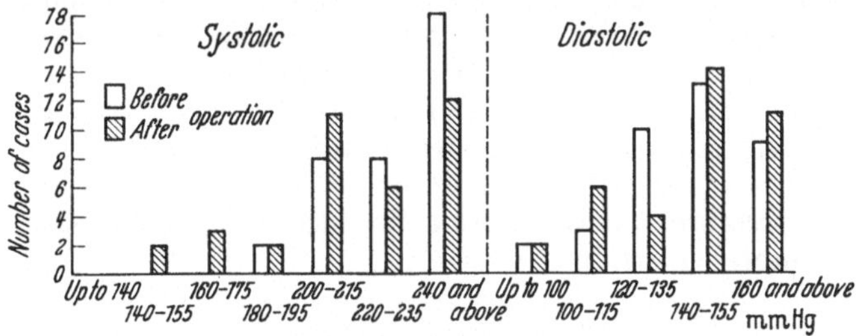

Fig. 3b. Blood pressure levels before and after operation in group II: a) systolic, b) diastolic

The response of the *eyegrounds* to surgery is outlined in Table 2. In groups I and II, taken together, the eyeground findings improved in 43% of cases, remained unchanged in 39%, and deteriorated in 18%. According to Peet's investigations, which to some extent, however, relate to more favourable cases, 82% of 88 patients suffering from angiospastic retinitis, with or without haemorrhages and exudate, showed an improvement 5—11 years after operation. There was a deterioration in only one case.

Table 2. *Eyeground findings after operation*

	No. of cases	No change	Improvement	Deterioration
Group I	24	11	13	0
Group II . . .	32	11	11	10
Groups I and II	56	22 (39%)	24 (43%)	10 (18%)

An improvement or a worsening in the state of the eyegrounds — as we and other authors have established — *is not always related to a decline or a rise in the blood pressure.* Even in cases where the blood pressure failed to drop, we often noted disappearance of retinal changes together with an objective improvement in vision. On the other hand, in certain cases angiospastic retinitis persisted although the blood pressure had been largely normalised. The improvement in vision and in the eyegrounds is indeed one of the most impressive results of sympathectomy, although in itself it has no prognostic significance as regards the pathological process viewed as a whole.

The size of the heart and the E. C. G.

In group I, the heart was of normal size in 10 cases and enlarged in 16 cases. 1—6 years after operation, in all the cases where the heart had been normal prior to surgery it had remained so and, in addition, a diminution in the size of the heart was noted in 8 (50%) of the cases of cardiac enlargement.

In group II, no diminution in the size of the heart was observed. *Cardiac decompensation is no contra-indication to sympathectomy.* In most cases, recompensation occurs after the post-operative fall in blood pressure, together with a decrease in the size of the heart and an improvement in the E.C.G.

Renal biopsy findings

Renal biopsy findings, based on material excised by ZENKER during the operation, revealed that, interestingly enough, surgical treatment proved successful (as regards the response of the blood pressure and the life expectancy) only where the organic renal lesions were slight, but not in cases of marked arteriolosclerosis.

Comparison of the renal biopsy findings with the clinical classification of the patients shows quite a good correlation (cf. Table 3). All mild-grade renal vascular changes belonged to group I, and all those of severe degree (grades 3 and 4) to group II. Only where the renal vascular changes were of grade 2 was the distribution as between groups I and II fairly even. Incidentally, the degree of renal insufficiency showed no discernible relationship to the renal biopsy findings. Most of our patients were compensated, although in some instances the renal vascular changes had already become quite pronounced.

Table 3. *Relationship between clinical and biopsy findings*

Renal vascular changes	No. of cases	Clinical groups				
		Ia	Ib	IIa	IIb	IIc
Normal (grade 0)	1		1			
Grade 1	2		2			
Grade 2	11	1	6	1	3	
Grade 3	14			1	13	
Grade 4	3				3	

Renal function

Patients suffering from renal insufficiency, either manifest or compensated by polyuria, generally fail to stand up to the strain of surgical intervention. In our experience, such insufficiency constitutes an absolute contra-indication to sympathectomy.

Follow-up examinations of hypertensives carried out 1—6 years after sympathectomy revealed the following correlations with renal function (cf. Table 4).

Table 4. *Renal function tests in 55 patients of groups I and II before and 1—6 years after the operation*

	No. of cases	Normal concentration over 1025	Subnormal concentration below 1025	Normal serum non-protein nitrogen	Excessive serum non-protein nitrogen
Group I . .	28	before operation 26	2	27	1
		after operation 27	1	26	2
Group II .	27	before operation 21	6	21	6
		after operation 15	12	19	8

In group I there was no deterioration in renal function or in the serum non-protein nitrogen values after the operation, whereas in group II diminished concentrating power and a rise in the serum non-protein nitrogen values was noted in numerous cases. A large number of patients in group II died of uraemia. As also reported by other authors, renal function does not necessarily deteriorate as the result of a fall in blood pressure. On the other hand, where no diminution in blood pressure occurs, renal function in most cases steadily worsens as time goes on, evidently as the result of increasing arteriolosclerosis; there is probably no connection between this deterioration in renal function and the operation itself.

Subjective complaints

The *subjective complaints* of hypertensive patients were in many cases relieved by the operation, *even in instances where surgery failed to produce a fall in blood pressure.* Table 5 lists the changes in

Table 5. *Changes in subjective condition following sympathectomy*

	Group I			Group II		
	Complete relief	Improvement	No improvement	Complete relief	Improvement	No improvement
Headache	3	5	2	3	4	3
Dizziness.	1	1				
Headache and dizziness	8	5	5	6	13	11
Total	12 (40%)	11 (37%)	7 (23%)	9 (22.5%)	17 (42.5%)	14 (35%)

the subjective condition of patients who underwent sympathecto-my. In group I, 77% of the patients obtained complete subjective relief or reported an improvement in their symptoms (headache and/or dizziness), while also in group II the percentage was as high as 65%.

Peet has reported similar results (1946). Of his 176 patients with symptoms described as unbearable, 72.8% obtained consider-able relief from the operation and only 27.2% felt merely a slight improvement or none at all.

Against these *benefits derived from the operation* as regards its effects on life expectancy, symptoms, visual acuity, and cardiac insufficiency must be set certain decided disadvantages.

One *unpleasant side effect* of the operation is the *disorders in orthostatic regulation* to which it gives rise. These were encountered chiefly in cases belonging to group I where there had been a marked fall in blood pressure. When the patient rose, a decline in the systolic and often also in the diastolic pressure occurred, together with tachycardia, a feeling of emptiness in the head, attacks of dizziness, transient scotoma or even collapse. The minute volume

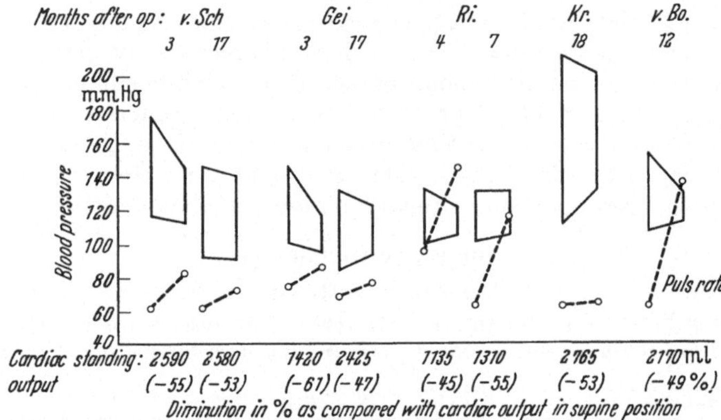

Fig. 4. Diminution in blood pressure and cardiac output in supine and standing position after operation

in the standing position diminished, sometimes to as low as 45%, and the pulse rate was liable to increase from 90 to as much as 140/min. (Sarre, cf. Fig. 4). Over a period of months, however, regulation of the cardiovascular system became more or less restored to normal. Fig. 4 illustrates how the results of the standing test improved in three cases after 7 to 17 months. The diastolic pressure no longer drops, but rises when the patient assumes the standing position; but even then a diminution in the minute volume is still generally apparent. Thus, a great many transitional stages occur before regulation is restored. This process of restoration is evidently dependent on the re-establishment of a proper vascular tonus.

Cerebral changes

Among our patients, consisting of 176 hypertensives who underwent surgery, 34 had suffered one or more apoplectic attacks prior to surgical intervention. Following sympathectomy, 18 (53%) of these died, including 7 from renewed apoplexy and 4 from other complications. Of the 16 survivors, 3 suffered another attack. 6 patients showed progressive mental deterioration or became more emotionally unstable. Some of them presented definite psychotic features. In addition, following sympathectomy 11 of the hypertensives had an apoplectic attack for the first time, from which 5 died.

Our own observations thus suggest that surgery constitutes a *far greater risk for cerebrosclerotic hypertensives* than for patients without cerebrosclerosis. The episodes observed by us were probably chiefly due to post-operative cerebral anaemia and/or acute fluctuations in blood pressure.

As a sequel to the operation, psychic lability has frequently developed among our patients — a condition aptly described by one patient as being "on top of the world at one moment and down in the dumps the next". Sometimes crises of depression occur. As a rule, the patients are easily fatiguable and lacking in initiative, although they tend to become unduly agitated by trivial matters. There are also cases in which the patient's original physical and mental agility gives way to a dull, languid, discouraged, and often hypochondriac temperament.

The intervention is, in fact, a major multitating operation which, though it does to some extent improve the patient's life expectancy, also exposes those responding with a marked fall in blood pressure to cerebral vascular disorders and mental impoverishment.

Indications

In the light of the results of follow-up examinations carried out on sympathectomised hypertensives, we regard the *operation as being indicated as follows:* generally speaking, only patients of group I should be operated on, and only in cases where the rapid progress of the disease, despite the patient's youth, gives reason to fear an unfavourable prognosis even where conservative therapy is employed (i. e. early forms of malignant hypertension). Contra-indications to surgery are:

1. Advanced cerebrosclerosis with signs of psychological and intellectual deterioration.

2. Severe coronary artery sclerosis, coronary infarction, but as a rule not cardiac insufficiency, which can be alleviated by conservative measures or by lowering the blood pressure.

3. Cases where renal function is decompensated or only compensated by polyuria, with or without a rise in serum non-protein nitrogen and with maximal concentrating capacity below 1020.

In view of the possibilities afforded today by medicinal therapy, even in cases of malignant hypertension, one should only decide to operate if these conservative measures have proved of no avail and if intolerable subjective symptoms and the rate of progress of the disease suggest a poor prognosis. Under such circumstances, the prospects are brightest for patients under 40 years of age belonging to group Ib, i. e. who are not yet suffering from any discernible vascular lesions. The fact remains that, of patients in stage Ib who underwent surgery, 92.2% were still alive after 5 years, as compared with only 57.1% of those receiving conservative therapy.

Adrenalectomy

In patients with hypertension it is impossible to maintain normal blood-pressure levels following adrenalectomy without giving adrenal hormones. Following bilateral adrenalectomy the blood pressure drops sharply in both experimental animals and man. Only by means of substitution treatment with cortico-steroids can it be adjusted to normal or higher than normal levels. Green, Nelson, Dodds and Smalley (1950) were the first to attempt total adrenalectomy in hypertensives. In 1958, Blake-more, Zintl and co-workers published a report on *116 patients*, in whom total or subtotal adrenalectomy had been performed together with sympathectomy, as compared with *114 patients* who had only undergone thoracolumbar sympathectomy. The mean post-operative follow-up period worked out at about 5 years. The patients were graded into groups I to IV according to Smithwick's classification; this corresponds roughly to the degrees of severity represented by our own groups listed earlier on. The composition of the cases was approximately the same in both instances, i. e. in the "Sympathectomy" and in the "Adrenalectomy" series (cf. Table 6). In each of the two series only those patients were operated on who were suffering from severe hypertension with diastolic pressures of over 120 mm Hg and who had failed to respond to conservative therapy. Patients with renal insufficiency were regarded as unsuitable for surgery and were therefore excluded from both series. The operative mortality was 0.9% for sympathectomy and 5% for adrenalectomy.

Table 6. *Smithwick classification*

Group	"Sympathectomy"	"Adrenalectomy"
I	2	0
II	38	31
III	19	31
IV	55	54
Total	114	116
Average	3.11	3.20

The distribution according to the severity of their hypertension by SMITHWICK classification in 114 patients who were treated by thoracolumbar sympathectomy ("sympathectomy") and 116 who were treated by total or subtotal adrenalectomy and a modified sympathectomy ("adrenalectomy"). It is apparent that the patients had hypertension of comparable severity and that many had very severe disease (grade IV).

Table 7. *The mortality and survival of patients who had had "sympathectomy" or "adrenalectomy" three to seven years previously*

	"Sympathectomy"	"Adrenalectomy"
Total patients	114	116
Living	83 (73%)	79 (68%)
Dead (total).	31 (27%)	37 (32%)
Operative mortality[1] .	1 (1%)	6 (5%)

The similarity of the mortality among the two groups of patients is apparent. Early in the series of patients with adrenalectomy, replacement therapy and adequate blood replacement were not as well understood and may have accounted for some of these deaths.

The results are presented in Table 7. Follow-up examinations carried out 3 to 7 years later (the mean being 4.2 years in the case of the adrenalectomised patients and 4.5 years in that of the sympathectomised cases) showed a survival rate of 68% in the adrenalectomised series and 73% in the sympathectomised series. Thus, when allowance is made for the difference in operative mortality, the long-term results will be seen to be almost identical (cf. Table 7).

---

[1] Survival less than 30 days post-operatively.

It is amazing that the major intervention of bilateral subtotal or total adrenalectomy did not yield better results than sympathectomy, although for obvious reasons the former operation led far more often to a lowering of the blood pressure to normal levels. 37% of the sympathectomised and 55% of the adrenalectomised patients had a normal blood pressure following the operation.

During the latter years of the observation period, generous recourse to steroid substitution therapy (cortisone or prednisolone) caused the patients' blood pressure to rise again somewhat.

It is interesting to note that in some cases, even where substitution therapy was given with low, barely adequate dosages, hypertension recurred (Thorn et al., 1952). Small doses, which in a normal case of Addison's disease would provoke no hypertension, are sufficient to cause a recurrence of hypertension in formerly hypertensive adrenalectomised patients, just as in hypertensives suffering from Addison's disease (cf. Table 8).

Table 8. *Basal blood pressure in patients following total bilateral adrenalectomy* (from Thorn et al. 1952)

Patient	Pre-operative blood pressure (mm Hg)	Blood pressure 3 months after operation (mm Hg)	Blood pressure 6 months after operation (mm Hg)	Blood pressure 12 months after operation (mm Hg)
W. Co.	160/100—350/150	128/98 —140/188	124/98 —140/104	—
W. Ch.	150/120—180/140	120/80 —150/110	124/84 —160/110	140/102—160/120
K. McC.	130/90 —184/120	150/80 —184/118	160/90 —200/150	150/90
C. Ha.	170/110—240/130	150/100—200/110	180/130—200/130	160/130—225/160
S. Ab.	220/120—250/160	150/100—224/136	170/90 —180/100	210/124—145/95
H. Ha.	130/90 —230/160	110/80 —150/104	130/105	160/120
A. Ma.	210/120—242/140	172/104—210/112	126/160—200/128	—
E. McC.	198/120—260/170	130/100—212/144	—	—
J. Ho.	130/92 —168/108	150/100	118/78 —138/88	142/90—172/100

It must therefore be concluded that in hypertensive patients the hypertension is not perpetuated solely by adrenocorticortical hyperfunction, but *that other factors must also enter into play* — factors which become immediately operative even when the smallest doses of cortisone are administered. Here, in as reliable a form as that provided by experimental means, we have evidence to show that the corticosteroids constitute only a concomitant factor. Hence, as Conn rightly states: "If the adrenal is important in essential hypertension, it is playing *a secondary, perhaps permissive, role* in allowing a pressor system to become activated". Following the operation, 21% of the adrenalectomised patients had an undesirably high blood pressure, although their signs and symptoms nevertheless showed some improvement. In both series the number of cerebrovascular accidents after the operation was the same. Orthostatic manifestations, however, were more pronounced among the sympathectomised patients.

The patients were maintained in a well-compensated state in response to daily doses of 25—37.5 mg cortisone, even during acute situations of stress due, for example, to infection, fever, or surgery.

From this painstaking comparison of *adrenalectomy* with splanchnicectomy and on the other hand sympathectomy alone, it becomes quite clear that this grave and major intervention affords *no improvement in the hypertensive's life expectancy*.

Summary

A report is given of the results of follow-up studies on 206 hypertensive patients sympathectomised by ZENKER using PEET's technique. The minimum observation period was 5 years. 306 hypertensives treated by conservative measures (largely still without effective anti-hypertensive drugs) served as controls. The patients were assessed according to the eyegrounds, diastolic pressure, and cardiac, renal, and cerebral complications. Surgery elicited beneficial results in those patients presenting only functional disorders, but poor results in those with organic disorders (e.g. coronary artery sclerosis, infarction, apoplexy, renal insufficiency). 5 years after the operation, 92.2% of the patients in Group I b (early stage of malignant hypertension, without organic complications) were still alive, as compared with only 57% of the non-operated cases. In Group II a—c (with organic complications) the results of surgery were moderate to poor.

Details are given of the changes in the eyegrounds, size of the heart, ECG, renal function, subjective symptoms, and side effects with cerebral disorders.

Renal biopsies showed that the operation yielded a good response in cases where the renal vessels had undergone only slight changes, but a poor response where the renal vascular lesions were already moderately severe to severe.

Contra-indications to surgery are advanced cerebral arteriosclerosis, severe coronary artery sclerosis, coronary infarction (but not cardiac insufficiency), and impaired renal function. The patients with the best prospects are those belonging to Group I under 40 years of age and without organic vascular changes.

Finally, reference is made to the long-term prognosis following total or subtotal adrenalectomy (with or without sympathectomy), an intervention which, according to data contained in the literature, does not improve the patient's life expectancy to a greater extent than sympathectomy.

Résumé

Nous rapportons les résultats d'observations faites pendant au moins 5 ans chez 206 hypertendus sympathectomisés par ZENKER selon la technique de PEET. 306 autres hypertendus non opérés et pour la plupart sans médicament hypotenseur actif, servirent de contrôle. On a jugé les malades au point de vue fond d'oeil, pression diastolique, complications cardiaques, rénales et cérébrales. L'intervention chirurgicale eut un résultat favorable chez les malades qui ne présentaient que des troubles fonctionnels, mais non pas chez les porteurs de lésions organiques, telles que sclérose coronarienne, infarctus, apoplexie, insuffisance rénale. 5 ans après l'opération, 92,2% des malades du groupe Ib vivaient encore (stade précoce de l'hypertonie maligne sans troubles organiques), tandis que parmi ceux qui ne furent pas opérés, 57% seulement étaient en vie. Les résultats opératoires furent médiocres ou défavorables dans le groupe IIa—c, qui était porteur de troubles organiques.

Les biopsies rénales ont montré que l'opération avait un bon résultat quand les vaisseaux rénaux ne présentaient que des modifications légères; le résultat était par contre mauvais si ces dernières étaient d'extension moyenne ou prononcée. Une sclérose cérébrale avancée, une sclérose coronarienne grave, un infarctus coronarien (mais non pas une insuffisance) ainsi que des troubles de la fonction rénale représentent des contre-indications opératoires. Les chances sont les plus favorables chez les malades au-dessous de 40 ans qui appartiennent au groupe I, c'est-à-dire sans lésions vasculaires organiques.

La question du pronostic éloigné après adrénalectomie totale ou subtotale avec ou sans sympathectomie a été aussi discutée. D'après les données de la littérature, ce traitement n'entraîne aucune amélioration de la survie en comparaison de la sympathectomie.

Literature

Blakemore, W. S., H. A. Zintel, W. A. Jeffers, A. M. Sellers, A. I. Sutnick, and M. A. Lindauer: Surgery (U.S.A.) **43**, 102 (1958). — Bowers, R. F.: J. Amer. Med. Ass. **154**, 394 (1954). — Bowers, R. F., and F. H. Knox jr.: A.M.A. Arch. Surg. **77**, 699 (1958). — Bowers, R. F., F. H. Knox jr., and B. R. Gendel: Surgery (U.S.A.) **34**, 664 (1953).

Hafkenschiel, J. H., and W. T. Fitts jr.: Trans. Amer. Coll. Cardiol. **5**, 107 (1955). — Hanley, H. G.: Brit. J. Urol. **29**, 359 (1957).

Morrissey, D. M., S. Brookes, and W. T. Cooke: Lancet (G.B.) **1953/I**, 403.

Newcombe, C. P., H. S. Shucksmith, and W. S. Suffern: Brit. Med. J. **1959/I**. 142.

Pfeffer, K. H., H. Nieth, and H. Schneider: Dtsch. med. Wschr. **80**, 956 (1955).

Sarre, H., and P. von Dittrich: Erg. inn. Med. (G.) **13**, 352 (1960). — Snellman, A., and M. Mustakallio: Acta chir. Scand. **109**, 219 (1955).

Thorn, G. W., J. H. Harrison, J. P. Merill, G. M. Criscitiello, T. F. Frawley, and J. T. Finkenstaedt: Ann. Int. Med. (U.S.A.) **37**, 972 (1952).

Whitelaw, G. P., and R. H. Smithwick: Angiology (U.S.A.) **2**, 157 (1951).

Zenker, R., H. Sarre, K. H. Pfeffer, H. H. Löhr, E. Koppermann, and P. Wisser: Erg. inn. Med. (G.) **3**, 1 (1952).

Discussion

HILDEN (to **REUBI**): One thing I want to emphasize: I think we have
all seen cases of malignant hypertension with poor kidney function after
treatment, but my experience during recent years has been that, especially
in renal hypertension, one should nevertheless make an attempt at treatment
in every case. I have very recently had a case with such poor kidney function
that I thought no treatment would prove of any avail, but she nevertheless
reacted very well to antihypertensive drugs. Her eyegrounds changed and
her renal function is being maintained at a level above 20%. I think one
ought not to exclude anyone or hardly anyone because of his kidney function,
particularly in cases of chronic renal disease. Now one comment on your
slides: Is the mean range of kidney function the same in these two groups?

REUBI: Yes, it was about the same.

HILDEN: Thank you. And now I should like very much to outline our
experience with malignant hypertension and with patients with exudates,
in relation to Dr. **SCHROEDER**'s work. I think it is very important to take
account of the death rate, which is the best way of assessing the results of
what we achieve or what we might or might not achieve. We often refer to
amelioration of the eyegrounds, and it is very important to look at the eyegrounds to see if our treatment is effective. But I want to emphasize that this
is for me not enough. It is not very difficult to move a fundus 4 down to 3 and
down to 2, but that is not enough; I think we have to lower the blood
pressure as much as possible, and to look at the heart size and electrocardiogram. That is to me the most important. In some cases I have been rather
misled by looking at the eyegrounds and seeing how nicely they were
improving, whereas at the same time the blood pressure was not very well
controlled.

HOOBLER: About Dr. **SARRE**'s paper, I would like to point out that if
we take the quantitative viewpoint concerning the effect of blood pressure
on prognosis, a reduction of 20—30 mm Hg mean pressure may be as
valuable to the patient with an initial level of, say 200 mm Hg, as to the
person who, after a 20 mm Hg blood-pressure fall, becomes normotensive.
Yet treatment results are often described in terms of the number of patients
who after therapy exhibit blood pressures in the normal range. A substantial
reduction, but not to normotension, by a treatment program goes unrecog-
nized if data are presented in this fashion. Also when post-operative statistics
are divided into groups with sustained blood-pressure reduction compared
to those who had no change in their hypertension, a lot may be learned
concerning the potential benefits of treatment. In a 5-year study of cases
who had had a cerebral accident prior to surgery, we found a greatly improved prognosis and almost no recurrence of cerebral attacks in the group
(about half of the cases) in whom the blood pressure was reduced by the
operation. Thus I would urge sympathectomy in patients with severe hypertension associated with a cerebro-vascular episode. In this group our results
have been much better than those reported by Dr. **SARRE**.

IMHOF: I would like to ask Dr. **SARRE** the following question: you are
dealing with a group treated from 1945 to 1955. Don't you think your results

would be much more in favour of the drug treatment which is getting more and more effective, if you were to compare your sympathectomised patients with a group treated from 1950 to 1960?

REUBI: I think it is a very important point which Dr. IMHOF has made. I was going to ask Dr. SARRE the same. I have got the impression that you were comparing sympathectomised patients with untreated patients, which means patients who had no effective medical treatment. Do you still consider that sympathectomy should be done on a certain choice of patients or do you believe it is unnecessary nowadays? Do you believe that there is one group of patients where surgical intervention is indicated more than medical treatment, or would you keep sympathectomy for those cases which do not respond to medical treatment? Or would you perhaps recommend the combination of both sympathectomy and medical treatment as the treatment of choice? I think that is one point which should be discussed.

SARRE: In view of the possibilities which medical treatment holds out today, I should not regard sympathectomy as being indicated unless and until vigorous treatment with antihypertensive agents had proved unsuccessful. This applies, for example, to severe cases of malignant hypertension refractory to every form of medicinal therapy. Thus, nowadays, the indications for surgery are very different from what they were, and far more restricted than 10 years ago. During recent years it has only been on rare occasions that I have referred a patient to the surgeon for sympathectomy.

REUBI: You would say that sympathectomy is a second-choice treatment?

SARRE: Yes.

REUBI: What do you think about that, Dr. HOOBLER?

HOOBLER: Well, it is very hard to answer your question. I would say that if a surgical operation had no mortality and had no residual pain or disability of any sort, it would be my choice in the treatment of hypertension, because if I followed this up with chlorothiazide only, I would have almost a permanent cure of at least half of the hypertensives. Now, unfortunately, this is not the case and therefore we have to consider the post-operative disability and the mortality rates, and always the human factor in not wanting to undergo anesthesia. This argues against surgery. However, from the standpoint of strict control of the blood pressure, no drug treatment that I know of, with the exception of chlorothiazide, perhaps, as consistently lowers the recumbent blood pressure and therefore the nocturnal risk of having some cerebral vascular difficulty. I see Dr. SCHROEDER beginning to object to this statement. However, I think many of us have failed to lower the recumbent blood pressure at night, even with the most intensive drug treatment. Perhaps he pushes treatment to a greater degree. I think we prolong life with drugs, but I think eventually we lose some patients treated by drugs, because the blood pressure control is never complete. When sympathectomy is successful, recumbent blood pressure is more apt to fall and, as I mentioned a moment ago, vascular accidents are largely prevented. Heart failure I think we can generally prevent with drugs, or we can tell when we are losing ground. Also progressive renal failure can be detected by appropriate measures, but the sudden stroke in the night cannot be anticipated and is most surely prevented by a successful sympathectomy. So the answer is a complicated one, but I think we are underselling sympathectomy at the moment, and if we did not have the complications associated with the operation, I would be a much stronger salesman for it than I am now.

HOOD: We have picked out the 380 cases of grades 3 and 4 in any of the classifications of KEITH and WAGENER, SMITHWICK, PALMER or HAMMARSTRØM and BECHGAARD, where treatment was introduced from 1950 to 1956. They have been treated along very much the same lines as Dr. SCHROEDER's patients, although maybe not fully as harsh and not using the home pressure method in the whole of the material, but only in selected cases. Results and experiences are very much the same as those of Dr. SCHROEDER. I would not like to bother you with details, but I would like to emphasize how the situation and the causes of death look now. First of all, there has been a tremendous shift, as you all know, because of the virtual disappearance of congestive failure. Then the expected death rate of uremia has gone steeply down, but we are now left, as Dr. HOOBLER pointed out, with two things and those more or less atherosclerotic in character: the myocardial infarctions and the cerebro-vascular lesions. Now, if we look at the myocardial infarctions, which numbered 21 cases, there was not a single case that occurred during the first 10 months of treatment, and in this severe type of case we usually introduced a real good sharp blood pressure reduction from the outset. The average age of the onset after the introduction of treatment was 35 months. As to lethal cerebro-vascular lesions, we have 60 of those in the material, and we would say that only 12 of these cases had a good nice regimen at the time of the stroke: 4/5 of the cerebro-vascular lesions occurred in cases which had a discontinued treatment or had an inadequate treatment performed by staff members who did not belong to the active group, or where a transitory reduction in the drugs or a complete going off the drugs had occurred. We have repeatedly observed massive haemorrhages to occur within 24 hrs to a fortnight after omission of the drugs. In other words, only 1/5 of the cerebro-vascular lesions occurred in those who at the time had a known real good medicamental regimen.

MILLIEZ: I am entirely in agreement with Dr. SARRE and Dr. HOOBLER on the question of surgical treatment for hypertension. I have had 120 patients operated on. The only real contra-indication is renal insufficiency: all the patients operated on who already showed pathological renal function died afterwards. I have never regarded a cerebro-vascular accident or a coronary artery lesion as contra-indications. Moreover, I have never had cause to regret an operation on a severe case of hypertension — even if the patient had had a cerebral or cardiovascular accident — provided, firstly, that renal function tests still yielded acceptable findings and, secondly, that the patient was less than fifty years old and had not been suffering from marked peripheral vascular sclerosis. In my view, one should attempt surgical treatment only in cases where six·months of rigorous and very thorough medical therapy have proved utterly unavailing. Among 120 patients, the operation yielded complete success, i. e. a return to normal blood pressure levels, in 25% of cases. The operative mortality was 4%, a figure accounted for by deaths among only the first 50 patients operated on. We instruct the operating surgeon to combine SMITHWICK's sympathectomy with total adrenalectomy on the one side and subtotal on the other, insisting that the remnant of adrenal tissue left in situ should be well vascularised. Under these circumstances, I have never encountered a case of permanent post-operative adrenal insufficiency nor, so far, have I ever seen a case in which adrenal function subsequently reverted to normal. Sympathectomy alone seems to me to yield good results in young women with severe hypertension desirous of completing a normal pregnancy or suffering from severe toxaemia of pregnancy; in such cases, it was possible to carry out SMITHWICK's operation during pregnancy.

PLATT: I would like to show two slides. Dr. HILDEN was saying that we should not judge the results merely by the death rate. This is the retina of a young man of about 25 years of age who had had acute nephritis about 5 years ago and was in a state of renal failure with blood urea of about 80 to 90 mg-% at the time that he came in. He was rapidly losing his sight completely, and the next slide will show you the same retina after treatment with pentolinium. Now it does show, of course, probably a partial optic atrophy which you nearly always get after treatment of a severe retinopathy, but that did not interfere with his sight at all, and he went back to work as a draftsman and worked for a year before he died of uraemia. There was no immediate significant change in his blood urea as a result of the treatment. We knew of course that we could not save his life for very long, but his sight completely returned and I think this result is worthwhile. Then the other thing I would like to say concerns something Dr. HOOBLER was saying and it was, of course, mentioned during the week, that BYROM has actually demonstrated arterial spasm in the brain in hypertensive rats, so it can exist.

ARNOLD: (Demonstration of three slides showing the funduscopic pictures during the treatment of a malignant hypertension: woman, 32 years old; normalisation of blood pressure since 6 months; the papilledema and the hemorrhages disappeared, the exudates were decidedly diminished after 6 months' treatment with guanethidine combined in the first three months with reserpine and in the last three with hydrochlorothiazide).

PLATT: With renal failure?

ARNOLD: No renal failure. Diastolic blood pressure over 140 mm Hg.

FERRERO: I would just like to make a point, i. e. the correlation between hypertensive patients under treatment and the electrocardiogram with respect to the left-heart strain patterns in a group of 26 patients treated for an average period of three years. We had the following correlations: In the 1st group: 5 cases did not respond well to the treatment for their hypertension; 2 of them had the same electrocardiogram, two others showed a worse record, and one case did better. The second group of 21 cases was treated with success: in $^2/_3$ of them the electrocardiogram improved or became normal. The first slide shows this. Before treatment blood pressure is 215 over 130, 2 years later 180 over 115; you see the better T waves in leads 1, 2, V 4, and V 6. This patient neglected the treatment after 59, and the electrocardiogram was worse; seven other cases did not show the same correlation between blood pressure and electrocardiogram. For instance, we had a patient with a very high blood pressure and a normal electrocardiogram, which remained exactly the same after treatment: in 1958 the blood pressure was 215 over 130, and you see a normal electrocardiogram; 2 years later, with a very normal blood pressure, 160 over 95, you see the same electrocardiogram within normal limits. The last slide shows you another type of correlation between electrocardiogram and blood pressure: it is a case of malignant hypertension, of 280 over 160, and you see it after one month of treatment: blood pressure goes down a little bit, 255 over 150, and the electrocardiogram is worse. These slides are presented just to show that, for a clinician, the blood pressure figures alone do not necessarily reflect the degree of hypertensive disease.

REUBI: I would like to ask whether there is anybody who has some experience with total adrenalectomy.

HOOBLER: We have had only one case. It did not get much better and required for maintenance enough cortisone to restore the hypertension.

SCHWARTZ: BLAKEMORE and ZINTEL performed bilateral and total adrenalectomy, supplemented by Adson-type interventions, in 44 hypertensive patients. The operative mortality here was higher than in the sympathectomised group, but on the other hand adrenalectomy led to a more marked decrease in blood pressure and produced a more clear-cut improvement in the electrocardiogram and eyegrounds.

HOOD: I would like to ask you, Dr. REUBI, a question concerning the slide where you showed a very rapid downhill slope of untreated patients in the renal function, and where your treated patients had some slope downhill, but not a very marked one. Now, these renal function studies were performed at a very much lower perfusion pressure, I would guess. It was not clear to me whether you allowed the blood pressure to go up slowly to pretreatment levels before you performed your second or third renal measurement during the active treatment, or whether you calculated what it would mean in terms of estimated renal resistance during the studies under continuous treatment.

REUBI: This is an important point. In earlier studies we could observe some sort of rebound when we stopped the treatment in order to perform the renal clearance tests. But I think we are not justified in interrupting the treatment, because we have to do the comparative examination while the blood pressure is kept down. All the cases I presented yesterday were actually studied under these conditions of continued treatment.

HOOD: Did you calculate the renal resistance ?

REUBI: No, I did not.

HOOBLER: Just one point. I suppose you are aware of the reports of MOYER and of CORCORAN concerning the gradual improvement in renal function after prolonged blood pressure reduction? Do you have any explanation for the disparity between their results and yours ?

REUBI: I think there is no essential disparity between MOYER's results and ours, but perhaps I should present some more slides which I did not show yesterday. We can observe almost every type of response in the treated cases. In some cases you may see merely an arrest of renal deterioration. In other cases there may be at the beginning a further drop in renal function and later a stabilisation at this low level. In yet other cases, you may have an initial drop, followed later by an increase. What I showed were only mean values. There is no doubt that in selected cases there may be a real improvement. But there is no doubt either that for the whole treated group there is still a decrease in glomerular filtration rate. I know there is some discrepancy between MOYER's figures and ours. MOYER's conclusions are perhaps a little too optimistic.

SCHROEDER: May I ask you a question, Dr. REUBI ? Examining some of your charts of blood pressure control, it appeared that strict normotension was not always achieved and that diastolic levels of 100 to 120 were sometimes maintained. Have you analysed your data to see whether those patients with strict normotension had an alteration in renal function different from those with residual hypertension ?

REUBI: I am sorry if you have got the impression that the cases assigned to the group of treated patients were not adequately treated, because we thought they were. As Dr. HOOBLER pointed out, I think the absolute values of blood pressure are not as important as their reduction in itself. Take a patient with a blood pressure of about 300/180 mm Hg before treatment: if you can bring it down to 180/110 mm Hg, I think that is quite a satisfactory response. Of course it is not normal.

SCHROEDER: May I disagree with that idea? Our results of therapy indicate definitely that normotension is not only desirable but necessary for reversal of the hypertensive process to occur. Of course one cannot always get it if the kidneys are badly diseased.

DAHL: There has repeatedly been discussion here concerning people who do not respond to medical therapy. I do not see such people. My results are similar to those of Dr. SCHROEDER, although numerically they are on a modest scale since therapy has not been our primary interest. We have continued to increase the dosage of drugs, sometimes to very large amounts, and thus far have been successful in modifying the blood pressure significantly. My experience is limited in numbers but includes patients with malignant hypertension. All patients have been hospitalized under very close observation and sometimes for long periods of time, because of the unique research facilities available in our establishment at Brookhaven. What has been the experience of others with wider clinical acquaintance in the field of therapy than my own?

PICKERING: I have patients who do not respond.

HILDEN: It is quite different to treat patients in the hospital than to treat them after they have been discharged. As regards patients in hospital, I would guess there would be very very few cases where we cannot bring down the blood pressure.

PEART: We have heard a great deal about how important it is — I think from Dr. HOOBLER and Dr. SCHROEDER — for the patient to take his blood pressure at home and how control is thus improved. I am prepared to believe this, but I would like to know if they could give us some figures as to the improvement in control. What percentage really are better with this regime? Are these better than the casual blood pressures which most of us tend to use in running an ordinary hypertension clinic? This is one thing I really would like to know, because if the case is successfully made out then I think it is very important to know the figures.

SCHROEDER: I would like to say a word on the point raised by Dr. DAHL. We have yet to see an untreated fresh hypertensive who was resistent to drugs. On the other hand, we have often seen hypertension become resistant after intermittent therapy. The best way to cause tolerance or resistance is to treat for a few days, stop, begin again, stop, and restart. Extreme resistance, even what appears to be total resistance to intravenous therapy with large doses, has been produced in this way. We have become so impressed with this phenomenon that we sought for drug-destroying enzymes in rabbit's livers. We do not stop therapy once started; we do not allow the blood pressure to escape control. I remember one patient, previously well controlled on drugs, whose diastolic pressure fell only 10 mm Hg for 15 min after 3.0 g hexamethonium chloride and 1.0 g hydralazine given rapidly into a vein; such resistance had developed as the result of his own lack of co-operation. A steady, continuous therapeutic pressure is essential for success. We cannot explain this phenomenon.

REUBI: Can anybody answer Dr. PEART's question.

HOOBLER: I think if the patient's blood pressure as determined in the clinic is adequately controlled, you do not need home readings, unless at home there are side-effects suggesting hypotension. I think frequently, when the patient's clinic blood pressures are very high, you cannot be sure what they might be at home.

Sometimes high clinic readings are associated with normal home readings; sometimes high clinic readings go along with high home readings and indicate failure of treatment. My guess would be that the difference between the casual office reading and the home reading on the average, with wide variations, is about 20 to 30 mm Hg. Would you like to comment on that, Dr. FREIS ?

FREIS: Yes, I agree. In the series of patients in the war veterans cooperative study, especially in patients on blocking agents, we would have concluded on the basis of clinic readings alone that the blockers were almost ineffective in the doses used; but they produced a very nice control of home blood pressures. This would mean that one advantage of home blood pressure readings, at least in our experience, is that they prevent the physician from overdosing on the basis of misleadingly high pressures in the clinic. We thereby largely avoid the discomforting side-effects which tend to discourage the patient from continuing his treatment. In addition, home pressures permit readjustment of dosage up or down according to the needs of the moment, as Dr. SCHROEDER has shown so well. Finally, the patient sees for himself the need for medication, which considerably increases his understanding and cooperation just as do home urine sugar determinations in the diabetic.

Hypertension and its associated vascular diseases

By

P. Imhof, I. H. Page and H. Dustan

Work of the past several years has brought some understanding
of the relationships between hypertension and its associated vascular diseases. These are important considerations, because hypertension causes premature death and disability which, in the case
of the malignant phase, result from arteriolar disease and, in the
"benign" form, from complications of arteriosclerosis. Clinical and
laboratory studies have shown the dependence on elevated arterial
pressure of necrotizing arteriolar disease, arteriolosclerosis, and
arteriosclerosis. In regard to clinical studies, the only presently
valid ones concern the clinical course of treated malignant hypertension, a syndrome which is usually fatal in 1 to 2 years if untreated. In "benign"essential hypertension, with its course of many
years, the appropriate studies have not yet been finished.

Hypertension and arteriolar disease

In 1938 Keith, Wagener, and Barker (*1*) described the
rapidly fatal course of malignant hypertension; 79% of their
patients were dead 1 year after the diagnosis was established.
Death usually results from uremia caused by renal arteriolar
necrosis and thrombonecrosis. Less frequent causes of death are
intracerebral hematoma, hypertensive encephalopathy, and cardiac
failure; atherosclerotic complications are rare.

Effective antihypertensive treatment profoundly changes the
clinical course of malignant hypertension. We have reported
results of therapy in 84 patients followed for periods ranging from
1 to 7 years (*2*). Seventy per cent survived 1 year; 50%, 3 years;
and 26%, 6 years. Of the 52 patients who died, only 9 succumbed
to malignant nephrosclerosis and, even in these, survival was
prolonged. Similar results of treatment have been reported by
Perry and Schroeder (*3*) and by Harington, Kincaid-Smith
and McMichael (*4*).

An explanation for the change in the clinical course of malignant
hypertension comes from a necropsy study of malignant nephro-

sclerosis by McCormack, Béland, Schneckloth and Corcoran (5). Among 100 cases studied, 19 had received antihypertensive drug treatment which in 14 had achieved sustained decreases in arterial pressure for many months; in the remaining 5, treatment periods had ranged from 3 days to 4 months. In the untreated patients, arcuate and interlobular arteries were thickened, with fragmentation and reduplication of the elastica. Arteriolar necrosis and thrombosis were common. In the treated group, evidence of acute vascular damage was greatly reduced or absent. In the 5 patients who had received short-term therapy, necrosis and thrombosis, while present, were much decreased, while in the 14 with long-term therapy these features were practically absent. Residual vascular disease was evidenced by thickening of arterial and arteriolar walls and occasional luminal obliterations by fibrous tissue. These findings show that reduction of arterial pressure in malignant hypertension suppresses renal arterial and arteriolar necrosis but does not reverse all signs of vascular disease; they also explain the decreased incidence of death from rapidly advancing uremia.

The relationship between hypertension and vascular disease has been studied in rats subjected to partial renal infarction and followed for periods of 1 week to 2 months; some received hydralazine, which kept arterial pressure at near normal levels (6). Untreated rats developed generalized vascular disease. If hydralazine was begun at the time of renal infarction, renal and extrarenal signs of vascular disease were minimal; if treatment was discontinued after one month, severe, acute vascular disease developed during the subsequent 4 weeks. When hydralazine was begun after one month of hypertension, examination 4 weeks later revealed healing and scarring of the vascular lesions. These experiments show that in the hypertensive rat, as in man, acute vascular lesions heal if arterial pressure is reduced. They also demonstrate that, in rats, development of vascular disease is, in part, a function of arterial pressure level; such a relationship has not yet been conclusively shown in essential hypertension.

Hypertension and arteriosclerosis

Premature arteriosclerosis is an accompaniment of hypertension; this explains the high incidence of arteriosclerotic complications in patients with "benign" essential hypertension. Development of arteriosclerosis seems to be a very slow process, and this may be the reason why arteriosclerotic complications are rare in malignant hypertension, where progression of arteriolar disease is so rapid that arterial disease does not have time to develop. When the malignant syndrome is successfully treated, arteriosclerosis eventually becomes manifest.

Types of fatal arteriosclerosis observed in treated malignant hypertension, as contrasted with untreated, are atherosclerosis and subintimal fibroplasia. The former affects the cerebral, coronary, and peripheral arteries; the latter, the renal interlobar and arcuate arteries. The importance of arteriosclerosis in shortening life in treated patients is seen in an analysis of causes of death (2). Fifty-two of our 84 treated patients died; 8 died of hexamethonium pneumonitis; 13, of cerebral hemorrhage or thrombosis; 7, of myocardial infarction; 2, of rupture of aortic aneurysm; 22, of renal failure — 9 of these followed an attenuated course of malignant nephrosclerosis and 13 lived months or years before renal insufficiency became incapacitating. This delayed renal failure, which seemed to result from subintimal fibroplasia of the interlobar and arcuate arteries, will be described later. In summary, of the 52 deaths, 35 were due to arteriosclerotic complications; 8 patients died of effects of treatment and only 9 succumbed in a fashion somewhat characteristic of malignant hypertension.

The atherosclerotic catastrophes in treated malignant hypertensive patients (e. g. cerebral hemorrhages, myocardial infarction, or rupture of aortic aneurysm) occurred between the 5th and 66th month of treatment. Only in the case of cerebral vascular disease did poor pressure control seem to contribute to the fatal complication. In 10 of 13 patients who died of cerebral hemorrhage, lying diastolic pressure levels remained above 110 mm Hg for months or years of treatment; in only 3 was arterial pressure persistently less than 110 mm Hg.

This clinical experience shows that treated malignant hypertensive patients, like those with "benign" essential hypertension, are prone to develop fatal, or incapacitating, atherosclerosis. The reason for this atherogenesis is not known, but a possibility can be proposed. Page (7) has suggested that elevated arterial pressure increases transmural lipid filtration and thus sets the stage for abnormal lipid accumulations and subsequent atherosclerosis. It follows, then, that elevated arterial pressure could result in abnormal accumulations of lipids in vessel walls even without abnormal plasma lipid values and that hypertension in the face of hyperlipemia and hypercholesterolemia should cause much greater vascular damage than it would when lipid levels are normal. In this regard, Bronté-Stewart and Heptinstall (8) found that hypertension greatly accelerates atherosclerosis in hypercholesterolemic rabbits, and MOSES (9) was able to produce arterial lesions in hypertensive, hypercholesterolemic dogs. This latter observation seems particularly significant, because dogs have no propensity for developing atherosclerosis spontaneously. To explore this possibility further, we studied the plasma protein fractions and cholesterol levels of hypertensive patients (10, 11). We found that many malignant hypertensive patients and essential hypertensives with atherosclerotic complications had slightly elevated amounts of β-globulin and cholesterol. The significance of such elevations cannot be determined until it is possible to maintain severely hypertensive patients normotensive or normocholesterolemic over many years.

Before potent antihypertensive drugs became available, little help could be given to azotemic hypertensive patients, even those with mild azotemia. Sympathectomy and pyrogen therapy were unsuccessful and sodium restrictive diets, while offering the most potential benefit, were often not followed rigidly enough to make them effective. The clinical impression was that presence of azotemia signified an irreversible vascular disease that would not benefit from reduction of arterial pressure. Experience of the past 9 years has proved this impression to be wrong, for moderately azotemic patients (blood urea up to 150 mg-%) often have their lives considerably prolonged by effective antihypertensive drug treatment. Of the group of malignant hypertensive patients which we have studied (2), 13 who were mildly or moderately azotemic prior to start of therapy improved greatly. Treatment resulted in remission of retinal hemorrhages and exudates and disappearance of papilledema; initially, renal function either improved slightly or showed no deterioration. Months, or a few years later, renal insufficiency became inexorably progressive. The difference between the course of this delayed renal failure and that of the attenuated form of malignant nephrosclerosis is apparent from the fact that the former group survived throughout 14 to 60 months of therapy (median survival was 27 months) while the latter group lived less than a year, 5 of these 9 patients having died within 6 months.

The necropsy study of MCCORMACK, BÉLAND, SCHNECKLOTH and CORCORAN (5) has explained the cause of this delayed renal failure. Of the 19 cases in whom antihypertensive drug treatment had been used, 14 had achieved considerable arterial pressure reduction but had eventually succumbed to delayed renal failure. Examination of kidneys showed almost complete absence of necrotizing arteriolar disease; instead, the interlobar and arcuate arteries had extensive subintimal fibroplasia, which in areas was so severe as to result in complete occlusion and segments of renal atrophy. Control of arterial pressure was not an important factor in the development of this vascular lesion, for in about half the patients satisfactory pressure levels had been obtained by treatment and in half, treatment had resulted only in orthostatic hypotension.

Causes of this arterial lesion are not apparent. It may be that hypertension initiates a vascular damage that is progressive even after arterial pressure has been reduced to normal or near normal levels. Whether it is peculiar to the renal vessels is not known, since other vascular beds have not been subjected to such intensive study. This subintimal fibroplasia is apparently not solely dependent on severe hypertension, for it has been described following partial renal infarction in rats even though hypertension was prevented by hydralazine administration and extra-renal signs of vascular disease were minimal (6).

Summary

Effective antihypertensive drug treatment prolongs the life of malignant hypertensive patients and suppresses the renal and extra-renal evidences of necrotizing vascular disease. Clinical and laboratory investigations have shown that renal arteriolar necrosis and thrombosis are a function of elevated arterial pressure.

Treated malignant hypertensives die, not of malignant nephrosclerosis, but of arteriosclerosis, either atherosclerosis or subintimal fibrous proliferation. Only so far as cerebral vascular disease is concerned does arterial pressure reduction seem important for the avoidance of arteriosclerotic complications.

Patients with mild to moderate azotemia prior to institution of treatment can live for many months without progression of renal damage and then develop fatal renal failure. This clinical course can be explained by a progressive subintimal deposition of fibrous tissue (in renal interlobar and arcuate arteries) that often results in segments of renal atrophy.

Résumé

Un traitement médicamenteux hypotenseur efficace prolonge la vie des malades présentant une hypertension maligne et supprime les manifestations rénales et extra-rénales de la maladie nécrosante vasculaire. Des investigations cliniques et de laboratoire ont montré que la nécrose artériolaire rénale avec thrombose est une conséquence de l'élévation de la tension artérielle.

Les malades présentant de l'hypertension maligne et traités meurent, non pas de néphrosclérose maligne, mais d'artério-sclérose (sclérose athéromateuse ou fibrose proliférative sous-intimale). C'est seulement en ce qui concerne les troubles vasculaires cérébraux que la réduction de la tension artérielle semble importante pour éviter les complications artérioscléreuses.

Les malades qui présentent une hyperazotémie discrète ou modérée au moment de l'institution du traitement peuvent vivre sans aggravation des lésions rénales pendant des mois, puis soudain présenter une insuffisance rénale fatale. Cette évolution clinique peut être expliquée par un dépôt progressif de tissu fibreux sous-intimal (dans les artères rénales interlobaires et arciformes) qui aboutit souvent à des zones d'atrophie rénale.

References

1. KEITH, N. M., H. P. WAGENER, and N. W. BARKER: Amer. J. Med. Sc. **197**, 332 (1939).
2. DUSTAN, H. P., R. E. SCHNECKLOTH, A. C. CORCORAN, and I. H. PAGE: Circulation (U.S.A.) **18**, 644 (1958).
3. PERRY, H. M., and H. A. SCHROEDER: A.M.A. Arch. Int. Med. **102**, 418 (1958).
4. HARINGTON, M., P. KINCAID-SMITH, and J. McMICHAEL: Brit. Med. J. **1959**/II, 969.
5. McCORMACK, L. J., J. E. BÉLAND, R. E. SCHNECKLOTH, and A. C. CORCORAN: Amer. J. Path. **34**, 1011 (1958).
6. MASSON, G. M. C., L. J. McCORMACK, H. P. DUSTAN, and A. C. CORCORAN: Amer. J. Path. **34**, 817 (1958).
7. PAGE, I. H.: Circulation (U.S.A.) **10**, 1 (1954).
8. BRONTÉ-STEWART, B., and R. H. HERTINSTALL: J. Path. Bact. (G.B.) **68**, 407 (1954).
9. MOSES, C.: Circulation Res. (U.S.A.) **2**, 243 (1954).
10. CORCORAN, A. C., L. A. LEWIS, H. P. DUSTAN, and I. H. PAGE: Ann. N.Y. Acad. Sc. **64**, 620, 1956.
11. CORCORAN, A. C., I. H. PAGE, H. P. DUSTAN, and L. A. LEWIS: Cleveland Clin. Quart. **23**, 115 (1956).

Prevention and treatment of
"atheromatous complications" of hypertension

By

G. SCHETTLER

The subject of this paper requires a certain amount of precision, inasmuch as the development of arterial atheroma constitutes only one among several causative factors of arteriosclerosis in man. The induration, loss of elasticity, and reduction in arterial lumen which together make up the clinical concept of arteriosclerosis may be brought about by various pathological-anatomical processes. In line with the Committee on Nomenclature of the American Society for the Study of Arteriosclerosis, arterial disease may be classified according to the following categories:

1. Degenerative arterial lesions
    a) atherosclerosis
    b) mediasclerosis (medial arteriosclerosis)
    c) arterionecrosis
2. Productive and/or hyperplastic arterial lesions
3. Inflammatory arterial lesions
4. Combined forms.

In relation to chronic arterial hypertension, only the first two categories are of interest to us, viz. degenerative arterial lesions and productive/hyperplastic arterial lesions.

While *specific* disorders of the arterial system due to hypertension do not exist as such, it is a fact that, in chronic arterial hypertension, productive and/or hyperplastic arterial lesions are extremely frequent. Hyaline degeneration of the arteries and arterioles is frequently encountered in chronic arterial hypertension, and arterionecrosis represents a pathological-anatomical substrate of so-called malignant hypertension. The development of Mönckeberg's medial arteriosclerosis is by no means necessarily associated with systemic hypertension, and its course is quite independent of the latter. The loss of arterial elasticity is reflected in a high pulse pressure, the systolic level being only slightly elevated. One may fairly speak here of arteriosclerotic hypertension, a form which is of no particular importance from either practical or clinical points of view. The atheromatous complications referred to earlier are, as stated, only one factor in the total process of arteriosclerosis. As such, they do not initiate the lesions of the vascular walls, but may exercise some influence over the course of the arteriosclerosis in individual cases. In arteries and arterioles of small diameter, the vascular lumen may be constricted by atheromatous beds of *intima*. Softening of tissue, ulcer formation, subsequent repair processes, thrombosis, sequestration, and haemorrhage not infrequently affect the clinical course and prognosis of arteriosclerosis. While none of these processes constitutes a specific result of hypertension, there can be no doubt that chronic arterial hypertension is, in importance and numerical incidence, the underlying disease which most frequently predisposes a patient towards premature severe arteriosclerosis. Even clinicians of earlier days such as HUCHARD and v. BASCH observed that "rises in the maximum blood pressure" very frequently paved the way for arteriosclerosis, and MARCHAND, to whom we owe the introduction of the term "atherosclerosis", recognised the clinical picture of a local rise in blood pressure as a pathogenic factor in arteriosclerosis. This general impression has since been confirmed by statistics. On the basis of morbidity statistics compiled in 1933 (albeit by incomplete methods), SYDENSTRICKER was able to demonstrate, with a high degree of probability, the existence of a direct connection between the level of the blood pressure and the extent of the clinical manifestations of arteriosclerosis. If we take the clinical diagnosis of systemic arteriosclerosis, we find that some 40% of patients suffer from hypertension. Allowing for other cases of arteriosclerosis not accessible to the clinician and for the fact that pre-existent cases of hypertension may later become normotensive or even hypotensive as a result of heart failure, it seems probable that the actual percentage is even higher.

According to WAKERLIN, 60% of all patients with fixed arterial hypertension exhibit signs of arteriosclerosis at the time their hypertension is first diagnosed in the clinic. The longer the hypertension persists, the greater is the likelihood of the arteriosclerosis becoming generalised. Statistics based on post-mortem findings also show that chronic arterial hypertension tends to promote arteriosclerosis. Studies based on some 22,000 autopsies performed at the Pathological-Anatomical Institutes of the Universities of Basle and of Marburg/Lahn, in collaboration with KÖHL, SOLTH, and WERTHEMANN, strongly suggest that the highest incidence of generalised arteriosclerosis and of coronary artery sclerosis occurs in association with hypertension. This applies with particular force to the severe forms of generalised arteriosclerosis and, more particularly, coronary artery sclerosis. Moreover, these lesions are encountered in younger age groups than is the case with normotensive subjects. Only in association with *diabetes mellitus* do we encounter a higher incidence of severe coronary artery sclerosis. Where hypertension and *diabetes mellitus* occur concomitantly, severe generalised sclerosis and coronary artery sclerosis are nearly always encountered from the age of 45 onwards. The combination of these two diseases is more frequent in women (7.6%) then in men (4.6%). To judge from the material available in Basle, it seems most probable that the combination of hypertension and diabetes occurs between the ages of 55 and 74.

Of 197 hypertensive subjects examined at autopsy by Rau in Freiburg, 30—40% were found to be suffering from severe aortic sclerosis; among 735 other cases without hypertension, by contrast, the incidence was only 5—10%, depending on age group. Even more striking were the differences in relation to coronary artery sclerosis — 50—80% among hypertensive subjects as against a mere 5% in other cases. According to Clawson and Bell, 45% of hypertensive hearts exhibit severe coronary artery sclerosis, 45% exhibit moderate sclerosis, and 10% show only slight changes. In about two-thirds of cases of sudden death from coronary artery sclerosis confirmed at autopsy, Rabson and Helpern observed cardiac hypertrophy resulting from previous hypertension. Other statistics on the connection between hypertension and coronary artery sclerosis have been supplied by Ackerman and co-workers, Davis and Klainer, Fishberg, Master and co-workers, Moschkowitz, Tobian, Anderson, and Keith.

An indirect pointer to the connection existing between blood pressure and arteriosclerosis is the fact that hypotensive subjects are less prone to arteriosclerosis and degenerative cardio-vascular disease than normotensive or hypertensive ones. Among persons with blood-pressure levels of 20 mm Hg below average, the mortality rate from coronary artery disease is some 25% lower than among normotensive and hypertensive subjects (Hunter). In our clinical experience, coronary infarction is very seldom encountered in cases of chronic hypotension; among 350 cases of infarction, we found a history of hypotension in only 4, i.e. in just over 1%. Cases of hypertension associated with chronic heart failure are, of course, not included. Page took the view at an early stage that hypotensive measures in cases of chronic arterial hypertension constituted the best prophylactic measure against arteriosclerosis in general and coronary artery sclerosis in particular. As far as this applies to coronary and cerebral vascular sclerosis, we would agree with this view; on the other hand, when dealing with the development of peripheral vascular disease on the basis of arteriosclerosis, chronic hypertension plays only a subsidiary part. By contrast once more, it must be assumed, in the light of anatomical, physiological, and clinical studies, that pulmonary arteriosclerosis is considerably aggravated by chronic hypertension.

The therapy of hypertension provides an example of the planned prevention of arteriosclerosis, with due regard to its aetiology and pathogenesis. All preventive and therapeutic measures, if they are to be effective, must take account of the multifarious origin of arteriosclerosis in man. Each one of the factors given here may be regarded as a point of departure for the prevention and treatment of arteriosclerosis. Among the many possible causes, we should like to mention some of the more important here.

Particular significance attaches to the connection between *diet* and *arteriosclerosis*. In the light of ethnological, clinical, and general morbidity and mortality statistics, it is to-day possible to discern two main trains of thought. One group, which counts ANCEL KEYS and NORMAN JOLLIFFE as its chief protagonists, takes the view that degenerative cardiovascular disease predominates among those peoples and ethnic groups which largely cover their calorie requirements with fats. Typical examples of such fatty diets are provided by the British and American countries, where up to 40 and 45% of the total daily calorie intake is made up of fats. At the other end of the scale are countries like Japan or Italy, where fats make up only 8—12% of the daily calorie intake. In addition, KEYS and other investigators of his persuasion assume a close connection between the fat content of the diet and the serum cholesterol and β-lipoprotein levels on one hand and fatal cardiovascular disease on the other. KEYS maintains that he knows of no patient or ethnic group with low fat consumption and low serum cholesterol levels which displays a high incidence of mortality from coronary artery disease.

There are, however, other investigators and research groups who are unable to follow this line of thought. Basing themselves on statistics from representative sections of various nations and ethnic groups, these authors have denied the existence of any direct connection between the fat content of the diet and the incidence of degenerative cardiovascular disease (YERUSHELMI and HILLEBOE, YUDKIN, STARE and co-workers, POLLAK). In a corporative study by PAGE and co-workers, the view was taken that nothing in findings to date could be held to justify altering the accepted

American diet, more particularly with regard to a drastic curtailment of fat intake. These investigators likewise rejected the demands made in various quarters for improving the quality of certain fats used.

Kinsell, Sinclair, Jolliffe, Malmros, and others take the view that human arteriosclerosis, and more particularly coronary artery sclerosis, is encouraged by a relative and/or absolute deficiency of essential or mainly unsaturated fatty acids. Sinclair regards arteriosclerosis in man as reflecting a definite deficiency in essential fatty acids. Even allowing for the metabolic effects of mainly unsaturated fatty acids (which may be regarded as definitely established), we have so far neither statistical nor sufficiently reliable empirical data regarding the significance of a dietary deficiency in essential fatty acids for the development of atherosclerosis. The ratio between mainly unsaturated or essential fatty acids to saturated fatty acids is alleged by some to play a decisive part in determining the origin and course of arteriosclerosis. However, even this interrelationship has not yet been confirmed by findings to date. We agree with the views of Page and co-workers and consider that, in Europe as in the U.S.A., no pressing grounds exist for drastically curtailing the fat content of the diet or for giving preference to fats and oils containing largely unsaturated fatty acids. It is not a simple matter of replacing "bad" saturated fats with "good" unsaturated ones. At the same time, in dealing with arteriosclerotic patients and those whose family history suggests a strong predisposition towards the disease, one may well make use of the beneficial effects of mainly unsaturated fatty acids in an attempt to reduce elevated levels of lipids and certain classes of lipoproteins. While the diagnostic and prognostic significance of the plasma lipids and lipoproteins is highly questionable, all authorities are to-day agreed on the important part played by these substances in the pathogenesis of arteriosclerosis. It is therefore a recognised principle in the treatment of arteriosclerosis to try and reduce elevated levels of plasma lipids, notably the plasma cholesterol, and to normalise pathological lipoprotein spectra. In this connection, the polyene acids have proved particularly effective. As the attached diagrams show, the addition to the diet of oils rich in polyene acids will reduce elevated serum lipid levels. Keys believes that 2 g of oils rich in polyene acids are sufficient to offset the effect of 1 g of fats rich in saturated fatty acids. According to our findings, a reduction in plasma lipids can be brought about with even smaller amounts of polyene acids. In all such studies, however, it must be remembered that neither the quantitative nor the qualitative composition of the plasma lipids and lipoproteins provides any reliable indication of the lipid or lipoprotein content of the arteries. WEITZEL and co-workers, for instance, were able to show, in the case of phenyl-ethyl-acetic acid, that the drastic reduction in serum lipids is not necessarily accompanied by a reduction in the lipid and lipoprotein content, nor by a regression in the sclerotic lesions of the arteries. Hens suffering from spontaneous atherosclerosis responded to phenyl-ethyl-acetic acid with a fall in serum cholesterol, yet the cholesterol and lipid content of the vessels tended rather to increase under this treatment, while the arteriosclerotic lesions were if anything aggravated. The effect of polyene acids on the composition of the lipids of the vascular walls and on the arteriosclerotic process has likewise not yet been sufficiently investigated, at least as regards arteriosclerosis in man. Nevertheless, in view of the vital pathogenic role of the serum lipids and lipoproteins in arteriosclerosis, we advocate the use of oils containing largely unsaturated fatty acids for those suffering from, or predisposed towards, arteriosclerosis. The percentage of fats in the total diet should not exceed 25% of the total calorie uptake. On this basis, the fat content of the average European diet would indeed have to be reduced for such patients. About half of the calories provided by fats should be supplied by fats and oils rich in polyene acids. In the case of obese subjects, an effort should be made to normalise bodyweight.

Even though some authors (e. g. KEYS) deny any connection between excessive weight and degenerative cardiovascular disease, the fact remains that morbidity and mortality statistics, supported by general clinical experience, strongly suggest that appreciable excess bodyweight is not unimportant in determining the onset and course of arteriosclerosis and more particularly coronary artery sclerosis. The combination of obesity with hypertension is especially unfavourable from this point of view, and in such cases weight-reducing measures are essential. The same applies to obese patients with metabolic disorders such as *diabetes mellitus* or gout; experience shows that such patients also tend to develop severe arteriosclerosis and coronary artery sclerosis at an early age. Concomitant chronic arterial hypertension is another factor likely to promote arteriosclerosis. Mention should also be made at this stage of those essential disorders of fat metabolism such as hypercholesterolaemia and hyperlipaemia, which sometimes occur according to a marked familial pattern, and in which severe coronary artery sclerosis tends to develop in youth and middle age. Premature severe coronary artery sclerosis is also encountered in severe cases of hypothyroidism. All measures calculated to exercise a beneficial effect on these underlying diseases may, in individual cases, fairly be regarded as preventive and therapeutic means of combating arteriosclerosis.

In treating arteriosclerosis, the patient's general mode of living should not be neglected. Important measures are regular physical exercise, adequate rest intervals, properly planned holidays, a regular night's sleep of at least eight hours, and the avoidance of excessive physical, mental, or emotional stress. Further details, which are outside the scope of this paper, will be found in our monograph on arteriosclerosis (Thieme, Stuttgart, 1960).

Prevention and treatment of arteriosclerosis by medicinal means. Active thyroid principles

Cases of congenital thyroid deficiency and hypothyroidism in children are typified by severe hyperlipaemia, hypercholesterolaemia, and elevated serum β-lipoprotein levels. In adults with hypothyroidism, the hyperlipaemia is less marked. Any improvement in thyroid function reduces the elevated lipid titres. The higher the initial titres, the more marked the reduction effected in the circulating serum cholesterol and the lipoproteins by the administration of dry thyroid substance (260—325 mg daily) (Strisower and co-workers). Once therapy is discontinued, the titres soon revert to their original levels. The serum cholesterol and cholesterol esters, the phosphatide quotient, and the β-lipoprotein titres of euthyroid subjects with coronary artery sclerosis also fall in response to L-thyroxine and L-tri-iodo-thyronine. In contrast to patients with myxoedema, however, the α-lipoprotein content does not rise in proportion. The acetic acid analogues of thyroxine and tri-iodo-thyronine, namely tetra-iodo-thyro-acetic acid (TETRAC) and tri-iodo-thyro-acetic acid (TRIAC) reduce the circulating plasma lipids, though the effects on the BMR are less marked. It has been found that the lipid-reducing effect of these related substances wears off after a time, with the result that the dosage must be increased. The effect of tri-iodo-thyro-propionic acid on the blood lipids is variously assessed. Bansi observed no cholesterol-reducing or other metabolic effects. By contrast, Moses and Danovsky, like Sachs and Arons, likewise Flynn and co-workers, all observed a beneficial effect on the circulating plasma lipids and lipoproteins. The details below show the fluctuations in serum lipid levels in a woman with genuine myxoedema. In view of this case, there can be no doubt as to the ability of tri-iodo-thyro-proprionic acid to reduce the serum lipid level. Despite the favourable effect of active thyroid principles on the serum lipids and lipoproteins, it must be admitted that clinical experience in the treatment of patients with *angina pectoris* and with coronary infarction is not encouraging.

47-year-old woman, menstruation normal, BMR — 26. Following I 131 uptake: 4% after 2 hrs, 7% after 24 hrs, 9% after 48 hrs, 6% after 72 hrs. PBI = 0.520%/l serum. Treatment with 3 mg tri-iodo-thyro-proprionic acid (Tritopion Hoechst) markedly reduced the (initially very considerable) hyperlipaemia. On the same dose of Tritopion, the serum lipid titres are now normal, the serum (previously highly lipaemic) is now clear, while the clinical signs of myxoedema, formerly marked, have now vanished. In the X-ray picture, the myxoedematous heart configuration has now become normal, with corresponding changes in the ECG.

The use of these substances is, of course, excluded in cases of acute coronary infarction. Their use also remains highly problematical in the case of subjects who have survived coronary infarction, since this therapy frequently provokes an increase in, or recurrence of, *angina pectoris* attacks. These attacks subside as soon as thyroid therapy is discontinued, recurring as soon as such treatment is resumed (OLIVER and BOYD, STRISOWER). Isolated cases have even been reported in which thyroid principles provoked new coronary infarction and even death. Admittedly, given the nature of the underlying disease, there is no proof of any connection between the two. At the same time, our own experience is also such as to discourage the use of thyroid principles — thyroxine and its analogues, TRIAC, TETRAC, and tri-iodo-thyro-proprionic acid — by euthyroid and especially hyperthyroid patients with coronary artery sclerosis. For patients with clear-cut thyroid hypofunction, by contrast, they form the method of choice. In patients with intermittent claudication, we have found that thyroid therapy, so far from effecting improvement, tends rather to aggravate the condition. We incline to agree with OLIVER and BOYD, who assume that the increase in coronary attacks and the reduced mobility are due to an increase in metabolism in the myocardium and the skeletal musculature, accompanied by increased oxygen requirement.

Sex hormones and arteriosclerosis

It is known that coronary artery sclerosis and obliterative peripheral arteriosclerosis are encountered far less frequently and in milder form in women with normal menstrual cycles than in men of comparable age groups. From this it has been deduced that lack of oestrogen favours the development of coronary artery sclerosis and so of coronary infarction. The anti-arteriosclerotic effect of oestrogens has been repeatedly confirmed in animal experiments.

Sex hormones also exercise an influence on the circulating plasma lipids and lipoproteins. The rise in plasma lipids with increasing age sets in later in women than in men, attaining the same levels as in men with the menopause and subsequently exceeding them. Similar findings exist as regards the lipoproteins. At the time of ovulation and immediately prior to menstruation, the cholesterol, phosphatide, and β-lipoprotein titres fall, rising again about the fourth day after menstruation and increasing during the luteal phase.

It therefore seemed logical to make use of the sex hormones for the prevention and treatment of arteriosclerosis in man. The first trials carried out were with androgens. Testosterone was repeatedly found to exercise a beneficial effect on peripheral vascular disease of various origin. However, this applied largely to patients with functional vascular disease and, in cases of obliterative arteriosclerosis, androgens would not appear to be indicated. Instead, numerous studies have been carried out with oestrogens (Furman and co-workers, Boyd and Oliver, Marmorston and co-workers, Adlersberg and co-workers, Stamler and co-workers). Oestrogenic substances will in fact reduce elevated serum cholesterol and β-lipoprotein levels, while the denser groups of α-lipoproteins and the phosphatides respond with an increase. Unfortunately, the "side-effects" of all the oestrogens so far used, including combined preparations (e. g. Premarin) are so pronounced that the long-term use of these substances in the treatment of peripheral and coronary vascular disease cannot be countenanced. Even minimal daily doses of ethinyl oestradiol are followed, in a high proportion of male patients, by gynaecomastia, partial or complete loss of libido, testicular pain, disorders of erection, while testicular biopsy reveals severe lesions of the germinal epithelium. In view of this, numerous oestrogen derivatives have been examined in an effort to find substances which would produce the same metabolic action, notably on the lipid and lipoprotein levels, but with less marked specifically sexual effects. One such preparation (Manvene) was first reported to have produced favourable results in patients who had survived myocardial infarction, but the side effects were again so considerable that this form of treatment must likewise be discouraged. Of particular importance are clinical reports on the effects of long-term oestrogen administration to patients with coronary artery disease (Oliver and Boyd, Stamler, Pick, and Katz). Oliver and Boyd administered 200 μg ethinyl oestradiol daily to 50 patients who had survived myocardial infarction. These studies extended over $2^1/_2$ years. At the end of nine months, it was found necessary to increase the daily dose to 300 μg in 5 men, in order to maintain the desired effect on the plasma cholesterol. A further 50 patients with similar manifestations were given a placebo preparation. Despite a clear-cut effect on the serum lipid and lipoprotein titres, no definite improvement in morbidity or mortality was observed among the coronary infarct patients as compared with the untreated controls. In another series of studies extending over $3^1/_2$ years, carried out at the Michael Reese Hospital by STAMLER and co-workers, there was again no definite proof of any beneficial effect of oestrogen therapy on morbidity or mortality rates in coronary artery sclerosis or coronary infarction. The daily dose in this case consisted of 10 mg Premarin. The authors express the hope that further studies now under way will produce more helpful results, while admitting that those achieved so far are not encouraging. Experiments are in progress aimed at reducing the specifically sexual effects of oestrogens by changing the molecule, and clinical results to date (CAVALLINI and MASSARINI; BANSI) merit our attention. The effects on the cholesterol balance observed by MER in animal experiments have still to be investigated in the clinic.

Vitamin A + E + B$_6$ in the treatment of arteriosclerosis

In experiments conducted on hens suffering for several years from spontaneous arteriosclerosis, WEITZEL and co-workers found that vitamin A effected considerable regression of the fat plaques, the total fat, and the cholesterol content of the aorta. The addition of vitamin E enhanced this effect. The effect of vitamin A on the fat and cholesterol metabolism also extended to the hepatic lipids but not to the serum lipids. Examination of the aorta showed an increase in vitamin A storage together with a clear-cut reduction in total lipids. Chemical analysis showed that the connective tissue of the aorta was unaffected by vitamin A + E. By contrast, vitamin B$_6$ had no effect on the aortic lipids but reduced the connective-tissue ground substance and, when given in large doses, the collagen tissue of the aortic wall. The combined administration of vitamins A + E + B$_6$ was therefore confidently expected to influence both the lipids and the connective tissue of the aorta. In fact, however, the combination of vitamins A + E + B$_6$ was found to have no greater anti-arteriosclerotic action than vitamins A + E alone; indeed, results suggested that the addition of vitamin B$_6$ tended rather to weaken the effect of vitamins A + E.

Following these experiments, the effect of vitamins A + E + B$_6$ was studied in "double blind" tests in 269 patients with peripheral arteriosclerosis, coronary artery sclerosis, and so-called cerebral

arteriosclerosis, over a period of 12 months. Those participating
in these studies included the University Medical Clinics of Cologne,
Leipzig, Marburg, Munich, and Tübingen, the University Medical
Policlinic in Heidelberg, and the Medical Clinic in Stuttgart-Bad
Cannstatt.

Subjective improvement (i. e. as regards *angina pectoris* attacks,
intermittent claudication, memory disorders, loss of concentration,
cerebral vertigo) was observed in 37% of patients following vitamins A + E, in 31% following vitamins A + E + B_6 in the double
blind test, in 39% following vitamins A + E + B_6 when administered openly, and in 26% of patients given placeboes. The subjective improvement achieved with vitamins A + E was largely
concerned with alleviation of the cerebral disorders; there was no
evidence that the *angina pectoris* disorders or the intermittent
claudication of arteriosclerotic origin responded any better to the
vitamins than to placebo treatment. Taking the symptoms of the
individual groups of patients with coronary artery, peripheral, and
cerebral vascular disease, there is no statistical evidence that
vitamin therapy produced any better results than placeboes.
Indeed, one cannot fail to be struck by the high rate of improvement effected by placeboes alone, namely 20% of cerebral symptoms, 32% of *angina pectoris* disorders, and 36% of cases of
intermittent claudication. Another striking factor is the difference
in results obtained between the groups given vitamins A + E + B_6
in open and in "coded" forms respectively. In the former instance,
there was a considerably higher improvement rate in cerebral
symptoms and *angina pectoris*. No objective evidence of improvement in arteriosclerotic manifestations was established, either by
circulatory studies (Brömser-Ranke method), positional tests,
ECG, mobility tests, or analysis of serum lipids and coagulation
factors (Kommerell and Berger). In other words, the subjective
results were not borne out by objective findings. Strangely enough,
the administration of vitamins A + E produced in some patients
considerable, macroscopically detectable, lipaemia, but this is not
the rule.

This study provides an interesting example of how hard it is
to test the pharmacological effects of a preparation on arteriosclerosis. It is interesting to note that the percentage improvement
obtained with placeboes conforms with the figures repeatedly
obtained in the treatment of *angina pectoris*.

The pharmacological effects on lipid metabolism cover absorption,
synthesis, intermediate metabolism, including catabolism, the state
of the lipids in the plasma and in various organs, and their excretion.

Prevention of fat and cholesterol absorption by means of silicic acid gel, mineral oils, or aluminium hydroxide gel is not a practical proposition. On the other hand, POLLAK, BEST, et al. found that β-*sitosterol* reduced the cholesterol, total lipid, and neutral fat titres and, to a lesser extent, the plasma phosphatides. Comparable effects were also observed in the lipoproteins. However, these results, reported by several authors, were confirmed by WILKINSON and co-workers in the case of human beings, and the practical worth of this therapy is gravely curtailed by the fact that daily doses of 18—25 g must be given in an emulsion.

The prevention of fat absorption with iodo-acetate and phlorhizin by means of phosphorylation is the subject of much dispute and is of little practical value. Nor have we any clinical study of the value of the blockade of pancreatic lipase by means of sodium-ethyl-sulphate. Promotion of cholesterol excretion via the bile by means of cholagogues and lipotropic substances is useless in view of the entero-hepatic circulation of the cholesterol. The breakdown of cholesterol in the intestinal tract by various *Coli* strains via cholestenon-coprostanon-coprostanol is impeded by antibiotics. This might account for the hyperlipaemia observed by us in patients treated with streptomycin or broad-spectrum antibiotics. We would also mention here the studies by ROSENHEIM and WEBSTER, who succeeded in promoting coprostanol formation from cholesterol with the aid of cerebrosides. These substances have no therapeutic importance in practice.

Attempts have been made to attack the endogenous synthesis of cholesterol and the neutral fats with *phenyl-ethyl-acetic acid*. Clinical therapy is based on animal experiments carried out by REDEL and COTTET, who succeeded in reducing elevated plasma cholesterol titres with phenyl-ethyl-acetic acid — results which were later confirmed in man. Favourable effects in hyperlipaemia and hypercholesterolaemia were likewise observed by PLEGER and TIRSCHEK, also by TRENKMANN. FRIEDRICKSON and STEINBERG, who observed inhibition of cholesterol synthesis in liver slices under the influence of phenyl-ethyl-acetic acid, failed to detect any plasma-lipid reducing effect on the part of phenyl-ethyl butyrate or phenyl-ethyl valerate. OLIVER and BOYD have reported the same phenomenon. Nearly all their patients complained of retching, vomiting, and nausea. We, too, were unimpressed by the clinical value of these substances, and in any case observed serious toxic side-effects. Two of our patients exhibited porphyrins in the urine, which compelled us to discontinue therapy. WEITZEL's findings, referred to earlier, also cast considerable doubt on the value of reducing the serum cholesterol level by phenyl-ethyl-acetic acid in the treatment of arteriosclerosis. From these studies, it must be concluded that substances which inhibit cholesterol synthesis do not necessarily possess anti-arteriosclerotic properties; on the contrary, such properties are more likely to come from substances which promote the metabolism and transportation of cholesterol. The rationale and clinical results of therapy with phenyl-ethyl-acetic acid have recently been discussed in detail by my collaborator, Wilz.

Nicotinic acid in the treatment of arteriosclerosis

According to investigations by Spies and co-workers, the sodium salt of nicotinic acid possesses potent vasodilator properties, and the substance has repeatedly been used in the treatment of arteriosclerotic vascular disease. In particular, nicotinic acid compounds have been tried in cases of functional vascular disease. Both oral and parenteral administration produce marked hyper-aemia of the skin, particularly in the upper extremities and the head, the effect on the lower extremities being much less marked. The mechanism of action consists of dilatation of the smaller blood vessels of the peripheral circulation (arterioles, capillaries, and venules), the opening up of small arteriovenous anastomoses, and the dilatation of collateral vessels. These effects set in 1—2 min after *intravenous* injection, rapidly attaining their maximum effect and subsiding again after about 10 min. *Intramuscular* injection delays the onset of action. Following *oral administration* of 100 mg of the sodium salt of nicotinic acid, the effect becomes clear-cut after about 10 min. A further effect of nicotinic acid compounds, observed *inter alia* by Altschul and co-workers, Steinmann and Schafroth, Parsons and co-workers, and Nieper, consists in the reduction of elevated serum cholesterol titres. Administration of 1—3 g of nicotinic acid daily (!) reduced the serum cholesterol level in proportion to the dosage given, the reduction effected being even more marked where the initial levels had been very high. Patients with familial history of hypercholesterolaemia frequently proved refractory. The falls in cholesterol effected ranged from 15—50% of the initial values. The nicotinic acid also reduced the titres of the total lipids, the total fatty acids, and the β-lipoproteins, but not the phosphatides. Unfortunately, the very high doses given almost always provoked severe subjective side-effects such as marked erythema, hot flushes, dizziness, nausea, retching, etc., with the result that attempts were made to achieve comparable results with smaller doses. Steinmann and Schafroth, like Nava and co-workers, have reported cholesterol-reducing effects with individual amounts of as little as 50—300 mg of nicotinic acid. In our own experience, such doses have failed to produce dependable results. Moreover, it seems certain that the lipid-reducing effect of nicotinic acid wears off after a time, thus forcing one to increase the dosage at regular intervals in order to maintain the metabolic effects desired. In animals, very large doses of nicotinic acid activate *fibrinolysis*, with typical changes in the thrombelastogram (IMHOF and co-workers; WEINER and co-workers; KOMMERELL and co-workers). The maximum effect sets in between 5 and 20 min after injection; within an hour, the levels have usually reverted to normal. After oral administration, the onset of action is delayed, the maximum level being obtained after about 1 hr and reverting to normal during the following hour. The reduction in the reaction time, demonstrable in the thrombelastogram, reflects the hypercoagulability of the blood; it is still clearly in evidence one hour after injection, and so lasts longer than the fibrinolysis. It is not yet clear whether this entails disadvantages from the therapeutic point of view, though clinical experience to date provides nothing to suggest that this is the case. Some authors advocate the prophylactic administration of anticoagulants to combat the increased coagulability. The therapeutic doses of nicotinic acid so far employed in order to reduce the lipid titres have failed to provide evidence that they activate fibrinolysis; on the other hand, it seems quite possible that the methods employed to date are not sufficiently sensitive to detect such activation. However this may be, great interest attaches to the clinical findings of STEINMANN and SCHAFROTH, who observed thrombo-embolic complications four times less frequently in hemiplegic patients given nicotinic acid than in corresponding patients not so treated.

The usefulness of nicotinic acid in coronary vascular disease has not yet been conclusively established. In peripheral vascular disease of arteriosclerotic origin, the improvement in cutaneous blood flow effected by nicotinic acid is not necessarily desirable inasmuch as it is usually achieved at the expense of the blood flow in the muscles (HENSEL and co-workers). In cases of intermittent claudication of arteriosclerotic origin, we failed to produce satisfactory results with either parenteral or oral administration of nicotinic acid.

The basic principles of nicotinic acid therapy in the treatment of vascular disease, with indications and contra-indications, were recently discussed by my collaborator NEIKES.

Surface-active substances in the treatment of arteriosclerosis

The serum lipids, as is known, are bound to proteins. The stability of these symplexes, the lipoproteins, is maintained by natural emulgators and is influenced by artificial emulgators. The natural stabilisers include the phospholipids (Ahrens and Kunkel). A high proportion of phosphatides, for instance, will maintain the clarity of sera containing large amounts of neutral fats; these undergo milky opacity on removal of the phosphatides. These clearing properties of the phosphatides have also been exploited in therapy. Attempts have been made, using lecithins of various composition and origin, to reduce elevated serum lipids by oral route and to improve the so-called cholesterol-phosphatide quotient (Steiner and Domansky; Gross and Kesten; and others). The effect of such substances is inconstant, and evidently wears off with time. Of interest is the lipid-reducing effect of highly purified phosphatide fractions (Klenk; Eikermann), as reported by various authors after oral doses of a few grammes and intravenous administration of milligramme amounts (Knüchel; Küchmeister; Leupold; Schettler and co-workers; Schön; Schrade and co-workers). Schrade, using a preparation containing large amounts of linolic acid (Lipostabil) by parenteral route, observed a definite clearing effect in cases of alimentary lipaemia. Fasoli and co-workers, using an ultracentrifuge, observed displacement of the β-lipoproteins in favour of the denser α-lipoproteins, while Lasch and co-workers noted an effect on coagulation activity. According to Leupold, the iodine index of the serum is also affected.

The serum albumins also produce stabilising effects on the lipids (Pollak). Highly purified human albumin is capable of dispersing lipaemia and has a clearing effect, which is not identical with that of the lipoprotein lipase induced by heparin. Heparin and heparinoid substances have also been tried in the treatment of arteriosclerosis. It is known that fatty meals may be followed by transitory lipaemia, which immediately clarifies in response to injection of heparin or heparinoid substances. This process of lipolysis is associated with the formation of glycerine and free fatty acids, whose concentration in turn influences the clarification process. Di- and mono-glycerides arise as intermediate products. In other words, heparin and heparinoid substances set in motion a clearing mechanism which is evidently regulated by lipoprotein lipase (Korn). Since the clarification factor is reduced in elderly persons and arteriosclerotics, attention was fastened on some defect in the clarification system for its possible significance in the pathogenesis of arteriosclerosis. It seemed worth while attempting to eliminate this defect with the aid of heparin and heparinoid substances. In addition to favourable reports (ENGELBERG, GRAHAM and co-workers; Lit. cf. GUBSER, also HEYMANN), there also exist negative accounts concerning the long-term use of these substances in arteriosclerosis and notably in coronary artery sclerosis (WILKINSON). Whereas the reduction of elevated neutral fat titres in the serum by heparin and heparinoid substances is generally recognised, the question of whether these substances are capable of influencing morphological vascular lesions remains a matter of dispute. In view of this, all the more importance attaches, in our view, to the favourable effect of these substances on visible xanthomas, as related in the following case report:

A. K., 54 years old, suffering from severe essential familial hyperlipaemia with disseminated xanthomas. For 9 years, vain attempts had been made, using Inocit, nicotinic acid, choline, pyridoxine, vitamin A + E, hyaluronidase, ACTH, and prednisone, to reduce the neutral fat content of the serum and to eliminate the xanthomas. Since the patient was a traveller by profession, a strictly low-fat regimen was impracticable. By means of long-term therapy with heparin and heparinoid substances, we succeeded in normalising the serum lipids, and the xanthomas, previously visible externally, vanished completely. In addition, the liver, originally greatly enlarged, resumed its normal size, and the heart pains, which took the form of anginal attacks, disappeared. Objectively, there is clear-cut improvement in the coronary vascular lesions, which were previously clearly discernible in the ECG.

Treatment was instituted in January 1958 with Elheparin, a heparinoid substance. The patient was given 4 × 5,000 U i.v. or i.m. weekly for 14 days. Following a mild attack of epistaxis, this treatment was discontinued. From March to December 1958, the patient was given doses of 3 × (later 2 ×) 300 mg depot-thrombocide i.m. weekly. Although the patient received no further heparinoid injections during 1959 and adhered to no special dietary regimen, the serum lipids have remained normal and the xanthomas have not so far reappeared. Nor has there been any recurrence of the subjective disorders. After one year's interruption in heparinoid treatment, the serum neutral fats gradually began to rise again, whereupon the patient was given doses of 300 mg depot-thrombocide once weekly. On this dosage, the neutral fat titres have remained normal. The patient feels well, and has remained free from skin lesions.

Equally good results were obtained in the case of this patient's 47-year-old sister, the serum neutral fat titres reverting to normal and the skin xanthomas regressing.

It remains to be seen whether long-term therapy with heparinoid substances will also prove successful in arteriosclerotic patients without xanthomas, i. e. those without serious disorders of fat metabolism. In patients with essential familial hypercholesterolaemia, the effects on the serum lipids and on coronary vascular disorders are disputed. Nor should it be forgotten that even relatively small doses of heparinoid substances, even below the coagulation threshold, may in the long run produce toxic reactions (cf. Studer and co-workers).

Summing up, it may be said that, while the drug therapy of arteriosclerosis affords certain promising aspects, we are still very far from having a key to any causal treatment. Indeed, given the multiple aetiology of arteriosclerosis in man, no panacea can reasonably be expected. More than in any other disease, the scheme of treatment for arteriosclerosis must take into account the entire mode of living of the patient, and it is not enough to wait until signs of sclerotic vascular disease have made their appearance before prescribing drugs.

Summary

After a review dealing with the susceptibility of hypertensive patients to early and severe arteriosclerosis, the prophylactic and therapeutic possibilities of dietary measures are discussed. The view is taken that, in laying down a practical dietary regimen for arteriosclerotic patients, there is no justification for confining the fats in the food intake exclusively to oils and fats rich in polyene acids. But in the case of arteriosclerotic patients with demonstrable disorders of fat metabolism, it is suggested that about half of the calories derived from fats should be supplied by oils rich in polyene acids. The percentage of fats in the total diet should not exceed 25% of the calorie uptake. In cases of obesity, efforts should be made to reduce the patient's body-weight. Important prophylactic measures against arteriosclerosis include treatment for such hypertension as may be present, as well as immediate measures to control metabolic diseases which tend to promote arteriosclerosis, e. g. diabetes mellitus, gout, essential hyperlipaemia, and hypercholesterolaemia.

Active thyroid principles, thyroxine and its analogues, are indicated only in the treatment of arteriosclerotic patients suffering from thyroid hypofunction.

Administration of oestrogens to male patients is only justified where extremely severe vascular lesions have already developed. The side effects of oestrogens are so pronounced as to outweigh their metabolic activity in normalising pathological lipid and lipoprotein patterns.

Double-blind studies failed to demonstrate any clear-cut effect when vitamins $A + E + B_6$ were employed to treat arteriosclerotic patients. Reference is also made to the effect of beta-sitosterol and phenyl-ethyl-acetic acid in hyperlipaemic cases of arteriosclerosis. In arteriosclerotic vascular diseases of the upper extremities, as well as in cerebral arteriosclerosis and patients who have survived an apoplectic attack, the sodium salt of nicotinic acid may render useful service; it also has specific effects on the lipid balance and on fibrinolysis. Artificial and natural emulsifying agents of the phospholipid type are capable of lowering elevated plasma lipid titres and more or less normalising pathological lipoprotein patterns. They also exert a clearing effect.

Preparations of the heparin and heparinoid type, which induce clearing, may eliminate vascular disorders in patients with essential hyperlipaemia and bring about the disappearance of xanthomas without recourse to further dietary measures. Clinical results are reported. The value of normalising pathological serum factors as a means of preventing and treating arteriosclerosis poses problems which are also referred to.

Résumé

Après avoir rappelé la tendance que présentent les hypertendus à faire une artério-sclérose précoce et sévère, l'auteur discute les possibilités prophylactiques et thérapeutiques du régime. Il estime que 25% seulement des besoins caloriques de l'artérioscléreux peuvent être constitués pour moitié par des huiles et graisses riches en acides gras non saturés. Chez les obèses, on s'efforcera d'obtenir une réduction du poids. D'importantes mesures prophylactiques au cours de l'artériosclérose sont le traitement d'une hypertension concommitante, ainsi que d'une maladie de la nutrition favorisant l'artério-sclérose, telle que diabète, goutte, hyperlipémie et hyper-cholestérolémie essentielles.

Les extraits thyroïdiens, thyroxine ou ses analogues, sont éventuellement indiqués dans le traitement des artérioscléreux hypothyroïdiens.

Les œstrogènes ne sont indiqués que dans les scléroses coronariennes graves. Les effets secondaires des œstrogènes limitent l'intérêt de leurs effets métaboliques (normalisation du lipido-protéinogramme pathologique).

Les vitamines A + E + B_6 n'ont aucun effet convaincant chez les artérioscléreux. L'auteur mentionne aussi l'action du sitostérol et de l'acide phényl-éthyl-acétique chez les artérioscléreux avec hyperlipémie. Au cours des troubles circulatoires artérioscléreux des extrémités supérieures, dans la sclérose cérébrale, et chez les sujets ayant survécu à un ictus apoplectique, le sel sodique de l'acide nicotinique peut être utile. On a observé avec cette substance des effets particuliers sur le taux des lipides et la fibrinolyse. Des émulsifs naturels ou artificiels du type des phospholipides peuvent faire baisser le taux des lipides plasmatiques et ramener le spectre lipido-protidique pathologique vers la normale. Ils possèdent en outre un effet de clarification (clearing effect). Les produits à "clearing effect" du type héparine ou héparinoïde peuvent amener, sans autres mesures diététiques, la disparition des troubles vasculaires chez les malades présentant une hyperlipémie xanthomatose essentielle. L'utilité de l'héparine dans la prophylaxie et la thérapeutique de l'artério-sclérose est enfin discutée.

References

ACKERMAN, R. F., T. J. DRY, and J. E. EDWARDS: Circulation 1, 1345 (1950). — ADLERSBERG, D.: Amer. J. Med. 23, 769 (1957). — AHRENS, E. H. and H. G. KUNKEL: J. exp. Med. 90, 409 (1949). — ALTSCHUL, R.: Circulation 14, 494 (1956).

BANSI, H. W.: Mkurse ärztl. Fortbild. 9, 454 (1959). — BANSI, H. W.: Med. Klin. 54, 673 (1959). — BASCH, R. VON: Über latente Arteriosklerose und deren Beziehung zu Fettleibigkeit, Herzerkrankungen und anderen Begleiterscheinungen. Vienna: Urban & Schwarzenberg 1893. — BELL, E. T. and B. J. CLAWSON: Arch. Path. 5, 939 (1928). — BEST, M. M., C. H. DUNCAN, E. J. VAN LOON, and J. D. WATHEN: Circulation 10, 201 (1954). — BEST, M. M., C. H. DUNCAN, E. J. VAN LOON, and J. D. WATHEN: Amer. J. Med. 19, 61 (1955).

COMESANA, F., A. NAVA, B. L. FISHLEDER, and D. SODI-PALLARES: Amer. Heart J. 55, 476 (1958).

DAVIES, D. and M. J. KLAINER: Amer. Heart. J. 19, 185 (1940).

EIKERMANN, H.: Fortschr. Med. 74, 381 (1956). — ENGELBERG, H., R. KUHN, and M. STEINMAN: Circulation 13, 489 (1956). — ENGELBERG, H., R. KUHN, and M. STEINMAN: Circulation 14, 498 (1956).

Fasoli, A., F. Salteri, and A. Cesana: Internat. Congr. Amer. Coll. of Chest-Physicians, Cologne Aug. 1956. — Fishberg, A. M.: Hypertension and Nephritis. 5th Ed. Philadelphia: Lea 1954. — Flynn, P. F., S. Splitter, H. Balch, and L. W. Kinsell: Circulation 20, 984 (1959) (lecture report). — Furman, H. F., R. P. Howard, L. N. Norcia, and E. C. Keaty: Amer. J. Med. 24, 80 (1958).

Graham, D. M., T. P. Lyon, J. W. Gofman, H. B. Jones, A. Yankley, J. Simonton, and S. White: Circulation 4, 666 (1951). — Gross, P. and B. M. Kesten: N. Y. St. J. Med. 50, 2683 (1950). — Gubser, J.: Medizinische 1956, 1190.

Heymann, A.: Internist 1, (1960) (in press). — Huchard and Jaques: Formes cliniques d'artériosclérose. Congr. franç. med. 10, 5 (1908). — Hunter, A.: J. Invt. Actuaries 70, 60 (1939).

Imhof, P., M. Imhof, E. Eichenberger, and H. Lauener: Schweiz. med. Wschr. 89, 736 (1959).

Jolliffe, N.: Circulation 20, 109 (1959).

Kernohan, J. W., E. W. Anderson, and N. M. Keith: Arch. intern. Med. 44, 395 (1929). — Kesten, H. D., and R. Silbowitz: Proc. Soc. exp. Biol. N. Y. 49, 71 (1942). — Keys, A., J. T. Anderson, and F. Grande: Lancet 273, 959 (1957). — Keys, A., J. T. Anderson, and F. Grande: Amer. J. clin. Nutr. 7, 444 (1959). — Keys, A., and P. D. White: Cardiovascular Epidemiology. New York 1956. — Kinsell, L. W., G. D. Michaels, R. W. Friskey, and S. Splitter: Lancet 274, 334 (1958). — Knüchel, F.: Therapiewoche 5, 570 (1955). — Kommerell, B. and H. D. Berger: Klin. Wschr. 38, 134 (1960). — Kommerell, B. and H. D. Berger: personal communication — Korn, E. D.: J. biol. Chem. 215, 1 (1955). — Küchmeister, H., H. Goldeck, and H. Hammers: Med. Klin. 51, 1455 (1956).

Lasch, H. G., K. Schimpf, and W. Winnewisser: Medizinische 1958, 944. — Leupold, F.: Bull. schweiz. Akad. med. Wiss. 13, 451 (1957). — Leupold, F.: Z. Kreisl.-Forsch. 47, 281 (1958).

Malmros, H. and G. Wigand: Lancet 273, 1 (1957). — Marchand, F.: Verh. Kongr. inn. Med. 21, 23 (1904). — Marmorston, J., O. Magidson, J. J. Lewis, J. Mehl, F. J. Moore, and J. Bernstein: New Engl. J. Med. 258, 583 (1958). — Master, A. M.: Circulation 8, 170 (1953). — Moschcowitz, E.: Virchows Arch. path. Anat. 283, 282 (1932). — Moses, C. and T. S. Danowski: Circulation 20, 988 (1959) (lecture report).

Nava, A., F. Comesana, E. Lozano, B. L. Fishleder, and D. Sodi-Pallares: Amer. Heart J. 56, 598 (1958). — Neikes, K.: Med. Welt. 1960 (in press). — Nieper, H. A.: Med. Welt 1960, 379.

Oliver, M. F. and G. S. Boyd: Amer. Heart J. 47, 348 (1954). — Oliver, M. F. and G. S. Boyd: Lancet 271, 1273 (1956). — Oliver, M. F. and G. S. Boyd: Lancet 272, 124 (1957). — Oliver, M. F. and G. S. Boyd: Lancet 273, 829 (1957).

Page, I. H.: Biol. Symposia 11, 43 (1945). — Page, I. H., F. J. Stare, A. C. Corcoran, H. Pollack, and C. F. Wilkinson: Fed. Proc. 18, 47 (1959). — Page, I. H., F. J. Stare, A. C. Corcoran, H. Pollack, and C. F. Wilkinson: Circulation 16, 163 (1957). — Parsons, W. B., F. W. P. Achor, K. G. Berge, B. F. McKenzie, and N. W. Barker: Proc. Mayo Clin. 31, 377 (1956). — Pfleger, L. and H. Tirschek: Wien. klin. Wschr. 68, 435 (1956). — Pollak, O. J.: Geriatrics 6, 182 (1951). — Pollak, O. J.: Circulation 7, 702 (1953). — Pollak, O. J.: Circulation 14, 309 (1956).

RABSON, S. M., and H. HELPERN: Amer. Heart J. **35**, 635 (1949). —
RAU, H.: Klin. Wschr. **34**, 167 (1956). — REDEL, J. and J. COTTET: C. R.
Acad. Sci. (Paris) **236**, 2553 (1953). — ROSENHEIM, O. and T. A. WEBSTER:
Biochem. J. **35**, 920 (1941).
SCHETTLER, G.: Klin. Wschr. **30**, 627 (1952). — SCHETTLER, G.: Dtsch.
med. Wschr. **78**, 264 (1953). — SCHETTLER, G.: Medizinische **1955**, 1247. —
SCHETTLER, G.: Therapiewoche **7**, 106 (1956). — SCHÖN, H.: Med. Klin.
54, 1394 (1959). — SCHÖN, H.: Med. Klin. **55**, 260 (1960). — SCHRADE, W.,
R. BIEGLER, and E. BÖHLE: Dtsch. med. Wschr. **83**, 1355 and 1396 (1958). —
SCHRADE, W., R. BIEGLER, and E. BÖHLE: Schweiz. med. Wschr. **89** 117
(1959). — SINCLAIR, H. M.: Lancet **270**, 381 (1956). — SOLTH, K., R. KÖHL,
G. SCHETTLER, and A. WERTHEMANN: Verh. dtsch. Ges. Path. **41** 64 (1958).—
SPIES, T. D., W. B. BEAN, and R. E. STONE: J. Amer. med. Ass. **111**, 584
(1938). — STAMLER, J., R. PICK, and L. N. KATZ: Ann. N. Y. Acad. Sci. **64**,
596 (1956). — STAMLER, J.: Internat. Symposium on Drugs Affecting Lipid
Metabolism. Milan 1960. — STARE, F. J., T. B. VAN ITALLIE, M. B.
MCCANN, and O. W. PORTMAN: J. Amer. med. Ass. **164**, 1920 (1957). —
STEINBERG, D. and D. S. FREDRICKSON: Proc. Soc. exp. Biol. (N. Y.) **90**,
232 (1955). — STEINER, A. and B. DOMANSKI: Arch. intern. Med. **71**, 397
(1943). — STEINMANN, B. and H. J. SCHAFROTH: Ther. Umsch. **16**, 147
(1959). — STRISOWER, B., J. W. GOFMAN, E. F. GALIONI, J. H. RUBINGER,
J. POUTEAU, and P. GUZVICH: Lancet **272**, 120 (1957). — STRISOWER, B.,
J. W. GOFMAN, E. F. GALIONI, J. H. RUBINGER, J. POUTEAU, and P. GUZVICH:
In: Hormones and Atherosclerosis. Ed.: G. Pincus. New York: Acad.
Press 1959. — STUDER, A., F. KOLLER, P. KAEGI, K. VOGLER, W. OBER-
HÄNSLI, and M. KOFLER: Bull. schweiz. Akad. med. Wiss. **13**, 239 (1957). —
SYDENSTRICKER, E.: Arteriosclerosis, a Survey of the Problem. New York:
1933.
TOBIAN, L.: Minn. Med. **38**, 784 (1955). — TRENCKMANN, H.: Ärztl.
Wschr. **11**, 423 (1956).
VOIGT, K.-D., E. GADERMANN, E. J. KLEINPIEN and C. SARTORI: Dtsch.
Arch. klin. Med. **204** 409 (1957).
WAKERLIN, G. E.: Ann. intern. Med. **37**, 313 (1952). — WEINER, M.,
W. REDISCH, and J. M. STEELE: Proc. Soc. exp. Biol. (N. Y.) **98**, 755 (1958). —
WEITZEL, G., H. SCHÖN, and F. GEY: Klin. Wschr. **33**, 772 (1955). — WEITZEL,
G. and E. BUDDECKE: Klin. Wschr. **34**, 1172 (1956). — WEITZEL, G., E. BUD-
DECKE, and H. KÖNIG: Hoppe-Seylers. Z. physiol. Chem. **310**, 139 (1958). —
WILKINSON, C. F. jr., E. BOYLE, R. S. JACKSON, and M. R. BENJAMIN:
Bull. N. Y. Acad. Sci. **31**, 198 (1954). — WILKINSON, C. F. jr.: Circulation
8, 444 (1953).
YERUSHALMY, J. and H. E. HILLEBOE: N. Y. St. J. Med. **1957**, 2343. —
YUDKIN, J.: Lancet **273**, 155 (1957).

For further literature see SCHETTLER, G., Arteriosklerose. Stuttgart:
Thieme 1960.

Discussion

STEINMANN: Dr. SCHETTLER has mentioned nicotinic acid. May I show you some slides concerning our treatment with nicotinic acid in hemiplegic patients? We treat them first with intravenous injections, later with 300 mg nicotinic acid daily for months. In the group treated with nicotinic acid one thrombo-embolic complication was seen in 46 patient months; in the control group without nicotinic acid there was one complication in about 13 patient months. In cases with auricular fibrillation the difference is even more pronounced. We compared our results with those of McDEVITT and WRIGHT who used long-term treatment with anticoagulants. As you can see, there is about the same ratio as in our results between the anticoagulants group and the control group, i.e. one thrombo-embolic episode in 44 patient months with, and in 12.5 patient months without, anticoagulants.

We first gave nicotinic acid in hemiplegic patients bearing in mind in particular its vasodilator effect on the cerebral vessels. After the fibrinolytic activity of the nicotinic acid became evident, it rather looked as if nicotinic acid had a preventory effect on thrombo-embolic complications. The doses of nicotinic acid used by us are not so high as the doses which must be given to achieve a reliable fibrinolytic effect. Therefore we cannot say with certainty whether the good prophylactic effect of nicotinic acid as regards thrombo-embolic episodes in our hemiplegic patients is only due to its fibrinolytic activity. We studied at the same time the influence of nicotinic acid on the serum cholesterol. Most of the other authors use higher doses for this purpose. With our rather small doses we saw an increase in low levels and a decrease in high levels of cholesterol, but not in all cases. Where the level prior to treatment with nicotinic acid was normal, it did not change markedly. Nicotinic acid seems to us to be worthy of further study.

HOOD: I have two questions. One to Dr. SCHETTLER: Now, as I got it, you yourself used a diet where you had a 25% total fat content, half of which you gave as vegetable oil. Now, what would that mean? On a 3,000 calory diet, 750 calories of fat; that means 375 calories as vegetable oil, which would be approximately 40 g of vegetable oil a day. Now that is entirely within reasonable limits, in practical terms, of a long-range therapy. We have studied a very large material of essential hypercholesterolemia and essential hyperlipemia on polyunsaturated fatty acids for several years, and we can easily have them take without any trouble up to 50 or 60 g a day, but the trouble is that the effect on the serum cholesterol is very slight at this dosage in our material; it worked out as a 30 mg-% decrease on a daily intake of 50 g. Really substantial decreases of total serum cholesterol or β-lipoprotein levels we did not get until we had a diet of about 75 g of vegetable oil a day on a low fat diet; and that was, in I would say at least 80% of our material, impossible to maintain for longer periods of time. That is a practical question. Now, the heparin question in hypertension is naturally a ticklish one. You could use more frequent lower doses, thus avoiding anticoagulant effects while still maintaining anticlearing effects. It should be possible to work it that way.

Then I have got a question that puzzles me, and that is this subintimal hyperplasia in the renal arteries. Now we have only seen a few cases of malignant hypertension which developed what you call a delayed uremia; those have, as far as I can remember, been exclusively cases of chronic pyelonephritis, where the progressive derangement due to infection was unaffected by the antihypertensive treatment, as one might expect. But what I am really puzzled about is that, in the works from the Cleveland Clinic group, focalized subintimal hyperplasia is estimated to occur as a cause of renal artery stenosis in about 20% of such cases.

Now, what I would like to know is: In this material of 84 malignant hypertensives, how many had an initial arteriography before treatment was started? Could you give me that figure?

IMHOF: Dr. HOOD, the obstructive renal artery lesion you are mentioning is a completely different disease from the one we are dealing with now. The obstructive renal artery lesion is a localized narrowing of the main stem and the main branches, whereas the subintimal fibroplasia we are describing is a diffuse lesion of the interlobar and arcuate arteries. Of course, some of our cases have undergone renal arteriography; this procedure seems to be noncontributory for the diagnosis of subintimal fibroplasia of the interlobar and arcuate arteries.

HOOBLER: With respect to Dr. IMHOF's paper, I would like to ask whether uremia or azotemia had a higher correlation with the subintimal fibroplasia which you described. With respect to the next paper, I would like to put in a credit word for MER-29, a drug which you ruled out. Many of us feel that it does lower cholesterol, and more interesting, it does relieve angina as well. I do not know why or how it does this, but it is an interesting drug. I was particularly interested in your report on the use of the heparin and was, as a matter of fact, so impressed that I would appreciate very much if you could give us more therapeutic details, because we all have cases such as these. Were you trying to indicate that nicotinic acid in a special dose, not too high, had a fibrinolytic action? If so, are there laboratory tests to demonstrate this action of nicotinic acid?

IMHOF: At the beginning of the treatment, 6 out of our 19 patients showed urea retention; at the time of death 15 had severe renal failure and most of them demonstrated the uremic syndrome. I believe that the relationship between azotemia and development of subintimal fibroplasia of the interlobar and arcuate arteries is an indirect one: patients with mild azotemia prior to institution of treatment have better chances of living for many months or years. Thus, subintimal fibroplasia has time to develop, in contrast to the more rapid course of severely azotemic patients. A quantitative relationship has not been established in this respect.

COTTET: I should like to ask Dr. SCHETTLER two questions. With regard to diets rich in non-saturated fatty acids, does he consider that such acids act as antidotes to saturated fatty acids? In the first place, I' d like to ask him if he thinks that at present one is justified in putting patients on permanent dietary regimens containing almost exclusively non-saturated fatty acids. Secondly, if I have understood him correctly, I think he said that, despite the very clear-cut hypocholesteronaemic effect of oestrogens, he had not observed any encouraging clinical results with them. If that is what he did say, then I'd like him to tell us what he thinks of the prognostic and diagnostic value of cholesterone, because in a work which we published recently (Société cardiologique), we studied patients who had had a myocardial infarction, patients suffering from angina pectoris, and classified them into cases with a cholesteronaemia of over 300 mg-% and those with a cholesteronaemia below 200 mg-%; and there is no doubt that there is a difference between the two groups of patients as regards the clinical course, the prognosis, the survival rate, and the incidence of coronary vascular accidents.

SCHETTLER: Concerning Dr. HOOBLER's question on the heparin treatment of hypercholesterolemia, I think that heparin has its indication only in cases with essential hyperlipaemia and in cases with very massive and very severe disturbances of fat metabolism. We could not find any good effects in cases with hypercholesteronaemia and with those of a *familial* type. I think this is very important to know. We administered 100 mg as a depot for one week over a period of one year. When not using a depot preparation, we administered twice a week between 100 and 200 mg of heparin, which is below the effective dose for coagulation. But, if I may repeat, we only saw good results in this small number of cases with essential hyperlipaemia.

With regard to the question of Dr. HOOD, we intend to reduce our diets from 3000 calories to 2300 and we give higher caloric diets only for persons who are working hard. If we apply diets with 2300 calories, we allow about 40 g (cc) of oil, 20 g of fats, and 20 to 30 g of hidden fats in the food. It is worthwhile to reduce diets and to reduce weight in patients with coronary attacks.

To Dr. COTTET: We do not know very much about the metabolism of high unsaturated fatty acids in correspondance to the saturated ones. I do not believe that there is a strict antagonism between these acids. According to American investigators, it is correct that the unsaturated fatty acids do enhance the excretion of bile acids, but one does not know in which way these substances are affected. And I think it is impossible to use a diet — your second question—which contains only unsaturated fatty acids. It is impossible, at least in Western Europe. Nobody will eat it, and I am sure in America it is the same. There are only small groups of phrenetic dietetic sects who use these diets.

Now the third point: the prognostic value of cholesterol and lipoproteins. I think that the diagnostic value of lipoproteins and cholesterol in cardio-vascular disease, in coronary disease, is very slight, but not their pathogenetic significance. I think it is true that high values of lipoproteins and cholesterol are harmful to the vessels.

COTTET: I agree with you.

Closing remarks

By

F. C. REUBI

Gentlemen, now that our meeting draws to its close, allow me first of all to say how much I have appreciated your kind collaboration. The pleasant atmosphere of this symposium, which each of you has helped personally to create, has, I feel, been particularly conducive to a free and frank exchange of views. Speaking for myself, I have derived a great deal from these debates of ours, and my reaction has been one of both humility and admiration: humility in face of the immense and complex problem with which we have been dealing; and admiration for the splendid work which is everywhere being undertaken with faith, conscientiousness, determination, and critical judgment.

While taking part in these discussions over the past few days, I have been struck once again by the number of pitfalls awaiting us whenever we try to tackle a problem as vast as that of hypertension. Since no doubt all of you at some time or other will have fallen into one of these traps, perhaps you will permit me to mention a few.

To begin with, there are the difficulties of method. These arise, for example, when we endeavour to determine adrenal hormone concentrations in the urine or in the blood. The discussion which followed the papers by Dr. GENEST and Dr. SCHWARTZ struck me as being very instructive in this connection. The same reservations have to be made when analysing renin or hypertensin. It would be a good thing if in future, when confronted with diverging results, authors were to carefully compare their techniques and try to discover why their findings do not tally before proceeding to interpret their results.

Another pitfall consists in seeing only one detailed facet of a problem without considering it in relation to the whole. Modern investigations are of such complexity that one is often compelled to concentrate on one particular aspect of a question. Where the results obtained prove interesting, one is tempted to exaggerate their intrinsic importance instead of trying to integrate them into the overall picture.

Often it is difficult to determine the causal connections between two phenomena observed at one and the same time, as for example in the case of hyperaldosteronuria and hypertension, or arteriolar necrosis and malignant hypertension. That the problem of arteriolar necrosis now seems to have been partly solved is due to the fact that it is possible to reproduce this lesion in animals by raising their blood pressure and to prevent its development in hypertensive patients by means of anti-hypertensive therapy. On the other hand, there is nothing to prove that essential hypertension is due to hyperaldosteronism. In the absence of experimental proof and clinical arguments, it might equally well be supposed that the hyperaldosteronuria is secondary to the rise in blood pressure.

I am quite convinced of the importance of experimental proofs in arriving at a correct interpretation of a given set of clinical facts; but it should not be forgotten that phenomena observed or provoked in the rat, the rabbit, or the dog cannot always be translated to human pathology. Dr. Gross has rightly emphasised how easy it is to produce hypertension in rats. On the other hand, we all know how comparatively unsusceptible dogs are to arteriosclerosis. Thus, the fact that a hypertensive dog shows very little tendency to nephro-angiosclerosis does not mean to say that in man the vascular lesions encountered are not partly due to elevated blood pressure. Again, the fact that rats treated with salt and corticosteroids develop hypertension and nephrosclerosis is no proof that essential hypertension in man is caused by an adrenal disorder.

However tempting, it is wrong to interpret a chronic metabolic or haemodynamic upset on the basis of short-term experiments. An experiment, by its very nature, is of limited duration. Now, the effects of a drug may be quite different depending on whether the results are determined immediately after a single intravenous injection or after months of continuous treatment. We have seen this in connection with the action of hypotensive agents on renal function and during the discussion following the paper by Dr. Freis. Though it is true that chlorothiazide begins by reducing the cardiac output, it ultimately leads to a decrease in peripheral resistance.

Finally, another grave danger to be guarded against is that of considering an hypothesis as an established fact. Science would hardly be conceivable without hypotheses. Every research worker has to fall back on them once he is in possession of a certain number of experimental findings, since only by forming an hypothesis can he obtain some idea as to the logical direction in which concentrate his efforts. Nevertheless, every hypothesis must be abandoned as soon as it no longer tallies with the objective findings. The survival of a mistaken hypothesis constitutes a severe handicap to scientific research. As for faulty hypotheses that have been set up as dogmas, suffice it to say that they doom all effort to frustration.

These few remarks of mine are so obvious that they no doubt strike you as superfluous. I should now like to turn to a few points which the past few days' discussions have perhaps helped to clarify.

I was particularly pleased that Dr. PICKERING and Dr. PLATT had an opportunity of giving us their points of view. Without wishing to repeat the arguments you have already heard, I have the impression that in the end there was some measure of reconciliation between diverging conceptions and that, at any rate, several misunderstandings were cleared up. Dr. PICKERING admitted that his hypothesis was open to certain criticisms and, in so doing, indicated that he was prepared to take account of them. Perhaps Dr. PLATT is right in suggesting that the mathematical method of analysis employed is not entirely satisfactory. Moreover, Dr. PICKERING agreed that a large number of different populations might be involved rather than one homogeneous population.

The vexed question of salt, the adrenals, and hypertension gave rise to an extensive exchange of views. There is hardly any disagreement on the whole as to the fact that hyperaldosteronism may possibly accompany essential hypertension. But opinions differ concerning the interpretation of this sign and the importance to be attached to it. My own feeling is that it is probably a secondary phenomenon and does not indicate the presence of a basic adrenal disorder. The same applies to the hypernatriuresis occurring in hypertension of every aetiology. However, the discussion did bring to light various unsuspected correlations between the activity of the adrenals and that of the renin-hypertensin system. Unfortunately, the whole question is complicated by the uncertainties involved in the techniques used. I am sure that the specialists will have derived great profit from this colloquium and that they now have a better idea than they did a week ago as to the direction in which to pursue their studies and the snags they must steer clear of.

The papers read by Dr. BECHGAARD and Dr. MILLIEZ gave rise to a most useful discussion on the definition of malignant hypertension. It was discovered, in fact, that there was no absolute clinical criterion of diagnosis and that each speaker had his own ideas on the subject. While we all ascribe major importance to the presence of high blood pressure side by side with Grade IV retinopathy, some of us pointed out that papilloedema might be absent in certain patients in whom other signs and symptoms (deterioration in general condition, massive albuminuria) indicated a diagnosis of malignancy. By contrast, Grade IV retinopathy may exceptionally be encountered in patients in whom the blood pressure is only moderately elevated.

On the other hand, there was unanimous agreement on the necessity of administering vigorous hypotensive treatment in all cases of severe or malignant hypertension, although Dr. Wilson stressed the shortcomings of such treatment from the theoretical standpoint. We were all impressed by Dr. Schroeder's results, which have been largely confirmed by other authors. However, it appeared that one problem — that of arteriosclerosis — has yet to be solved. From the work undertaken by Dr. Page and his team, it is evident that certain patients with malignant hypertension, treated with apparent success by means of hypotensive agents, succumb to vascular complications of the atheromatous type or subintimal fibroplasia. Nor does it seem that hypotensive therapy has any significant influence on the slow progression of benign nephro-angiosclerosis.

As to the choice of, and indications for, the various antihypertensive drugs, it is generally agreed that the saluretics and guanethidine constitute the major acquisition of recent years. The mode of action of chlorothiazide still does not seem to have been definitely elucidated. Darenthin (bretylium tosylate) has disappointed most of those who have used it. Nevertheless, we have good reason to be satisfied with the progress achieved by pharmacologists during the last 10 years. That is why I should like to endorse the optimistic views expressed by Dr. Plummer and to conclude these remarks by quoting his statement to the effect that: "The hope for further life-enhancing drug therapy seems bright indeed".

Gentlemen, it is time for us to part. I sincerely hope we shall have an opportunity of meeting again in the not too distant future and of resuming our discussions where we have now left off.

The editors acknowledge with gratitude the valuable assistance of Mr. H. D. Philps, M. A., Dr. W. Hatzinger, Miss S. R. Naegeli, Miss B. Pfeifer, and Miss U. Sturzenegger.

REPRINT FROM

ESSENTIAL HYPERTENSION

AN INTERNATIONAL SYMPOSIUM

CHAIRMAN
F. C. REUBI · BERNE
EDITED BY
K. D. BOCK · BASLE — P. T. COTTIER · BERNE

SPRINGER-VERLAG / BERLIN · GÖTTINGEN · HEIDELBERG / 1960
PRINTED IN GERMANY
NOT IN CIRCULATION

THE MOSAIC THEORY OF HYPERTENSION

BY
I. H. PAGE

WITH 3 FIGURES

REPRINT FROM

ESSENTIAL HYPERTENSION

AN INTERNATIONAL SYMPOSIUM

CHAIRMAN
F. C. REUBI · BERNE
EDITED BY
K. D. BOCK · BASLE — P. T. COTTIER · BERNE

SPRINGER-VERLAG / BERLIN · GÖTTINGEN · HEIDELBERG / 1960
PRINTED IN GERMANY
NOT IN CIRCULATION

INHERITANCE OF HIGH BLOOD PRESSURE

BY
G. W. PICKERING

REPRINT FROM

ESSENTIAL HYPERTENSION

AN INTERNATIONAL SYMPOSIUM

CHAIRMAN
F. C. REUBI · BERNE
EDITED BY
K. D. BOCK · BASLE — P. T. COTTIER · BERNE

SPRINGER-VERLAG / BERLIN · GÖTTINGEN · HEIDELBERG / 1960
PRINTED IN GERMANY
NOT IN CIRCULATION

THE NATURE OF ESSENTIAL HYPERTENSION

BY
R. PLATT

WITH 5 FIGURES

REPRINT FROM

ESSENTIAL HYPERTENSION

AN INTERNATIONAL SYMPOSIUM

CHAIRMAN
F. C. REUBI · BERNE

EDITED BY

K. D. BOCK · BASLE — P. T. COTTIER · BERNE

SPRINGER-VERLAG / BERLIN · GÖTTINGEN · HEIDELBERG / 1960
PRINTED IN GERMANY
NOT IN CIRCULATION

POSSIBLE ROLE OF SALT INTAKE
IN THE DEVELOPMENT OF ESSENTIAL HYPERTENSION

BY
L. K. DAHL

WITH 2 FIGURES

REPRINT FROM

ESSENTIAL HYPERTENSION

AN INTERNATIONAL SYMPOSIUM

CHAIRMAN

F. C. REUBI · BERNE

EDITED BY

K. D. BOCK · BASLE — P. T. COTTIER · BERNE

SPRINGER-VERLAG / BERLIN · GÖTTINGEN · HEIDELBERG / 1960

PRINTED IN GERMANY

NOT IN CIRCULATION

RENAL HEMODYNAMICS, WATER AND ELECTROLYTE EXCRETION IN ESSENTIAL HYPERTENSION

BY

P. T. COTTIER

WITH 5 FIGURES

REPRINT FROM

ESSENTIAL HYPERTENSION

AN INTERNATIONAL SYMPOSIUM

CHAIRMAN
F. C. REUBI · BERNE

EDITED BY

K. D. BOCK · BASLE — P. T. COTTIER · BERNE

SPRINGER-VERLAG / BERLIN · GÖTTINGEN · HEIDELBERG / 1960
PRINTED IN GERMANY
NOT IN CIRCULATION

ADRENOCORTICAL FUNCTION AND RENAL PRESSOR MECHANISMS IN EXPERIMENTAL HYPERTENSION

BY
F. GROSS

WITH 12 FIGURES

REPRINT FROM

ESSENTIAL HYPERTENSION

AN INTERNATIONAL SYMPOSIUM

CHAIRMAN
F. C. REUBI · BERNE
EDITED BY
K. D. BOCK · BASLE — P. T. COTTIER · BERNE

SPRINGER-VERLAG / BERLIN · GÖTTINGEN · HEIDELBERG / 1960
PRINTED IN GERMANY
NOT IN CIRCULATION

POSSIBLE RELATIONSHIP BETWEEN SALT METABOLISM AND THE ANGIOTENSIN SYSTEM

BY

W. S. PEART

WITH 7 FIGURES

REPRINT FROM

ESSENTIAL HYPERTENSION

AN INTERNATIONAL SYMPOSIUM

CHAIRMAN
F. C. REUBI · BERNE
EDITED BY
K. D. BOCK · BASLE — P. T. COTTIER · BERNE

SPRINGER-VERLAG / BERLIN · GÖTTINGEN · HEIDELBERG / 1960
PRINTED IN GERMANY
NOT IN CIRCULATION

ADRENOCORTICAL FUNCTION
IN ESSENTIAL HYPERTENSION

BY
J. GENEST, W. NOWACZYNSKI, E. KOIW, T. SANDOR,
and P. BIRON

WITH 8 FIGURES

THE SIGNIFICANCE OF HYPERALDOSTERONURIA IN HYPERTENSION

BY
J. WARTER, J. SCHWARTZ, and R. BLOCH

WITH 3 FIGURES

REPRINT FROM

ESSENTIAL HYPERTENSION

AN INTERNATIONAL SYMPOSIUM

CHAIRMAN

F. C. REUBI · BERNE

EDITED BY

K. D. BOCK · BASLE — P. T. COTTIER · BERNE

SPRINGER-VERLAG / BERLIN · GÖTTINGEN · HEIDELBERG / 1960

PRINTED IN GERMANY

NOT IN CIRCULATION

THERAPEUTIC ASPECTS OF SALT RESTRICTION

BY

A. GROLLMAN

REPRINT FROM

ESSENTIAL HYPERTENSION

AN INTERNATIONAL SYMPOSIUM

CHAIRMAN
F. C. REUBI · BERNE

EDITED BY

K. D. BOCK · BASLE — P. T. COTTIER · BERNE

SPRINGER-VERLAG / BERLIN · GÖTTINGEN · HEIDELBERG / 1960
PRINTED IN GERMANY
NOT IN CIRCULATION

MECHANISM OF HYPOTENSIVE ACTION OF SALURETICS

BY

E. D. FREIS

WITH 1 FIGURE

REPRINT FROM

ESSENTIAL HYPERTENSION

AN INTERNATIONAL SYMPOSIUM

CHAIRMAN
F. C. REUBI · BERNE
EDITED BY
K. D. BOCK · BASLE — P. T. COTTIER · BERNE

SPRINGER-VERLAG / BERLIN · GÖTTINGEN · HEIDELBERG / 1960
PRINTED IN GERMANY
NOT IN CIRCULATION

THE NATURAL HISTORY OF BENIGN HYPERTENSION

BY
P. BECHGAARD

WITH 4 FIGURES

REPRINT FROM

ESSENTIAL HYPERTENSION

AN INTERNATIONAL SYMPOSIUM

CHAIRMAN

F. C. REUBI · BERNE

EDITED BY

K. D. BOCK · BASLE — P. T. COTTIER · BERNE

SPRINGER-VERLAG / BERLIN · GÖTTINGEN · HEIDELBERG / 1960
PRINTED IN GERMANY
NOT IN CIRCULATION

THE NATURAL COURSE OF MALIGNANT HYPERTENSION

BY

P. MILLIEZ, P. TCHERDAKOFF, P. SAMARCQ, and L. P. REY

PHARMACOLOGY OF NEW HYPOTENSIVE DRUGS

BY
A. J. PLUMMER

WITH 4 FIGURES

REPRINT FROM

ESSENTIAL HYPERTENSION

AN INTERNATIONAL SYMPOSIUM

CHAIRMAN
F. C. REUBI · BERNE
EDITED BY
K. D. BOCK · BASLE — P. T. COTTIER · BERNE

SPRINGER-VERLAG / BERLIN · GÖTTINGEN · HEIDELBERG / 1960
PRINTED IN GERMANY
NOT IN CIRCULATION

BRETYLIUM AND GUANETHIDINE (CLINICAL RESULTS)

BY
T. HILDEN

COMBINED DRUG THERAPY OF HYPERTENSION

BY
S. W. HOOBLER and P. LAUWERS

WITH 4 FIGURES

REPRINT FROM

ESSENTIAL HYPERTENSION

AN INTERNATIONAL SYMPOSIUM

CHAIRMAN
F. C. REUBI · BERNE

EDITED BY
K. D. BOCK · BASLE — P. T. COTTIER · BERNE

SPRINGER-VERLAG / BERLIN · GÖTTINGEN · HEIDELBERG / 1960
PRINTED IN GERMANY
NOT IN CIRCULATION

EFFECTS OF THE ADMINISTRATION OF SALURETIC DRUGS IN THE TREATMENT OF ARTERIAL HYPERTENSION

BY
C. BARTORELLI

WITH 5 FIGURES

REPRINT FROM

ESSENTIAL HYPERTENSION

AN INTERNATIONAL SYMPOSIUM

CHAIRMAN
F. C. REUBI · BERNE
EDITED BY
K. D. BOCK · BASLE — P. T. COTTIER · BERNE

SPRINGER-VERLAG / BERLIN · GÖTTINGEN · HEIDELBERG / 1960
PRINTED IN GERMANY
NOT IN CIRCULATION

SURVIVAL RATES IN SEVERE HYPERTENSION INTENSIVELY TREATED WITH HYDRALAZINE AND GANGLIONIC BLOCKADE

BY
H. A. SCHROEDER and H. M. PERRY, jr.

REPRINT FROM

ESSENTIAL HYPERTENSION

AN INTERNATIONAL SYMPOSIUM

CHAIRMAN
F. C. REUBI · BERNE

EDITED BY

K. D. BOCK · BASLE — P. T. COTTIER · BERNE

SPRINGER-VERLAG / BERLIN · GÖTTINGEN · HEIDELBERG / 1960
PRINTED IN GERMANY
NOT IN CIRCULATION

THE LATE EFFECTS OF HYPOTENSIVE DRUG THERAPY ON RENAL FUNCTIONS OF PATIENTS WITH ESSENTIAL HYPERTENSION

BY
F. C. REUBI

WITH 5 FIGURES

REPRINT FROM

ESSENTIAL HYPERTENSION

AN INTERNATIONAL SYMPOSIUM

CHAIRMAN
F. C. REUBI · BERNE

EDITED BY

K. D. BOCK · BASLE — P. T. COTTIER · BERNE

SPRINGER-VERLAG / BERLIN · GÖTTINGEN · HEIDELBERG / 1960
PRINTED IN GERMANY
NOT IN CIRCULATION

LATE RESULTS OF SURGICAL THERAPY (SYMPATHECTOMY AND ADRENALECTOMY)

BY
H. SARRE

WITH 4 FIGURES

REPRINT FROM

ESSENTIAL HYPERTENSION

AN INTERNATIONAL SYMPOSIUM

CHAIRMAN
F. C. REUBI · BERNE
EDITED BY
K. D. BOCK · BASLE — P. T. COTTIER · BERNE

SPRINGER-VERLAG / BERLIN · GÖTTINGEN · HEIDELBERG / 1960
PRINTED IN GERMANY
NOT IN CIRCULATION

HYPERTENSION
AND ITS ASSOCIATED VASCULAR DISEASES

BY
P. IMHOF, I. H. PAGE, and H. DUSTAN

REPRINT FROM

ESSENTIAL HYPERTENSION

AN INTERNATIONAL SYMPOSIUM

CHAIRMAN

F. C. REUBI · BERNE

EDITED BY

K. D. BOCK · BASLE — P. T. COTTIER · BERNE

SPRINGER-VERLAG / BERLIN · GÖTTINGEN · HEIDELBERG / 1960

PRINTED IN GERMANY

NOT IN CIRCULATION

PREVENTION AND TREATMENT OF "ATHEROMATOUS COMPLICATIONS" OF HYPERTENSION

BY

G. SCHETTLER